Black and Blue

Black and Blue

The Origins and Consequences of Medical Racism

JOHN HOBERMAN

University of California Press

BERKELEY   LOS ANGELES   LONDON

University of California Press, one of the most distinguished university presses in the United States, enriches lives around the world by advancing scholarship in the humanities, social sciences, and natural sciences. Its activities are supported by the UC Press Foundation and by philanthropic contributions from individuals and institutions. For more information, visit www.ucpress.edu.

University of California Press
Berkeley and Los Angeles, California

University of California Press, Ltd.
London, England

© 2012 by The Regents of the University of California

Library of Congress Cataloging-in-Publication Data

Hoberman, John M. (John Milton), 1944-
   Black and blue : the origins and consequences of medical racism /
John Hoberman.
      p.   cm.
   Includes bibliographical references and index.
   ISBN 978-0-520-24890-8 (hardback)
   ISBN 978-0-520-27401-3 (pbk)
   1. Discrimination in medical care—United States.   2. Minorities—
Medical care—United States.   3. African Americans—Medical care—
United States.   4. Health services accessibility—United States.   I. Title.
   RA563.M56H63   2012
   362.1089'96073—dc23

                                                          2011045598

Manufactured in the United States of America.
21   20   19   18   17   16   15   14   13   12
10   9   8   7   6   5   4   3   2   1

In keeping with a commitment to support environmentally responsible and sustainable printing practices, UC Press has printed this book on Rolland Enviro100, a 100% post-consumer fiber paper that is FSC certified, deinked, processed chlorine-free, and manufactured with renewable biogas energy. It is acid-free and EcoLogo certified.

This book is dedicated to the African American doctors of the past century who, despite the cruelties and indignities of racist exclusion from American medicine, have persisted in their humanitarian mission to serve patients of all races.

Contents

Acknowledgments   ix

1. THE NATURE OF MEDICAL RACISM: THE ORIGINS AND
   CONSEQUENCES OF MEDICAL RACISM   1
   Introduction   1
   "Avoidance and Evasion"   3
   Judging How Physicians Behave   7
   Judging Physician Conduct: Privacy and the "Halo Effect"   8
   The Oral Tradition   11
   Physicians Share the Racial Attitudes of Their Fellow Citizens   12
   The Medical Liberals   14

2. BLACK PATIENTS AND WHITE DOCTORS   18
   The African American Health Calamity: The Silence   18
   Medical Vulnerability and Racial Defamation   24
   How Do (White) Physicians Think about Race?
   Evidence of Medical Racism   32
   Resistance to the Critique of Racial Bias in Medicine   37
   Medical Liberalism and the Medical Literature   41
   The Physician's Private Sphere   52
   Playing Anthropologist   55
   From Racial Folklore to Racial Medicine   66

3. MEDICAL CONSEQUENCES OF RACIALIZING
   THE HUMAN ORGANISM   71
   Racial Interpretations of Human Types and Traits   71
   Introduction   71
   Racial Interpretations of Black Infants and Children   71
   Racial Interpretations of the Black Elderly   81
   Racial Interpretations of the Black Athlete   83
   Racial Interpretations of Black Musical Aptitude   85
   Racial Interpretations of Losing Consciousness   87

Racial Interpretations of the Nervous System 92
Racial Interpretations of Pain Sensitivity 97
Racial Interpretations of Heart Disease 98
Racial Interpretations of Human Organs and Disorders 106
Racial Interpretations of the Eyes 107
Racial Interpretations of Black Skin 109
Racial Interpretations of Human Teeth 110
Racial Interpretations of "White" and "Black" Disorders 112
Black "Hardiness" 120
Physical Hardiness 121
Emotional Hardiness 125
Conclusion: How Human Organ Systems Acquire Racial Identities 130
Racial Folklore in Medical Specialties 130
A Century of Racial Pharmacology: From Racial Folklore to Racial Genetics 130
The Role of Racial Folklore in Obstetrics and Gynecology during the Twentieth Century 139

4. MEDICAL APARTHEID, INTERNAL COLONIALISM, AND THE TASK OF AMERICAN PSYCHIATRY 146
Introduction 146
"Africanizing" the Black Image 154
American Psychiatry as Racial Medicine 158
The Racial Primitive in American Psychiatry 160
The Task of Black Psychiatry 176
Colonial Medical Status 193

5. A MEDICAL SCHOOL SYLLABUS ON RACE 198
Introduction 198
The Doctor-Patient Relationship 200
The Problem Patient 202
Medical Authors' Aversion to Race 204
Race and Medical Education: The Search for "Cultural Competence" 207
Two Official Versions of "Cultural Competence" 212
Physicians' Beliefs about Racial Differences: A (Belated) Study 216
A Medical Curriculum on Race 217
Practical Advice for Physicians 221
Social Class, Misdiagnoses, and Therapeutic Fatalism 222
"Cultural Competence" as Knowledge of Stereotype Systems 224
Raceless Humanism: "Medical Humanities" and the Evasion of Difference 226
Medical Curriculum Change Is Possible: The Case of Abortion Training 229

Notes 235

Index 279

Acknowledgments

Like any work of research produced over a long period of time, this book has been made possible by the efforts of many people and institutions. Much of the research was done at the Francis A. Countway Library of Medicine at Harvard Medical School, the John Crerar Library at the University of Chicago, and the Life Sciences Library at the University of Texas at Austin. I am grateful to those who have built and maintained these wonderful collections. This work has benefited greatly from years of classroom discussions with the University of Texas students who have taken "Race and Medicine in African-American Life" since 2001; some of their stories are in the book. Many colleagues, friends, and correspondents have generously contributed to this project by providing information, ideas, invitations, introductions, good conversation, and comments about the manuscript. I would like to offer my special thanks to Rachel Brown Ater, MSW, Carl C. Bell, MD, Deborah Bolnick, PhD, Khiara Bridges, PhD, David Broad, PhD, Robert Eisenberg, MD, Adriane Fugh-Berman, MD, John Hartigan, PhD, Edward Havranek, MD, Crystal Hlaing, MD, David Hoberman, PhD, Eric P. Hoffman, PhD, Michelle Holmes, MD, Joel Howell, MD, PhD, Sherman A. James, PhD, Shannon Jones, III, MPA, Jay Kaufman, PhD, David J. Malebranche, MD, Jonathan Marks, PhD, David Morris, PhD, Thomas Murray, PhD, Robert S. Schell, MD, and John Valentine, PhD.

This book was made possible by Stan Holwitz, former Associate Director of the University of California Press. Stan's belief in the importance of investigating race relations in American medicine never wavered, and I will be forever grateful for his loyalty and support. Following Stan's retirement, Naomi Schneider, Executive Editor for the Social Sciences at UC Press, took on the project and saw it through to completion. I am very grateful for her commitment and tenacity. Thanks also to Stacy Eisenstark,

Acquisitions Coordinator; Hannah Love, Associate Editor for Health; and Kate Warne, Managing Editor. Heather McElwain did a fine job as copy editor of the manuscript. I am also grateful to Michael Bohrer-Clancy, Project Manager at Macmillan Publication Services North America, for supervising the final production of the book.

Finally, I thank my wife Louisa for her companionship and her understanding of the research-oriented life. It is a life she has known first hand. During the long years of work on *Black and Blue*, she inspired me once again by remaking her professional life with a courage and determination I have always admired. It is a pleasure to acknowledge how much she has done on behalf of this book and everything else we are fortunate to have.

1. The Nature of Medical Racism

The Origins and Consequences
of Medical Racism

INTRODUCTION

The idea that discredited (and even disgraceful) ideas about racial differences might play a role in medical diagnosis and treatment is a possibility that some doctors find profoundly disturbing. The racially biased treatment of patients would appear to be a grievous violation of medical ethics and a direct threat to the dignity of the profession. Yet, in the course of the last two decades, the medical literature has published hundreds of peer-reviewed studies that point to racially motivated decisions by physicians either to deny appropriate care to black patients or to inflict on them extreme procedures (such as amputations) that many white patients would be spared.[1] "How are we to explain, let alone justify, such broad evidence of racial disparity in a health care system committed in principle to providing care to all patients?" the socially active physician H. Jack Geiger asked in 1996. His reply to his own question offered two possible explanations. The first option was to attribute the observed disparity to "unspecified cultural differences" or decisions made by black patients who did not understand that they needed medical care. The second and more discomfiting explanation was, as Dr. Geiger phrased it, "racism—that is, racially discriminatory rationing by physicians and health care institutions." Confronting the data that he had felt compelled to present to the medical community, Dr. Geiger could not bring himself to categorize the documented behavior of his medical colleagues as racist. Indeed, he added, "if racism is involved it is unlikely to be overt or even conscious."[2] For this conscientious physician, medical racism that implied individual culpability was still somehow unreal, a specter to be exorcized rather than a threat to be acknowledged and confronted.

Black and Blue is the first systematic description of how doctors think about racial differences and how this kind of thinking affects the treatment of their patients. While some fine studies of medical racism have appeared, they have not examined the thought processes and behaviors of physicians in any sort of detailed way. In effect, these studies have not seen fit to enter into the physician's private sphere where specific racial fantasies and misinformation distort diagnoses and treatments. Nor have they shown much interest in identifying the specific origins of racially motivated diagnoses and treatments of black patients that have ranged across the entire spectrum of medical sub-disciplines, from cardiology to obstetrics to psychiatry. It is true that American physicians have been "major perpetrators of racialist dogma," as a monumental history of American medical racism states.[3] *Black and Blue* moves beyond such general claims about racially motivated medical behaviors and describes how mainstream medicine devised racial interpretations that have been applied to every organ system of the human body.

The studies to date have occasionally noted but failed to describe the oral traditions that convey medico-racial folklore and persist over generations of medical students and doctors. As we shall see, the physician-authors who have taken the trouble to write about the racial dimension of medicine confirm that the medical profession has never embarked upon this kind of self-scrutiny in a serious manner. Interestingly, the medical profession's lack of interest in confronting the racial complexes of doctors has created little activism among even the most concerned medical observers beyond ritualized expressions of concern. While these white "medical liberals" profess to be "troubled" by this topic, their efforts at raising consciousness have been episodic and have never acquired the political traction that might catalyze a more effective reckoning with the racially motivated and medically harmful behaviors that have been proven beyond a doubt to exist. It is, therefore, no accident that this book-length examination of the racially motivated mental habits and professional mores of doctors is the work of an outsider to the medical profession.

At the same time, I would point out that this history and analysis of medical racism is the work of a grateful outsider. The criticism of the medical profession presented in this book is not motivated by personal dissatisfaction with doctors. On the contrary, physicians have served me well throughout a long life that has included an open-heart surgery that saved me from a debilitating future of congestive heart failure. My father was a physician-scientist, and his commitment to his patients was inspiring. I learned about medical racism in the library while doing research for another book. I was stunned by the overt racism that appeared in medical journals such as the *Journal of the American Medical Association* or the *American Heart Journal* during the first half of the twentieth century. So was my father, who received his M.D. in 1946, a man of anti-racist principles, who knew the famous African American physician Charles Drew in Boston before the latter's premature death in 1950. As a Jew who had experienced anti-Semitic insults, my father was aware of the reality of bigotry in American society. But the medical racism of American physicians during his lifetime had somehow passed him by.

"AVOIDANCE AND EVASION"

"The general awkwardness surrounding racial issues in our society bleeds into medicine," the prominent African American cardiologist Clyde Yancy observed in 2009.[4] This awkwardness about practicing and discussing race relations has long been a fact of medical life the profession has been slow to recognize or deal with in a deliberate or systematic way. The political conservatism of the medical establishment was evident even during the civil rights movement, as the national leadership of the American Medical Association (AMA) deferred to the racist exclusionary policies of state medical societies and refused to intervene on behalf of black physicians who sought membership in the AMA and the professional status they had long been denied.[5]

Today the great majority of doctors are likely to regard information about medical racism as of little relevance to their professional lives. This is hardly surprising, given that large majorities of white Americans take little or no interest in the special problems their African American fellow citizens experience. There has long been, and there remains, a widespread conviction among whites today that the disadvantages blacks face are of their own making, since formal racial equality was established by the civil rights and voting rights laws and affirmative action initiatives, all of which date from the 1960s. And there is no reason to assume that the racial views of doctors differ in any significant ways from those of the general population.

My own firsthand exposure to how physicians receive news about medical racism occurred on a chilly evening in New York City in November 1999. A friendly bioethicist had arranged for me to attend a discussion of the medical profession's treatment of African Americans at the New York Academy of Medicine at Fifth Avenue and 103rd Street in Manhattan. The host, as I recall, was the vice president of the academy. He stood before a seated group of his medical colleagues and told them what the medical literature had by now demonstrated beyond a doubt: American medicine was failing to serve the African American population in a racially equitable manner. The question before them, he said, was whether or not they as a profession were going to choose to "own" this issue, to take responsibility for the uncomfortable reality of racially unequal medical treatment.

Fifty professionally and financially comfortable physicians listened to this pitch in their chairs. I saw no one on the edge of his or her seat. While it was clear that the speaker took this matter seriously, the tone of his comments did not convey a sense of urgency or an expectation of medical activism from those who sat before him. On the contrary, it was clear that making the effort to repair this injustice and take more responsibility for the health of black people was being presented, not as an ethical obligation, but as an option. The ethical obligation was real to the speaker, but one sensed that he did not really expect his colleagues to rally to this cause.

American medicine's disengagement from the black population is only one dimension of the much larger racial disengagement that characterizes American society as a whole. Ignoring African Americans or relegating them to marginal status has been a deeply rooted American habit. In his classic *An American Dilemma* (1944), Gunnar Myrdal commented that, in the literature on American democracy he had read, "the subject of the Negro is a void or is taken care of by some awkward, mostly un-informed and helpless, excuses." Ralph Bunche, whose extraordinary career as a black academic foreign policy expert and international diplomat culminated in the 1950 Nobel Peace Prize, told Myrdal in 1940 that "consciously or unconsciously, America has contrived an artful technique of avoidance and evasion" to separate itself from its Negro citizens.[6]

A generation later the famous black psychologist Kenneth B. Clark explained white racial detachment as a form of emotional self-defense on the part of whites. "The tendency to discuss disturbing social issues such as racial discrimination, segregation, and economic exploitation in detached, legal, political, socio-economic, or psychological terms as if these persistent problems did not involve the suffering of actual human beings," Clark wrote in *Dark Ghetto* (1965), "is so contrary to empirical evidence that it must be interpreted as a protective device." The "purist approach rooted in the belief that detachment or enforced distance from the human consequences of persistent injustice is objectively desirable," and he added, is "a subconscious protection against personal pain and direct involvement in moral controversies."[7] For many people, the most threatening controversy that might personally implicate them is racism. Maurice Berger has pointed out that, in an age of political correctness, "most people will do almost anything to preserve the comfortable illusion of themselves as free of prejudice."[8]

The sheer magnitude of the African American health disaster can produce both emotional detachment and a dehumanizing sociological reduction of black life to its bleakest essentials. The recitation of endless statistics documenting medical racial disparities depersonalizes the human dimension of what is happening to black people. Our attention is displaced from the specific behaviors and predicaments of doctors and patients into an abstract dimension of enormous and hopelessly complicated social processes that can only be imagined. What is more, as one Indian-British physician has noted, "documenting inequalities may have little impact on reducing them."[9]

The statistical depersonalization of black people and its association with disease were recognized as far back as 1951 by James Baldwin, long before sociology became the conceptual language of race relations during the heady days of the Great Society in the mid-1960s. The Negro, he wrote, "is a social and not a personal or human problem; to think of him is to think of statistics, slums, rapes, injustices, remote violence; it is to be confronted with an endless cataloguing of losses, gains, skirmishes; it is to feel virtuous, outraged, helpless, as though his continuing status among us were somehow analogous to disease—cancer, perhaps, or tuberculosis—which must be checked, even though it cannot be cured."[10] The black person exists in the form of various social disasters, human life conceived as numerical formulas, and threatening but incurable disease processes. The black individual remains invisible and unknown, and this too has its consequences. For as Baldwin points out, "The privacy or obscurity of Negro life makes that life capable, in our imaginations, of producing anything at all,"[11] including all of the dysfunctional behaviors that physicians and many others customarily associate with black people.

The traditional detachment of the medical profession from identifying and solving its racial problems has been evident in the medical literature and in the work of medical authors who are at liberty to range farther and deeper into social and personal issues than is possible in medical journals. David Satcher, a young black physician who became surgeon general of the United States in 1998, pointed out in 1973 that: "Much has been written about the doctor-patient relationship and its many challenges and ramifications. However, almost nothing is written about the effects of race on this relationship."[12] (In his pioneering commentary on doctor-patient race relations, David Levy made the same point about the pediatric literature in

1985.[13]) Then, as now, the great majority of doctors were white men whose ignorance and naïveté regarding their black patients had long been evident to black physicians. The estrangement from blacks that resulted from this mind-set has expressed itself in many ways. In 1940, *Time* reported that "few white doctors dare to operate on their 'massively' infected Negro patients" afflicted with tuberculosis.[14] At this time black doctors noted with chagrined amusement that, "The average young white physician enters practice with the idea that all Negroes have syphilis or tuberculosis."[15] A generation later the medical anthropologist George Devereux described his observations of "White-Negro doctor-patient pairs" and the diagnostic errors that resulted from the doctor's "'tactful' reluctance to examine closely the most distinctive portions of a racially alien patient's body."[16] White dermatologists may be alternately alarmed about or unaware of the characteristics of black skin and the emotional consequences of skin problems for patients.[17] White doctors sometimes underestimate the intelligence and self-control of black patients and treat them accordingly.[18] The cumulative effects of such naïveté are often evident to blacks but are less evident to the white medical community that does not monitor and report on such incidents.

The writings produced by white physician-authors reflect the social distance from African Americans they share with a large majority of their fellow citizens. As the black sociologist Orlando Patterson noted in November 2009, "in the privacy of homes and neighborhoods we are more segregated than in the Jim Crow era." Various degrees of segregation occur within "the disciplined cultural spaces of marriages, homes, neighborhoods, schools and churches."[19] Hospitals and clinics are disciplined cultural spaces that are subject to the same racial tensions and estrangements that occur within the other "disciplined" social venues. It is, therefore, not surprising that physicians who write about race relations within these medical spaces tend to avoid direct confrontations with uncomfortable racial issues. For example, a collection of 80 reflective columns by doctors taken from the pages of the *Journal of the American Medical Association* during the 1980s contains many profound and moving stories that together constitute the most sympathetic portrait of the medical profession I can imagine. Of the hundreds of people who appear in these stories, there is exactly one African American patient, a humble sharecropper in sweltering Alabama who is grateful to find a white medical student who is willing to talk to him. An elderly black hospital orderly is sympathetically presented as incarnating one of the classic folkloric images of black humanity: the musical Negro. From these dozens of medical authors, there are a handful of references to "slum children," inner-city "juvenile delinquents," and a six-year-old West

African child who dies despite the best efforts of the American physician who tries to save him. There are no black doctors or nurses. All but a few picturesque and stereotypical examples of black humanity were apparently absent from the recollections of most of a hundred physicians.[20]

Paul Austin's *Something for the Pain* (2008), a candid, caustic, sensitive, and sophisticated memoir of his many years as an emergency room (ER) doctor in North Carolina, refers to race rarely, carefully, and allusively. The tone of a young black mother's voice has "a brittle edge" until the doctor's gentle manner wins her over. The author refuses to give a racial edge to the hostility of a despairing young black man whose mother lies dying in the ER.[21] Thoughtful writing of this kind reminds us of medicine's color-blind ideal; and it is likely that some physician-authors avoid the topic of race out of fidelity to the dream of medical care that transcends color.

The problem with color-blind writing about medicine is that it ignores the long history and persisting reality of racially motivated medical behaviors that can alienate, injure, and sometimes kill black patients. Another genre of medical writing focuses on the brutal conditions experienced by doctors who practice medicine in the ghetto. *Doctors Talk About Themselves* (1988) describes the emotional impact on doctors of dealing with the dregs of humanity who show up in inner-city ERs: "You see such awful things that are totally beyond any experience you have ever had. You ask, 'How can people live like this?'" In this "snake pit" the cynicism that has been widely observed in older medical students becomes complete, as beleaguered and resentful physicians absorb "every conceivable kind of abuse" from their black clientele.[22]

Finally, there is medical writing that ignores the race issue entirely. Jerome Groopman's 2007 bestseller *How Doctors Think* does not contain a single sentence that addresses the question of how doctors think about race. Groopman confirms that there is a great deal of potentially useful thinking that doctors do not do. He knows that social context and the doctor's emotions matter. But he is unwilling or unable to connect these commonsensical principles to real-life scenarios that involve interactions between patients and physicians across the racial divide.

JUDGING HOW PHYSICIANS BEHAVE

Making judgments about what goes wrong between white doctors and black patients requires a sense of realism and humility on the part of those who observe and analyze these relationships. White professionals in other occupations—professors, for example—should be subject to the same kind of scrutiny of their professional conduct. An important difference is that academics do not as a rule have access to the intimate details pertaining to the minds and bodies of their students. Nor are professors traumatized in the line of duty in the ways that ER doctors or oncologists and other physicians can be. Relations with students are seldom fraught with fateful consequences that might result from a professor's incompetence. In addition, most university students are courteous and cooperative people who can be expected to conduct themselves in a reasonable manner and in their own best interest. The patient population that doctors serve is not so easily managed. My father retired from practicing outpatient medicine in his late seventies when he became exasperated with the noncompliant behavior of the patients he encountered at a hospital in the Bronx, many of whom must have been black or Hispanic. Noncompliance, such as a refusal to take prescribed medications or to stop smoking or drinking, is a massive problem for doctors. Noncompliant students, on the other hand, will either change their behaviors or fail their courses and vanish from their professors' classrooms.

JUDGING PHYSICIAN CONDUCT: PRIVACY AND THE "HALO EFFECT"

The detection of racially motivated diagnoses and treatments by physicians remains an ineffectual statistical exercise that has been repeated in hundreds of papers in medical journals over the past two decades. The systematic use of diagnostic and treatment protocols by doctors who track outcomes and adjust care is modern medicine's best hope for improving the services it offers patients. But peer-reviewed evidence of racially biased medicine has produced no reforms remotely comparable to what is now being done at many hospitals to improve survival rates among diabetics and preterm infants. Frequent calls for "further research" into the causes of racial health disparities simply defer the possibility of intervention into racially motivated behaviors into the indefinite future.

So the fundamental questions here are: Why has the medical profession never systematically studied how physicians produce racially motivated diagnoses and treatments that can cause medical harm? And how has traditional, and often defamatory, racial folklore been absorbed into medical practice in specific forms that have infiltrated medical specialties from cardiology to obstetrics to psychiatry?

Traditional norms discourage the analysis and assessment of physician conduct or even misconduct. The medical community, like some other professional groups, has been reluctant to discipline its members for unprofessional and even harmful conduct. As one physician-author noted in 1988, "doctors are unwilling to blow the whistle on other doctors. It's somehow bad manners or breaking the faith of the medical profession to report a bad doctor."[23] In this sense, the practice of medicine, like police work, is more of a fraternal order than a scientific community that recognizes and acts upon its responsibility to monitor and correct the deviant and dangerous misconduct of its practitioners.

Another powerful factor that shields doctors from scrutiny is the "halo effect" that wraps physicians in an aura of benevolent power. "Doctors," a *New York Times* writer noted in 2009, "have a degree of professional autonomy that is probably unmatched outside of academia. And that is how we like it. We think of our doctors as wise men and women who can combine knowledge and instinct to land on just the right treatment."[24] The combination of benevolent intent and the power to heal has traditionally conferred upon doctors "a degree of professional autonomy" that can make them appear as sages who have earned a status that puts them beyond the judgments of observers who do not belong to the guild.

The physician's authority and autonomy can promote a socially conservative identity that resists both personal self-examination and social reforms. Social conservatives may not see the causal relationship between self-scrutiny and a willingness to promote social change, including the profound social changes that antiracist policies require. Even today, social conservatives (and others) retain the option of preserving the traditional racial hierarchy and its racist folklore inside their heads, while conforming to antiracist public norms that enforce public civility and a degree of racial integration within "disciplined" workplaces such as hospitals and clinics. There can be no doubt that many doctors choose this option, thereby disciplining their social conduct but not their racial imaginations.

Given the degree of autonomy traditionally accorded to doctors, requiring them to examine their own feelings about race, and perhaps change their behaviors, will be regarded by many of them as an invasion of privacy. Whether doctors are entitled to this privacy depends on what privacy may conceal. If it is true that "few people are free of unconscious fantasies about imagined racial characteristics," as one prescient physician wrote in 1985, then the existence of unconscious fantasies with potential medical consequences challenges the right to privacy of the doctor who harbors them.[25] According to the prominent physician and author Sherwin Nuland, "conscious and unconscious prejudice pervades rounds, teaching conferences, and even decision-making."[26] In a word, it can be medically dysfunctional for physicians to preserve and act upon their "private" racist fantasies and beliefs.

Another traditional aspect of physician privacy is the right of doctors to be apolitical and uninvolved in public policy. As two proponents of medical curriculum reform wrote in 1994: "Although organized medicine may occasionally take a stand on matters of public policy and bioethics, such positions are often weakened by medicine's long-standing position that individual physicians cannot be expected to act contrary to their own moral beliefs."[27] While this position appears to defend acts of conscience, some physicians will find it difficult to distinguish between their moral beliefs and their intuitions about racial differences. Those who believe that the traditional Western racial hierarchy is an expression of natural law may well reject the positive (man-made) laws that mandate racial equality. In such cases, how will apolitical and social policy–averse physicians establish relationships with black patients? These patients are, after all, people who require sympathetic racial attitudes on the part of those who treat them.

The racially "conservative" physician thus finds himself in a difficult position, caught between the demands of modern racial etiquette and his own private beliefs about racial traits and differences. It is, therefore, not surprising that the medical school instruction in "cultural competence" that is designed to resolve such conflicts has encountered much resistance for this and other reasons. It is easy, for example, to argue that an already crowded medical curriculum simply has no room for "touchy-feely" instruction in human relations that displaces courses in the "hard" medical sciences. Many doctors who are asked to expand their emotional repertories to include new attitudes toward blacks and other racial groups will reject this as an unreasonable and unrealistic demand on their emotional resources that amounts to a violation of personal privacy.

For this reason the very idea of asking doctors to examine their own feelings for the purpose of better serving their patients already represents radical reform. Integrating the race issue into this process is a further complication that many doctors will interpret as mandated political correctness and unrelated to improving medical treatment. Another factor involved in requiring medical professionals to engage in self-examination is the emotional stress that is often a part of medical practice. The ER doctor Paul Austin has thought deeply about the emotional costs of his medical practice and reached some conclusions that depart from the stereotype of the "caring" and "compassionate" physician. Compassion "isn't an emotion. It's an action. A discipline." Similarly, "emotional distance may not always indicate a failure of empathy." Austin recognizes both the practical value and the costs of emotional distance, which can promote emotional survival but also repress feelings in ways that can eventually harm both the physician and his patients.[28]

Doctors may also find the task of introspection time-consuming and impractical. "Frequently physicians think that dealing with emotions is opening a Pandora's box, that they'll be asked about things they can't do anything about, and that it will take a lot more time—especially if the feelings are about sadness or anger."[29] Inside this Pandora's box lurk the devastating consequences of poverty and family trauma that impact the lives of black patients in a disproportionate way. And it is true that the doctor can do little or nothing in a direct way about social conditions or dysfunctional relationships. What the doctor can do is to study his or her own responses to traumatized people. This process should make it possible to distinguish between the unique identity of the patient and the racial folkloric traits conveyed by the oral tradition described later in this book.

The idea of providing or requiring psychotherapy for racially prejudiced physicians has been heard in the past and has gone nowhere as a way to prevent medical racism. "For psychiatrists who lack the empathy needed for work with all groups of people," David Levy wrote in 1985, "psychoanalysis has been recommended to erase distorted perspectives concerning race or at least to enable them to become more aware of when their irrational attitudes might impede the treatment process."[30] Two decades later the same proposal appeared in *Academic Medicine:* "When they are not brought to the level of consciousness, physicians' personal attitudes, biases, fears, emotional reflexes, psychological defenses, and moods can interfere with their abilities to arrive at an accurate diagnosis, prescribe appropriate treatment, and promote healing."[31] From the perspective of many white physicians, therapeutic intervention will be construed as an intolerable intrusion. From the perspective of many black patients and physicians, the therapeutic option may be regarded as the least the profession can do to protect them from racially motivated mistreatment. Once again the professional's right to privacy confronts the patient's right to unbiased treatment.

THE ORAL TRADITION

Physicians' "private beliefs" about racial differences can have effects that extend beyond their own medical practices. The physician's private sphere also takes the form of an oral tradition that conveys racial folkloric beliefs from one generation to the next. In 1983, for example, a paper in the

American Heart Journal raised the question of "whether a 'traditional' diagnostic belief exists that blacks simply do not develop myocardial infarction." That "traditional" belief did, in fact, exist, and has persisted, as this book will demonstrate. Interestingly, this author is unsure as to whether this belief was real, and he suggested that "a broad survey of physicians' beliefs and attitudes on these issues" would be in order.[32] Three decades later, this and other surveys of physicians' beliefs about racial traits still have not been done. While the racial history of American cardiology does appear later in this book, the survey proposed in 1983 would have done far more to improve the care of black heart patients.

Medical students, too, can participate in this process. As a former student wrote to me in 2005: "One of my MCAT class teachers is finishing his 3rd year at [University of Texas] Southwestern Medical School now. He tells us interesting things about the patients he sees. For example, he has observed that African Americans are genetically more athletic than other races (overall), but they also have a much greater risk of having high blood pressure and certain types of cancer."[33] We may assume that the genetic reductionism that prompted this medical student's imaginative claim about athletic genes continues to thrive alongside other bits of uninformed gossip in "the oral culture of medical training." For this reason all medical personnel should keep in mind that medical gossip thrives, "not so much at the bedside (medicine's preeminent metaphor) but via its more insidious and evil twin, 'the corridor.'"[34] African Americans know and fear this oral tradition as "the silent curriculum" that many white doctors carry around in their heads. But the positive image of the medical profession, along with the racial imbalance of power that conceals much black suffering, has effectively shielded the oral tradition from public scrutiny.

PHYSICIANS SHARE THE RACIAL ATTITUDES OF THEIR FELLOW CITIZENS

The pervasiveness of the oral tradition raises an important question about doctors' racial beliefs: Do the racial attitudes of physicians differ from those of the general population? Recent sociological findings indicate that while "whites have largely abandoned principled racism . . . they have not necessarily given up negative racial stereotypes" or "negative sentiments and beliefs about African Americans."[35] The prominent black sociologist William Julius Wilson reported in 2009: "The idea that the federal government 'has a special obligation to help improve the living standards of blacks' because they 'have been discriminated against for so long' was supported by only

It is important to recognize the role that political conservatives have played in promoting the "halo effect" that protects this powerful, and predominantly white, professional community. It has been an axiom of political conservatism, and its traditional emphasis on white male authority, that physicians are beyond criticism regarding the racial attitudes that a majority of white Americans share. The conservative social policy analyst Byron M. Roth, for example, found "questionable the charge that blacks suffer disproportionate health problems because racism taints American medicine. Doctors and nurses are among the least likely candidates upon whom to pin the label of bigotry."[40] The psychiatrist and conservative ideologue Sally Satel has made a public career of promoting the mistaken argument that "political correctness is corrupting medicine."[41] In fact, and as this book demonstrates, the medical profession is a predominantly conservative professional community that has tended to resist "politically correct" norms and policies.

THE MEDICAL LIBERALS

As is so often the case in American policy debates, the conservative attack on "politically correct" medicine has not been matched by a comparably vigorous response from the "liberal" side. The grand document of medical liberalism is *Unequal Treatment: Confronting Racial and Ethnic Disparities in Health Care* (2003), a publication of the prestigious Institute of Medicine, the health arm of the National Academy of Sciences.[42] In his contribution to this volume, H. Jack Geiger portrays doctors as the helpless victims of a stereotyping process that is "automatically triggered and operates below the level of conscious awareness." Once again medical racism remains for this author a hypothesis rather than a documented reality: "[F]urther research is necessary," he says, "to clarify whether sociocultural and educational incongruity between providers and patients translates into misunderstandings about patients' preferences and expectations, and to evaluate the extent to which stereotyping, discrimination and bias exist in the hospital setting."[43] The fact that these hypothetical misunderstandings and stereotypes had already been thoroughly documented inside and outside of the medical literature appears to be unknown to this author. Only ignorance of the history of medical racism in the United States can account for naïveté on this scale. A similar essay by a team of medical ethicists repeats Geiger's claims about "well-meaning" medical personnel and the unfortunate consequences for minority patients of "clinician errors" that cannot be blamed on doctors who are the victims of their own "unconscious" biases.[44]

one in five whites in 2001, and has never exceeded support by m
one in four since 1975. Significantly, the lack of white support for
is not related to background factors such as level of education an
In short, a large majority of the white population is either unwillin
able to see African American problems in their historical context
only limited knowledge of what the black experience has been like.

The research I have done for this book confirms that physician
the racial attitudes of their fellow citizens. Indeed, their intimate ir
ment with medically afflicted black bodies and minds may even cre
intensify feelings about the racial differences they perceive. There is
no evident reason to assume that doctors feel greater sympathy tow
possess a greater understanding of African Americans that most whi
On the contrary, it is probable that many doctors, like police office
exposed to more than their fair share of extreme and unattractive beh
of the troubled and the indigent, a disproportionate number of whom
be black. These experiences do not produce racial goodwill. Conseque
as one African American physician commented in 1990: "The proble
not that medical providers are ethically deficient compared with the pu
it is that we are no longer any better. Our ranks include racists and vi
ally every other variety of impaired citizenry."[37]

Medical authors have occasionally wondered about how they as a gr
compare to the general public regarding racial prejudice. "As health p
fessionals," two physicians wrote in 2002, "we need to become aware
any deep-seated attitudinal biases that parallel those of the general pu
lic and the media and confuse our best clinical intentions."[38] A year lat
H. Jack Geiger, who has been disinclined to acknowledge the existence
systemic medical racism, noted "the persistence and prevalence of raci
beliefs and discriminatory behaviors in contemporary American society
and reluctantly conceded that doctors are not "fully insulated from att
tudes toward race, ethnicity, and social class that are prevalent (thoug
often unacknowledged) in the larger society." At the same time, Geiger
assertion that "most physicians" possess a "conscious commitment t
anti-discriminatory principles" appears to claim that the racial enlighten
ment of doctors exceeds that of the general public.[39] It is worth noting tha
Geiger's emphasis on doctors' relative immunity from prejudice aligns
him with racism-denying conservatives who have directed caustic attacks
on medical liberals such as himself. From the conservative perspective,
even taking seriously the possibility of systemic medical racism expresses
an unwarranted and offensive lack of confidence in the (white) medical
profession as a whole.

And what about the effects of the medical school experience on students' attitudes toward patients who are resented for one reason or another? "One of the few areas of universal agreement concerning students' development," *Academic Medicine* reported in 1996, "is that medical training can make students and residents more cynical and insensitive."[45] But not when it comes to race at Harvard Medical School, these ethicists report. Among the medical students they observed, "political correctness appears to be the normative order in public discussion. Medical students with whom we spoke note they never hear overtly negative racist comments in the hospital or among classmates. This sensitivity is new to the late twentieth-century generation of medical students and faculty in our study area."[46] Yet in the same year the Institute of Medicine volume appeared, another author in *Academic Medicine* who studied other medical students cites "a derogatory term widely used by students and faculty members to refer to patients from the skid row area of the city."[47] A decade earlier, *Academic Medicine* had observed that medical students sometimes saw patients as "sources of frustration and antagonism—evocatively recast as 'hits,' 'gomers,' 'geeks,' and 'dirtballs.' They become 'the enemy,' with students feeling justified in their use of negative labels and corresponding behaviors."[48] Are Harvard medical students really immune to the racist banter more realistic observers have noted? The credulity of the Harvard ethicists, who take at face value medical students' assurances about their generation's racial enlightenment, perfectly complements Geiger's dogged resistance to the idea that physicians should be held responsible for racially motivated decisions that derive from unconscious impulses.[49]

Medical liberals who adopt the exculpatory approach to physician responsibility are in no position to contest the claims of conservatives who argue that medical racism is a minor issue or does not exist at all. The *Unequal Treatment* report first issued in 2002, the product of a committee chaired by a former president of the American Medical Association, Alan Nelson, is a thoroughly moderate document. The strongest language in Dr. Nelson's speech to the Institute of Medicine on March 22, 2002, reads as follows: "Bias, stereotyping, prejudice, and clinical uncertainty on the part of health care providers may contribute to racial and ethnic disparities in health care. While indirect evidence from several lines of research support this statement, a greater understanding of the prevalence and influence of the processes is needed and should be sought through research."[50] Here, as elsewhere, medical liberalism was still treating the effects of "stereotyping, prejudice, and clinical uncertainty" as hypothetical, and there is the usual call for additional research, an implicit claim that the medical status of African Americans—and the behavior of their doctors—was still too complicated to understand.

Even this tepid call to action was too much for Dr. Sally Satel, whose response to this document appeared in *The Wall Street Journal* under the title "Racist Doctors? Don't Believe the Media Hype."[51] The authors' refusal to call doctors racists was irrelevant to this conservative ideologue; the real offense of the Committee on Understanding and Eliminating Racial and Ethnic Disparities in Health Care was to have even considered the possibility that American doctors might be capable of racially motivated misconduct on a scale exceeding the misdeeds of a few bad apples.

One antidote to tentative medical liberalism and obstinate conservative denial is historical knowledge of the relationship between American medicine and the black population over the past century. The publication of a massive history of modern medical racism in 2002, while noted in the press, should have had a greater catalytic effect than it did.[52] That it did not shows that historical documentation of medical racism is not enough, because these narratives can easily promote the mistaken view that medical racism was a phase that modern medicine has left behind. Understanding how this illusion has prevailed becomes possible once we realize what modern doctors do not know about the racial attitudes and behaviors of their twentieth-century predecessors. Without this knowledge doctors will be literally unable to imagine their own capacity for racially motivated behavior. They will remain unaware of how the "hidden curriculum" of medical training perpetuates racial folklore that can do harm. They will continue to interpret traits and conditions of environmental origin as evidence of a "black" racial essence. In short, a medical profession that remains unaware of the racist legacy of American medicine cannot even begin to pursue meaningful reform.

The author of this book agrees with the Harvard ethicists that this situation requires "a critical perspective that has largely been ignored by most research to date." And anyone who doubts that doctors are capable of ignoring entire dimensions of their own medical experiences need only read Jerome Groopman's *How Doctors Think*. For even as he ignores the race factor in medicine, the author of *How Doctors Think* has a lot to say about the limitations of current medical thinking. Do doctors' feelings about patients or their social backgrounds affect their thinking? "Nearly all of the practicing physicians I queried were intrigued by the questions but confessed that they had never really thought about how they think." What Groopman and his colleagues "rarely recognized, and what physicians still rarely discussed as medical students, interns, residents, and indeed throughout lives, is how . . . emotions influence a doctor's perceptions and judgments, his actions and reactions." "I cannot recall a single instance," he says, "when an attending physician taught us to think about social context."[53]

No medical culture that is so devoid of introspective activity regarding human emotions and social realities can understand the consequences of its entanglement with America's racial traumas. It is my hope that *Black and Blue* will enable physicians, and those who study the world of medicine, to understand how our racial complexes have infiltrated medical thinking and practice, and how a disengagement from these complexes might begin.

2. Black Patients and White Doctors

THE AFRICAN AMERICAN HEALTH CALAMITY:
THE SILENCE

The ongoing medical calamity experienced by the African American population since the Emancipation of 1865 has never provoked the public outrage or the political mobilizations associated with other forms of racial injustice and suffering. Jim Crow segregation, the repression of black voting rights, the demoralizing poverty of the inner cities, and police brutality against blacks have all galvanized movements or urban uprisings. A professed concern about the state of the black family produced the Million Man March of 1995 and the enormous publicity that surrounded it. Yet comparable expressions of protest against the traumatic medical history black Americans endure have not happened. The outrage that followed revelations in 1972 about the Tuskegee Syphilis Experiment, an unethical study carried out on poor black sharecroppers over a period of forty years, did not produce anything like an organized movement. This brief firestorm of publicity also demonstrated the limited usefulness and double-edged character of such information in a racially polarized society. For what the black population learned about the one truly infamous example of American medical racism simply deepened a long-standing mistrust of the white medical establishment that had already established itself as a black oral tradition. For that reason the aftereffects of the exposé may have killed more African Americans than the experiment did. The Tuskegee scandal left behind a damaging emotional legacy rather than an organized response to the tremendous toll of premature death and preventable disease that has afflicted African Americans over many generations. The unhappy fact is that the most intense black feelings about the state of black health that achieve public expression are the widely believed conspiracy theories about government plots to exterminate black people by spreading the AIDS virus. The credence that is invested in such stories derives from a larger set of fears about black vulnerability to assorted dangers that can appear paranoid to most whites. Yet the fact is that what blacks believe about African American health and illness is often associated with ostensibly bizarre urban rumors that draw upon deeply entrenched memories of medical abuse and other traumas.

The sheer magnitude of the African American health crisis has been documented repeatedly, exhaustively, and—in important ways—fruitlessly. The number of annual "excess deaths" occurring in the African American population as of 2002 was estimated to have been 83,570.[1] Measured over decades, this points to a toll numbering in the millions. African Americans die of heart disease, strokes, cancers, liver disease, diabetes, childbirth, tuberculosis, and premature birth at much greater rates than non-Hispanic whites.[2] "The average length of a Negro's life in the South at present is 35 years," Booker T. Washington wrote in 1915. By 1947 black life expectancy had risen to 57 years as opposed to 66 years for whites.[3] As of 1998 whites were still living six years longer than blacks (70 versus 76 years). During the 1990s the "years of healthy life" gap stood at about eight years.[4] These are the statistics underlying the discussion about whether African Americans live long enough to collect the Social Security payments they make over their working lifetimes.

How can we account for the lack of urgency attending a major public health emergency that is covered regularly in the media but that fails to ignite in the way some other crises do? Why, for example, have American physicians chosen not to regard black health issues as a public health emergency?

One reason for the low public profile of the black health crisis is its apparent intractability. As one observer put it back in 1990: "The poor ranking of America's black population in the indices of poor health is a scandal of such long standing that it has lost the power to shock."[5] Or as a *Health Affairs* editorial commented in 2005: "The very persistence and intractability of these symptoms may constitute an insidious disincentive to act."[6] The flood of research papers documenting the medical suffering of the black population has become a kind of dirge, an endless tale of woe and victimization that can create an impression of overwhelming hopelessness and thus paralyze the will to enact policies that might begin to reverse the dire conditions that are described. The recitation of endless statistics documenting the racial health gap can also have the effect of depersonalizing and obscuring the human reality of what is happening to people. Our attention is displaced from the behaviors of doctors and patients into an abstract dimension of enormous and hopelessly complicated social phenomena that can only be imagined or, at best, theorized.

The bureaucratic language in which the data on racial health disparities are presented promotes this sense of anonymous forces acting on people who remain invisible. The soporific and euphemizing effects of public health jargon conceal what can go wrong in relationships between medical professionals (regardless of their race) and their black clients. Indeed, a major argument of this book is that these relationships are often profoundly affected by traditional ideas about racial differences that have survived to a much greater degree than the medical establishment is willing to concede. This false assumption about physicians' immunity to racially motivated thinking helps to account for the limitations of the instructional programs in "cultural competence" that some medical schools now offer in their attempts to sensitize medical students to the needs and circumstances of minority patients.

Playing down or denying the urgency of the medical problems of black people is also accepted because it can serve the emotional interests of both whites and blacks. Even racist whites have found opportunities for feeling magnanimous about their concern for black health. The white Christian masters of antebellum slave plantations, for example, saw themselves as medically conscientious guardians of their black wards, even if their primary motive was to maximize the efficiency of the labor force. The mistaken idea that these slaves had enjoyed excellent health under the supervision of their white overseers became a staple of post-emancipation racial mythology.

The severe health problems that afflicted the liberated and impoverished black population following emancipation were now interpreted as one more pernicious effect of the freedom that had created social conditions in which the allegedly filthy hygienic habits and disease-spreading sexual licentiousness of black people could flourish. Black health problems became a major source of racist resentment. As the *Journal of the American Medical Association* commented in 1909: "In former times they lived a healthy out-door life, and, if for no other reason, in the commercial interests of their owners they were well fed, clothed and lodged. In the last half-century, however, they have left their open-air life and gravitated into the cities, without any one to overlook their physical well-being. Their happy-go-lucky disposition has led them to ignore all principles of sanitation—even if they had an opportunity of becoming acquainted with them. . . ."[7] The medical misery of black people was rationalized as a natural consequence of the "disposition" that had brought about a state of degradation for which whites bore no responsibility. The only responsibility incumbent upon white health authorities was to do everything possible to make sure that unhealthy blacks did not infect the white population.

A half century after this *JAMA* commentary, Dr. Robert A. Hingson of the Case Western Reserve University School of Medicine in Cleveland told the readers of the nation's only black-edited medical journal that the very survival of African Americans had been made possible by "the humanitarian and scientific ministrations of a compassionate nation," in which the (white) medical profession had played a principal role. This anesthesiologist's report on black and white mortality during obstetrics and surgery suggests that he was more compassionate than most of his peers toward the plight of the black patients who were dying under anesthesia in much greater numbers than their white counterparts. He even quotes Franklin D. Roosevelt on the unmet needs of the nation's poor. At the same time, he appears to have been oblivious to the entrenched medical racism of his own profession, which he believed bore no responsibility for the medical problems of his black patients. "We shall leave it to the sociologist to determine the damage the scars of history have left upon the black man," he writes. Separating the medical profession from the damage done to black people in this way expresses a tenacious and self-protective institutional instinct that still prevails over the self-critical approaches to the racial health disparities that have emerged since Hingson pointed to the "racial melancholia" that "all physicians, and especially all psychiatrists" recognized as a syndrome affecting the black population in the 1950s.[8] The persistence of this self-defensive posture among white physicians is evident both in the medical literature and from other sources that describe dysfunctional relationships between white doctors and black patients.

The desperate conditions created by urban poverty have ensured a constant flow of disordered or self-destructive black patients to emergency rooms staffed by white and foreign-born physicians who draw their own conclusions about racial character: "I did a year of training in general medicine at a university-affiliated, inner-city hospital," says one doctor, "and it was the worst year of my life. The place was a snake pit." Constant exposure to the self-destructive behaviors indulged in by what appear to be disproportionate numbers of an ethnic group can have a devastating effect on how doctors feel about such people: "The patients were there either because they abused drugs, or had an illness like diabetes that they wouldn't take care of, or were alcoholic, or had gotten beaten on the head while they were robbing a store. Almost all of them had self-inflicted illness. It's very hard to get real sympathetic with people who make themselves sick."[9] These scenarios, in which disorderly, recalcitrant, and criminal individuals demoralize the physicians who attempt to help them, can reinforce in doctors' minds some deeply rooted ideas about intractable social pathologies from which some blacks seem unable to escape.

Negative images of black patients among white physicians have not been limited to the most deranged or irresponsible black patients who show up in the nation's emergency rooms. American medicine's traditional strategies for minimizing white responsibility for black health problems have always included a more general denigration of the intelligence and emotional stability of blacks who seek medical care. During the first half of the twentieth century, white doctors' impatience with "the Negro patient" became a familiar theme in the medical literature. "He is an unwieldy, unwilling, unsatisfactory patient," *JAMA* reported in 1899.[10] The principal "obstacles to negro practice," according to a 1908 *JAMA* extract from the *Mississippi Medical Monthly*, were "a delight in fooling the doctor if possible; an utter inability to understand and follow directions; the interposition of outsiders, who dissuade from obedience to instructions; the undying fondness for filling his belly; his morbid dread of water; his poverty and filth, and fondness for night prowling and sexual excesses."[11] Over the next half century a medical folklore made up of many such assessments of "the Negro patient" appeared in the medical literature. These accounts presented blacks as particularly exasperating examples of what came be known as "noncompliant" patients who lack the intelligence or the self-discipline to follow doctors' orders.

The other and ostensibly different type of "Negro patient" who provoked medical commentary during the era of Jim Crow was the docile simpleton who displayed a striking medical naïveté or a slavish version of compliance that evoked the submissive Sambo stereotype. White doctors commented on his "optimism" or stoicism or "the absence of worry" in such people. "Complications are accepted as being foreordained and unavoidable. The majority of them bear pain, impairment of function, and the destruction of tissue with little complaint or apprehension," two urologists write in 1935.[12] "His idea of the medical world," a syphilis expert wrote in 1910, "is that there is a remedy for every disease and that all that the doctor does is to select the right medicine."[13] Dr. R. A. Vonderlehr, a participant in the Tuskegee scandal, commented in 1936: "The average negro is a most congenial person and he has a tendency to agree with almost everything that one wishes him to agree with."[14]

A sometimes fatal consequence of this disconnect between doctor and patient has been a tendency among blacks to neglect symptoms and delay visits to the doctor. "The average negro," an Arkansas doctor wrote in 1926, "does not call for medical aid until he thinks himself seriously ill. He first tries all kinds of charms, herbs and teas, thereby cheating himself of his best opportunity of recovery." This doctor also notes "much confusion in medical terms. They have no such words as stools, urine, etc., in their vocabulary."[15] A cardiologist comments in 1927 on how differently blacks and whites describe chest pain: "That which the white man speaks of in a striking, graphic manner, the negro refers to as 'misery in the stomach' or 'misery in the chest.'"[16] Speaking a medical language of their own, such black patients appear to have received little sympathy from the white physicians who could not understand them. Today such problems persist but are wrapped in a depersonalizing jargon that speaks of "the complex interaction between physician and patient" or "problems in communicating with their physicians." This terminology can make physicians and patients equally disoriented participants in a process that may seem beyond remedy or the responsibility of either party.

Comments about the black patient's tendency to ignore symptoms and delay treatment have appeared in the medical literature for the last century. But the tone in which such behaviors are described in today's medical journals has changed from one of impatience and contempt to a more politically correct humane understanding of circumstances and motives. Sarcasm and exasperation have been replaced by the somber (and often stultifying) idiom of public health professionals and their recognition of sociological factors bearing on black health problems that offer an alternative to simply blaming the victims.

In summary, the American medical establishment has never mobilized on behalf of a medically traumatized African American population. The early twentieth-century white public health officials and doctors who feared the black population in the South as an infectious "reservoir of disease," due to the ravages of tuberculosis and syphilis, were primarily concerned about protecting the health of their own racial community. As the chief health officer of Savannah, Georgia, warned in 1904, it was necessary to reduce disease among blacks, because "in doing this we protect ourselves."[17] "They knead our bread and rock our babies to sleep in their arms, dress them, fondle them, and kiss them," a physician from Florida reminded the American Public Health Association in 1912; "can anyone doubt that we may not escape this close exposure?"[18] The Southern white population did, in fact, escape the feared consequences of their close exposure to their black servants; widespread fears of infection proved unfounded. But the hysterical element inherent in this sort of white thinking about black disease has manifested itself in various forms up to the present day.

For decades afterward, the stereotype of the irresponsible "Negro patient," whether sullen and recalcitrant or ignorant and docile, served to rationalize the black man's subordinate status and relieve both the white physician and society at large of the responsibility for taking on "Negro" medical problems as a serious social project. Doctors' judgments about perceived black immorality prompted them to turn their backs on the Negro patient: "Some physicians of the day were overtly judgmental and spoke of blacks as having earned their illnesses as just recompense for wicked life-styles."[19] Over the past century the razor-slashed, shot-gunned, and overdosed black men and women who have come staggering into hospital emergency rooms after their bouts of Saturday night mayhem have left behind a racial stigma in the minds of the many doctors who have treated them. The tardiness and medical noncompliance of the far greater number of black people who simply do not trust white medical institutions have persuaded many medical personnel that efforts to promote black health face insuperable obstacles. In his classic study of the Tuskegee experiment, James H. Jones points out: "Private physicians had long agreed that the [syphilis] problem was serious, but most despaired of being able to do anything about it, preferring instead to exchange stories on the difficulties of treating black patients."[20] Over the past two decades the medical establishment has adapted to the challenge of widening "racial health disparities" by embracing epidemiological research and clinical studies while omitting the most candid accounts of difficult patients. These publications dress up medical suffering and hardship, as well as failed doctor–patient relationships, in a psychological and sociological jargon that excludes or strictly limits any deeper (and necessarily historical) discussion of racially biased ideas and behaviors among medical personnel.

MEDICAL VULNERABILITY AND RACIAL DEFAMATION

African Americans, including physicians, have long had their own reasons not to draw special attention to their health problems. The medical defamation of black people by whites in positions of authority has taken many forms over the past two centuries and has done incalculable damage to race relations in general and to black confidence in a medical system that has always been controlled by whites. In addition, medical folklore about blacks has played a major role in the history of American racism and its campaign to stigmatize black people as both immoral and inherently inferior.

During the era of slavery, the campaign of defamation aimed primarily at justifying plantation slavery on physiological and psychological grounds. Slave owners and the plantation physicians who served them found it convenient to talk about black slaves' "efficiency as laborers in [a] hot, damp, close, suffocating atmosphere—where, instead of suffering and dying, as the white man would, they are healthier, happier and more prolific than in their native Africa." This physiological rationale for putting slaves into the heat of the cotton fields was accompanied by a psychological rationale—regarding the slaves' deficient willpower—that justified keeping them under the control of whites.[21] An elaborate system of racist ideas about black anatomy and physiology gave chattel slavery an ostensibly scientific foundation and remained influential well into the twentieth century.

The most destructive defamatory campaign lasted for decades after emancipation and portrayed blacks as a disease-ridden and biologically degenerate race. A 1915 article in the *Southern Medical Journal*, to choose from one of many examples, called the Negro "a hive of dangerous germs, perhaps the great disease-spreader among the other subspecies of *Homo sapiens*."[22] Predictions that syphilis and tuberculosis would eventually bring about their extinction were common before and after the turn of the century. In his influential *Race Traits and Tendencies of the American Negro* (1896), Frederick L. Hoffman had welcomed the news that contemporary rates of "constitutional and respiratory diseases" would henceforth limit the growth of the black population. "It is sufficient to know," he writes, "that in the struggle for race supremacy the black race is not holding its own. . . ."[23] Many African Americans were thus made aware that millions of whites, including some doctors, were looking forward to their extinction as a race.

The Social Darwinism of this era constantly evoked the idea of a racial competition that African Americans were fated to lose. In the context of this deadly serious contest, black medical problems became nothing less than harbingers of racial extinction. Constant reports of high rates of syphilis among blacks reinforced folkloric ideas about their sexual immorality that attained the status of dogma for many white physicians and further intensified black hostility toward the medical profession. "It is the prevailing opinion," one doctor writes in 1915, "that practically every negro who has reached middle life is syphilitic, an opinion which finds support in the exceedingly lax moral standards of the race."[24] Here is the heritage of medical defamation that makes today's African Americans reluctant to protest against the legacy of medical racism by declaring, "Look how sick we are!"

Public discussions of black medical inferiority forced black leaders, and black doctors in particular, into the position of having to defend the biological integrity of the "race" and even the capacity of Negroes to benefit from medical therapies—a campaign that persists up to the present day in the case of certain medications. The Urban League's official publication declared in 1924, for example, that "the Negro possesses 'biologic fitness'" and, contrary to the belief of some white doctors, is also capable of responding to the treatment for pulmonary tuberculosis.[25] In 1932, a white member of the American Social Hygiene Association welcomed "the willingness of Negro leaders to face statistics relative to actual health conditions. A few years ago the Negro was inclined to interpret statements and figures regarding syphilis and gonorrhea as a racial indictment."[26] Black people understood that defamatory claims about black sexual behavior were poisoning race relations and alienating black people from white doctors.

Describing the medical problems of black people without causing offense has been a long-standing problem. A black physician writing in the Urban League magazine in 1941 strives for balance by acknowledging the seriousness of the "Negro health problem" while refusing to accept the familiar claims about the sickliness of his people. "The health of the Negro *is* a problem," he writes, "but, before submitting proof, let us define the premise. *The health of the Negro*, as used by the intelligent and honest observer and narrator is not by assertion or implication a derogatory statement. Certainly, it is not intended to place undue emphasis upon his susceptibility to disease or his maladjustment in the complex pattern of American life." The challenge for Dr. Roscoe C. Brown of the U.S. Public Health Service was to confront two ideological adversaries. On one side were the white doctors who made a policy of exploiting black health problems to promote the idea of racial inferiority and the ideal of segregation. On the other side were those of his fellow blacks who resented public discussions of the state of their health and favored "a more euphemistic and optimistic declaration of racial parity in health status and life expectancy."[27] In 1945 the first African American physician to earn a masters degree in public health, Dr. Paul B. Cornely, struck a blow for the medical integration of all Americans by declaring that "there is [no] such an entity as a 'Negro Health Problem,' for the health achievements and problems of this racial group are merely expressions of the total health situation of the country."[28] A decade later Cornely was able to report some incremental progress in the desegregation of an American medical system that was still refusing to embrace racial integration.[29] But the era of real militancy directed against the de facto racism of the American Medical Association and its segregated medical system was yet to come.

Open resentment of pessimistic and unflattering descriptions of black health problems emerged along with other expressions of black self-assertion during the 1960s. On occasion these reactions reversed white claims about black infirmity and exhibited a rhetorical inflation that distorted reality. On March 24, 1961, for example, Malcolm X, invoking the spectacle of biblical wrath, told a white audience at Harvard Law School the following: "Your people are being afflicted with increasing epidemics of illness, disease, and plagues, with which God is striking you because of your criminal acts against the twenty million ex-slaves."[30] The same need for compensatory illusion appeared a year later when a black doctor told the annual meeting of the National Medical Association that slavery had been "the greatest biological experiment of all times" and a eugenic boon to black Americans.[31] In a different vein, the Reverend Martin Luther King, Jr accused the American Medical Association in 1966 of promulgating a racist "conspiracy of inaction" against black people. Amidst all of the apolitical and now routine celebrations of Dr. King, this prescient analysis and protest against institutional medical racism has been forgotten.[32] By 1968 Paul Cornely had taken note of the radical moment and warned that racial health disparities were adding "fuel to the smoldering Negro revolution which explodes intermittently."[33] During the 1966 riots in Chicago, blacks had burned down a health clinic on the city's West Side. In 1969 *Newsweek* informed its readers that "slum dwellers themselves wryly refer to municipal hospital clinics as 'the butchershop' or 'the plantation.'"[34] It is no accident that these gritty details appeared, not in a medical journal, but in a newsmagazine that was uncensored by the editorial policies of medical editors.

The point here is not that the highly credentialed Paul Cornely had become a radical. On the contrary, his conduct as a black physician and public health official remained self-disciplined and professional throughout this period of growing black dissatisfaction with the medical care white authorities chose to make available to Negro patients. What matters here is Cornely's professional deportment, his adherence to the standards of what I wish to call "the black physician as gentleman," the black medical man of this era who constantly had to control his anger as he devoted himself to caring for black patients in circumstances that racist practices made difficult or impossible. This self-control included not alienating the

white medical establishment on which black doctors were deeply dependent. While some of these men must have imagined a social protest movement that would relieve the medical misery of the black masses, the public
expression of such anger and demands for relief do not begin to appear
until the militant rhetoric of the 1960s offered political cover to black doctors who were moved to protest.

Black physicians have been a beleaguered and often disdained minority
within the medical profession, and this marginal status has limited their
ability to challenge the white medical establishment. During the early decades of the twentieth century, blacks and whites alike questioned both
their competence and their motives. Black doctors were also blamed for the
state of black health: "The Federal Government inadvertently contributed
to the embarrassment of the Negro physician when it perennially issued
statistics that showed the Negro death rate to be from 5 to 7 times higher
than that of the general population. These figures could be interpreted in
one of two ways. First, that the Negro was biologically different or inferior,
a conclusion reached by Dr. Stoddard of Harvard and later by Dr. Putnam
of Princeton. Second, that the treatment the Negro received was patheti-
cally inadequate. The latter conclusion would reflect on the competence of
Negro physicians who took care of these people. . . ."[35]

Even in their own medical schools, the black historian and journalist
Carter G. Woodson wrote in 1933, black medical students were made to
feel inferior "in being reminded of their role as germ carriers." Nor could
black doctors be effective if their own people did not believe they were
competent, since they "had difficulty in making their own people believe
that they could cure a complaint, fill a tooth, or compound a prescription."[36]

The self-assertive attitude among blacks that advanced during the civil
rights decade also changed attitudes toward black physicians. In 1970 *Time*
reported that African Americans were feeling an "increasing sense of security visiting a black rather than a white doctor. This is a complete reversal
of the older pattern: blacks used to take their minor ills to a black doctor,
but seek a supposedly superior white practitioner for major medical matters because there were few black specialists."[37] This attraction of black
middle-class patients to the "great white father image" was still being discussed in the African American medical press in 1985.[38] The black population was still emerging from a period that included the marginalizing and
humiliation of its medical personnel, who still lacked the prestige to mount
an effective campaign against the consequences of medical racism. In fact,
the professional status of the black physician can still be called into question. As one of my African American students wrote in 2001: "Patients

discriminate against physicians. Blacks prefer a white doctor on the white or so-called 'good' side of town."

The ability of African Americans to campaign against the causes of their medical misfortunes has also been limited by the sheer volume of disease and disability, along with the accompanying demoralization, with which they and their doctors have had to contend up to the present day. Listening to physicians who care for the black poor at Meharry Medical College, it is easy to conclude that impoverished African Americans in particular have come to accept impairment by severe medical problems as a way of life. Under the doctors' attitude of realism one senses an undercurrent of resignation. "I think we are losing the war in terms of prevention," says one doctor. "It's a socioeconomic thing. Most poor people don't have adequate access. They don't have good insurance, good education. They don't come unless it impairs their ability to work. By that time the damage has already been done." A second black doctor addresses the issue of group demoralization head on: "The biggest issue," he says, "is self-esteem. I don't think our hopes go as far as white people's. Our teachers don't expect us to do more. We have a tendency to let things get worse. We get caught up in crime, drugs, prison."[39] Given the emotional burden of group suffering on this scale, any sense of collective grievance that might be mobilized in the form of public protest becomes overwhelmed by doctors' and patients' immediate needs to cope and survive, whether physically or emotionally. This emotional burden is compounded by the shortage of black medical personnel in many parts of the country. "We have one black surgeon in Savannah, no black nephrologists, one black gastroenterologist, two black pediatricians, both women, no black dermatologists," a black physician commented in 1999.[40] A young black professional once told me how difficult it was for him and his wife to find a black pediatrician in as large a metropolitan area as Austin, Texas. The stresses and discomfiting situations black clients seeking black physicians experience are seldom noted in the accounts of black health issues produced by public health officials. Here, too, African Americans are expected to adapt to circumstances and endure a variety of difficult situations that are otherwise reserved for poor whites and other people who exist on the margins of society.

Contemplating this long history of medical ordeals suggests that some African Americans have, to one degree or another, become resigned to medical infirmity, because the fatal combination of poverty and institutional medical racism has made medical hardship a fact of life. Today, the memory of these hardships persists in the form of an estrangement from the medical profession that will be described throughout much of this book. But it is also important to recognize the value to black people of an adaptive response to medical hardship that amounts to more than a habituation to silent suffering. Medical hardship has played a significant role in the creation of an African American doctrine of survival—a cultural ideology that portrays black people as resilient and dignified survivors rather than as downtrodden victims.

Self-assertive expressions about black resilience can also cross the line into a kind of compensatory make-believe. In his remarkable anthology of African American testimonies *Drylongso* (1980), the black cultural anthropologist John Langston Gwaltney records the following declaration from a poor African American woman who had survived many hardships: "Most black people think that they are mentally and physically better than white people, and I think that they are physically superior to white people. I think it goes back to slavery-time. I think that only the strongest of us were able to survive, so that gave us better stock to start with."[41]

Eugenic fantasies of this kind have long served as emotionally satisfying responses to defamatory claims about the biological and mental health of blacks. The imaginary racial advantage can also take the form of a presumed superior resistance to disease. In 1970, for example, *Time* reported that almost half of the African American population believed that "whites are more apt to catch diseases" than blacks, a folkloric belief that has always been contradicted by the public health data.[42] *Jet* magazine reported in 1984 that having a "touch of diabetes" had helped blacks survive the ordeals of slavery, yet another variation on the eugenic interpretation of black enslavement.[43] A medically disadvantageous use of black "hardiness" is what the journalist Ellis Cose has called "an ethic of toughness" that "makes it very hard to admit that you are in pain or need help either physical or psychological." Dr. Jean Bonhomme, president of the National Black Men's Health Network, calls this trait "pathological stoicism," and he regards it as a health threat.[44]

Stoicism of this kind can affect African American attitudes toward coping with depression. One study found that almost two-thirds of African Americans regard depression as a "personal weakness," and that the same proportion "reported they believed prayer and faith alone would successfully treat depression 'almost all of the time' or 'some of the time.'" A quarter said they would "handle" clinical depression alone, and only a third said they would take antidepressant medication if it were prescribed by a doctor, as compared to 69 percent of the general population.[45]

The stoic approach to depression incorporates several mutually related themes that have shaped African American responses to disease and medical hardship. Medical stoicism on the part of blacks is in part an abstention from participating in a medical culture that whites have created and controlled. The African American cardiologist Richard Allen Williams pointed out the following thirty years ago: "A person with chest pains may be so angry at the medical system that he may refuse to go to the hospital and may die at home. If such behavior occurs on a large scale, the effect that it will have on morbidity and mortality statistics is obvious."[46] The medical and public health literatures, which seldom look at patient behavior as a product of historical experience, treat this sort of recalcitrance as a kind of passive negligence, while others will see such recalcitrance as self-assertive and even self-protective behavior.

Medical stoicism has been embraced because it expresses a toughness or "hardiness" that can serve as a source of racial pride. Such feelings, as we have seen, can inspire eugenic fantasies of black racial superiority. "The fact," the black writer George Schuyler said in 1927, "is that in America conditions have made the average Negro more alert, more resourceful, more intelligent, and hence more interesting than the average Nordic. Certainly if the best measure of intelligence is ability to survive in a changing or hostile environment, and if one considers that the Negro is not only surviving but improving all the time in health, wealth, and culture, one must agree that he possesses a high degree of intelligence." At a time when the ideas of Sigmund Freud were taking the eastern seaboard of the United States by storm, Schuyler ridiculed the psychiatric fashions and emotional insecurities of "sophisticated whites" by alluding to the psychological hardiness of his fellow blacks: "It is difficult to imagine," he wrote, "a group of intelligent Negroes sprawling around a drawing-room, consuming cigarettes and synthetic gin while discussing their complexes and inhibitions."[47]

The idea that black emotional hardiness makes psychiatry unnecessary for black people exemplifies the stoic attitude that prompts some African Americans to make fewer rather than more demands on the medical system. Medical stoicism, an ethos of self-reliance, self-defensive eugenic thinking, and a doctrine of black hardiness, is a belief-system that encourages African American estrangement from the medical system. "The experience of inferior racial status has not transformed the Negro into a super human being," the black psychologist Kenneth B. Clark wrote in 1965.[48] But some African Americans have believed otherwise, persuaded that the extraordinary hardships of the African American experience must have produced a race of strong and tenacious survivors. This tension between the eugenic and tragic interpretations of the African American experience has persisted into our own era.

Calling racial health disparities a civil rights issue has become one argument health care reformers use. The Reverend Al Sharpton's declaration in 1998 that the black health crisis is "the new civil rights battle of the 21st century" did not galvanize African Americans because—unlike the O. J. Simpson verdict—it cannot be reduced to a single dramatic event that symbolizes the experience of shared oppression.[49] Even the Tuskegee revelations, and the sordid details they revealed, failed to produce that kind of community outrage. The preceding pages have offered an explanation of why open revolt against medical racism has not taken place. The relevant factors include the sheer magnitude of the black health crisis and the demoralization it has caused among black laypeople and physicians alike; the mind-numbing jargon that smothers human suffering in sociological abstractions in the medical and public health literatures; the racial imbalance of power that has limited the power and influence of black physicians; the enduring reputation of "the Negro patient" among physicians, not excluding some black and foreign-born physicians; the long history of estrangement of African Americans from the medical system in general; African Americans' reluctance to draw attention to health problems that have been exploited for the purpose of defaming them as a race; and the belief in black hardiness and the medical stoicism it can encourage.

HOW DO (WHITE) PHYSICIANS THINK ABOUT RACE? EVIDENCE OF MEDICAL RACISM

Over the past twenty-five years the most prestigious American medical journals have produced massive evidence confirming that racially biased diagnosis and treatments are a fact of life in American medicine.[50] These analyses document racially biased behaviors and have prompted one official investigation and no disciplinary proceedings. Other professionals serving the public, such as policemen or professors, are not granted such immunity from scrutiny of their professional conduct. The racially motivated habits whose effects are presented in the medical literature as statistical data are so ingrained that some doctors do not deviate from them even when they know their interactions with black patients are being recorded for observation.[51] Their personal eccentricities and the specific harms they cause to their patients remain anonymous, buried in the statistics that make it into print. Concealed behind the sterile terminology about racial "disparities" and "cultural differences" are an unknown number of biased behaviors that in other social venues might be regarded as negligence or violations of the law.

What evidence do we have that doctors employ racially motivated thinking when dealing with patients of color? The abundant data that indicate differential diagnosis and treatment for a wide range of diseases and disorders are one type of evidence. Their crucial disadvantage is that they portray collective behavior rather than the more detailed scenarios of private professional conduct that do not appear in the medical literature. The motives for some physician behaviors can be deduced on the basis of what is known about the history of racialist thinking by physicians. Deductions of this kind are indispensable to understanding racially motivated medical thinking and behavior, given the dearth of current survey data about physicians' racial thoughts and fantasies. But they are open to the objection that what we know about doctors' racial complexes from the overt medical racism of the past may not apply to modern practitioners who have supposedly absorbed socially sanctioned disapproval of racist speech and behaviors and conduct themselves accordingly. This book's methodology is based on the premise that, to the contrary, significant aspects of the medical racial folklore of the pre–civil rights period have persisted and adapted to modern circumstances to a greater extent than many have assumed possible in an age of officially mandated racial equality and racially civil public discourse.

There is, in fact, no reason to assume that medical students and doctors are less likely to absorb and act upon the racial fantasies that still suffuse modern societies. In 2001, for example, three white medical students at the University of Alabama at Birmingham were exposed by the news media after they wore blackface to a Halloween party. One was dressed as Stevie Wonder, the second as a character from the *Fat Albert* cartoon show, and the third as a black woman.[52] The medical school officials who handled this case, with whom I communicated, resolved this matter by accepting public apologies and devoting a day to racial sensitivity training. The idea that this behavior demonstrated character defects that might make these individuals unfit to practice medicine apparently did not figure in the process that finally certified them as fit to treat black patients. This incident also raises the question of where cultural stereotyping ends and biological race fantasies begin. Blackface signifies a fantasy of racial transformation, just as cross-dressing signifies a fantasy of gender transformation. These medical students found gratification in taking on the identities of a blind singer, a comical cartoon image, and the generic black female who has traditionally ranked at the bottom of our racial hierarchy. These future physicians regarded playing with distorted versions of the black body as a kind of entertainment. One can only wonder what the experience of public humiliation and a day of racial sensitivity training may have done to temper or redirect their fantasies about black bodies in ways that might serve the interests of the African American patients who will some day consult them for medical treatment.

The most thoroughly documented racial disparities concern the diagnosis and treatment of heart disease, the leading cause of death in the United States among blacks as well as whites. This book argues that the medical folklore about blacks and cardiovascular diseases that was so evident throughout the twentieth century has distorted some doctors' responses to heart disease in black patients. The absence of this historical perspective in the current medical literature demonstrates the naïveté of medical authors who regard racially differential diagnosis and treatment of heart disease as a mysterious phenomenon whose causes have somehow eluded our understanding. Reading our way back through the relevant medical publications on coronary disease will help to clarify the mystery. At this point let us survey the findings about racially disparate treatment of patients requiring therapy for heart disease that have appeared since the late 1980s.

As of 1989 white patients were undergoing one-third more coronary catheterizations and more than twice as many coronary angioplasties as black patients.[53] In 1993 researchers confirmed that "white patients consistently underwent invasive cardiac procedures more often than black patients."[54] In a 1996 editorial in the *New England Journal of Medicine*, H. Jack Geiger expressed deep concern about the unequal treatment of heart disease: "Perhaps most consistent—and most disturbing—are the repeated findings that blacks with ischemic heart disease, even those enrolled in Medicare or free-care systems, are much less likely to undergo angiography, angioplasty, or coronary-artery bypass grafting (CABG)."[55] A 1997 report came to similar conclusions regarding bypass surgery; the author called this finding "disturbing, because we also found that they were not due to differences in the severity of disease or to coexisting illnesses."[56] A 2000 report confirmed that "medical therapies are currently underused in the treatment of black, female, and poor patients" who have suffered acute myocardial infarction. "This variation was not explained by severity of illness, physician specialty, hospital, and geographic characteristics"[57]— possible confounding factors this study ruled out, leaving physician bias as the most probable explanation for why black patients were offered fewer therapeutic procedures. A 2005 survey of racial differences in the management of acute myocardial infarction covering between 1994 and 2002 found that racial differences in care had persisted rather than diminished during this period.[58]

Racially differential practices have also been found to affect the treatment of early-stage lung cancer. One research team wrote the following in 1999: "Our analyses suggest that the lower survival rate among black patients with early-stage, non-small-lung cancer, as compared with white patients, is largely explained by the lower rate of surgical treatment among blacks."[59] The same conclusion was reiterated in 2006: "Black patients obtain surgery for lung cancer less often than whites, even after access to care has been demonstrated. They are likely not to have surgery recommended, and more likely to refuse surgery."[60] It is historically conditioned fear that causes some black patients to refuse surgery even when it would be in their best interest to consent. The medical literature refers to these decisions as examples of "patient preferences," as though these decisions to reject surgery were free and autonomous acts on the part of empowered medical consumers. In fact, blacks' fears of surgery persist because the medical profession has never addressed the consequences of its racist history in a way that might reassure African Americans who feel estranged from the medical system.

Heart and cancer surgeries are generally regarded as desirable procedures that benefit patients, and that is why racially differential access to them is unjust. There are other kinds of surgery that are undesirable when better alternatives exist, and here too black patients have borne an extra burden of suffering. The effects of a hysterectomy, for example, are likely to be more of an ordeal for a black woman than for her white counterpart, since "black women are more likely to get the more invasive kind of hysterectomy, which doesn't require a large incision. The vaginal operation is more expensive and harder, and studies have shown it is used more on women higher on the socioeconomic scale."[61] It was reported in 1996 and 1998 that black patients with diabetes and circulatory problems were less likely than whites to have leg-sparing surgery and were more likely to undergo the amputation of these limbs. Yet precisely the reverse was true of a more beneficial type of operation, since blacks were less than half as likely as whites to get hip replacements.[62] Here, too, "patient preferences" dissuade some black patients from undergoing hip or knee surgeries because they "report less confidence in the efficacy" of such operations.[63] Accepting such "patient preferences" as autonomous decisions is mistaken, since the black patient's lack of confidence in the procedures is an expression of mistrust rooted in a group history of traumatic experiences involving the medical profession.[64]

Evidence of racially differential thinking by physicians has also appeared in studies of emergency room analgesia.[65] Making judgments about doctors' unequal provision of pain relief to members of different racial or ethnic groups is complicated by three related factors—the subjective nature of pain perception, those cultural factors that may influence an individual's response to the experience of pain, and folkloric ideas about racially differential responses to pain.[66] Doctors' judgments have been affected by a traditional medical folklore about racial differences in pain sensitivity, in particular the idea that black people do not feel pain as acutely as whites do. "I can find no evidence to support the belief that the Negro does not feel pain as well as the white person," one cardiologist wrote in 1942, and this assertion made him a dissenter among his peers.[67] But historical knowledge of this kind is rare among today's medical researchers. The author of a 1993 *JAMA* article that found Hispanic patients got less pain relief than whites comments: "The mechanism by which ethnicity influences pain management decisions is unclear." He and his colleagues, he reports, were now involved in "an attempt to discover whether physicians assess pain differently in patients of different ethnic groups."[68] The abundance of published evidence confirming that physicians for many years have based pain assessments on racial distinctions appears to have been unknown to him. It did not occur to this author to look for evidence of what he was looking for in the medical literature that preceded him. And, even if he had sought and found it, he might have assumed that today's physicians, unlike their predecessors, are too enlightened to think of pain thresholds as a racial trait.

Confirming the likelihood of racially discriminatory behaviors by physicians in a statistically convincing way is complicated and requires controlling for so-called confounding factors. The fact that the diagnoses and treatments offered to black and white patients may not be identical does not in and of itself demonstrate biased judgments or behaviors on the part of physicians. Other factors, such as biological or cultural differences, may account for these discrepancies. Economic and educational status can have enormous effects on health quite apart from how physicians behave. Poverty and illiteracy are powerful predictors of medical problems regardless of a patient's race or ethnicity or of how doctors respond to that person's medical problems. Racially motivated behaviors on the part of doctors may be absent or difficult to identify precisely because they coexist with other plausible contributing factors, such as unemployment or dietary habits, for which doctors do not bear a direct responsibility.

Conscientious physicians and medical scientists acknowledge confounding factors even as they may propose a diagnostic or therapeutic scenario that documents medically discriminatory behavior. For example, the author of one of the studies of heart disease previously cited cautions that "racial variation in rates of coronary revascularization may have resulted in part from differences in the prevalence of disease, the severity of disease, and other clinical factors."[69] If heart disease occurs more often in one group than another, then that in itself might account for different numbers of procedures in the respective patient populations. Similarly, if the severity of a disease differs in blacks and whites for biological reasons—glaucoma, for example, is a more serious disorder in blacks than in whites—then different treatments may be appropriate. Determining whether the appearance of more (or more severe) disease in one racial group is due at least in part to biological factors remains difficult and controversial for reasons we will examine next.

RESISTANCE TO THE CRITIQUE OF RACIAL BIAS IN MEDICINE

American medicine has reacted ambivalently to the hundreds of studies that have documented racial disparities in health care. On the one hand, medical journals publish the reports that confirm the disparities, and these reports are sometimes accompanied by editorial commentaries that describe the disparities as intolerable and call for action to reverse them. At the same time, these medical authors have developed a rhetorical strategy that allows them to deplore racial health and treatment disparities without taking responsibility for them. Even the liberal white doctors who actually care about racial injustice in medicine have found ways to formulate their analyses of physician behaviors in such a way as to avoid threatening their own self-images and exposing the profession to critical scrutiny by outsiders.

Ambivalence about confirming the existence of medical racism has also been evident in the federal agencies responsible for monitoring and improving public health. In 1985 the Department of Health and Human Services (HHS) released its Report of the Secretary's Task Force on Black and Minority Health, documenting many health disparities. In 1999, Congress instructed the Agency for Healthcare Research and Quality (AHRQ) to publish an annual report, beginning in 2003, to document "prevailing disparities in health care delivery as it relates to racial factors and socio-economic factors in priority populations." The first National Healthcare Disparities Report (NHDR) was released in 2003, the second in 2004, and a third (and more complete) report in 2005.[70] The National Academies' Institute of Medicine issued a similar report in 2002.[71] The chairman of the committee that wrote the report, a former president of the American

Medical Association (AMA), commented: "The real challenge lies not in
debating whether disparities exist, because the evidence is overwhelming,
but in developing strategies to reduce and eliminate them." At the same
time, the National Academies' news release, summarizing the implications
of the report, made notable use of the exculpating rhetoric and euphemizing vocabulary alluded to previously: "The report says that although it is
reasonable to assume that the vast majority of health care providers find
prejudice morally abhorrent, several studies show that even well-meaning
people who are not overtly biased or prejudiced typically demonstrate unconscious negative racial attitudes and stereotypes. In addition, the time
pressures that characterize many clinical encounters, as well as the complex
thinking and decision-making they require, may increase the likelihood
that stereotyping will occur."[72]

This is the standard medical liberal's interpretation of the individual
doctor's racially motivated behavior. According to this account, the "vast
majority" of medical personnel are committed antiracists; "well-meaning"
people succumb to "unconscious negative racial attitudes and stereotypes"
that are hidden from them and for which, therefore, they cannot be held
responsible until they are made aware of them. The stereotyping of patients originates in external circumstances such as "time pressures" that
exacerbate the already formidable challenges of "complex thinking and
decision-making." There is, of course, some truth to this interpretation,
including the essential point that a person can be unaware of his or her
racial attitudes and their consequences for other people. But this is also a
children's book version of medical reality that has been sanitized to preserve the self-image of the medical profession. The racial goodwill of the
"vast majority" of white practitioners is taken for granted. Their racially
motivated behaviors originate in unconscious attitudes and hectic schedules that do not allow them to be their true and racially wholesome selves.
The black patients who may have been subjected to racially motivated negligence are absent from a drama that is focused on the needs of its white
dramatis personae.

A similarly evasive strategy is evident in the influential and expanding
field of biomedical ethics, which has effectively taken a pass on the issue
of medical racism. The fifth edition of the standard text, Beauchamp and
Childress' *Principles of Biomedical Ethics* (2001), devotes exactly one and
one-half pages to the "unfair distribution of health care based on race."
Its approach is entirely sociological; we are presented with the familiar
data about lower black rates of cardiac surgery and organ transplantation
and nothing on the psychology or possible misbehaviors of the individual

physician.[73] Here, too, medical professionals are exempted from scrutiny that might challenge their image as uniformly humane and impartial caregivers. Similarly, *The Oxford Handbook of Bioethics* (2009) includes nothing about race and medical ethics.

Despite its self-exculpating agenda, the liberal perspective on health disparities and medical racism is self-critical when compared with right-wing responses to criticism of the medical profession's treatment of minority patients. Resistance to even acknowledging the reality of racial health disparities can appear in state or federal agencies when the ideological winds in government are blowing in from the conservative end of the political spectrum. The deputy administrator for the Wisconsin Division of Public Health, Kenneth Baldwin, stated the following in 2001: "I'm not willing to say or place [*sic*] racism as a reason for [the] health disparity. I think it would be naïve to say that, when there is no one answer to the problem." This official preferred to identify poverty as the explanation for differential health outcomes and suggest that race was irrelevant to higher rates of black morbidity and mortality.[74]

The same preference for nonracial explanations for racial health disparities came to public attention in 2004 when political appointees in the Department of Health and Human Services (DHHS) of President George W. Bush were found to have altered a federal report on health disparities based on the 2002 Institute of Medicine report. The original version of this report issued in July 2003 concluded that racial disparities are "pervasive in our healthcare system."[75] This finding was too much for DHHS conservatives, so the version released in December 2003 was edited to present a more upbeat interpretation of the data. For example, "A report by the special investigative division of the Congressional Committee on Government Reform found that the word 'disparity,' mentioned 30 times in the 'key findings' of the [initial] draft, was used only twice in the key findings of the final version."[76] M. Gregg Bloche, a physician and bioethicist who had served on the Institute of Medicine Committee, commented in 2004: "In playing down our conclusion, the rewrite broke with the great weight of scientific opinion. . . . By insisting that the AHRQ researchers treat the existence of racial disparities as an unproven hypothesis rather than an established premise for their report, those who ordered the rewrite imposed their politics on federal science." The conservatives went so far as to demand that the AHRQ researchers do the virtually impossible—control for enormously complex confounding factors such as the effects of social class and education—or eliminate all claims about disparities from the report. When leaks from DHHS forced the DHHS Secretary, Tommy Thompson, to release the original and uncensored version, he called the initial release of the altered report a "mistake."[77]

Why did DHHS conservatives want to suppress data about racial health disparities? M. Gregg Bloche pointed to their disdain for government-sponsored social engineering and the related emphasis on personal responsibility: "A coherent vision motivated the proponents of the rewrite. This vision stresses the centrality of personal responsibility, both for our health and for our circumstances more generally. To call the rewrite's supporters racially insensitive oversimplifies matters."[78] The conservatives' other urgent priority was to suppress any claim that doctors were guilty of racially motivated misconduct. That is why the rewritten version, while acknowledging that "some socioeconomic, racial, ethnic and geographic differences exist," also states the following: "There is no implication that these differences result in adverse health outcomes *or imply moral error or prejudice in any way* [emphasis added]."[79] Like the medical liberals, these medical policy conservatives were deeply invested in protecting the image of white physicians. This required them in turn to make the absurd claim that physicians are somehow immune to the effects of racial prejudice. In reality, a doctor who was incapable of falling into "moral error" would have to be a godlike creature. It is this element of hard-bitten denial that separates the obdurate conservative from the medical liberal whose ideas about the physician's intrinsically benign temperament are less extreme and are more open to correction on the basis of evidence.

One critic of Secretary Thompson's decision to release the original health disparities report was Dr. Sally L. Satel, a psychiatrist who specializes in the treatment of drug addiction and is affiliated with the conservative American Enterprise Institute. "Secretary Thompson succumbed to political pressure that was applied by members of Congress who are identified with ethnic causes," she charged.[80] The idea that racial health disparities do not originate in prejudice or injustice has been a fundamental premise of the ideologically driven views on race and medicine that Satel has published over many years. While conceding that some "lingering bias" may persist in the medical system, Satel's position is that "many race-related differences in health care are not what they seem." Physicians and public health professionals who see racism in medicine are "indoctrinologists" who demonstrate a "stubborn reluctance to acknowledge that each person has some responsibility for preserving his or her own health—an attitude that threatens to reverse the gains made by public health in the past century." She opposes any federal spending on research that is based on the idea that racism might affect African American health. Finally, she argues that racially differential treatment of whites and blacks results in part from anatomical differences between the races that disadvantage black patients.[81] In summary, Satel's argument against what she regards as politically correct medicine amounts to a comprehensive defense of American physicians against the idea that racially motivated behaviors play any significant role in their relationships with black or other minority patients.

MEDICAL LIBERALISM AND THE MEDICAL LITERATURE

The conservative exculpation of physicians differs from the medical liberal's version in that the liberal analysis of physician behavior is more open-minded, far more concerned with ensuring social justice, and somewhat more willing to expose doctors' behavior to critical scrutiny. Still, the liberal consensus that has emerged over the last two decades almost always gives physicians the benefit of the doubt. These authors assume that American physicians are simply too conscientious to be capable of racially discriminatory diagnosis and treatment. They find it implausible that doctors would be as capable of absorbing and acting upon racial folklore as other people are.

The medical literature's response to overwhelming evidence of racially biased (and potentially deadly) behaviors has thus combined two strategies. On the one hand, there are the hundreds of peer-reviewed reports of racially differential diagnosis and treatment. At the same time, the presentation of these data employs a rhetoric of alibis, euphemism, and denial.[82] The purpose of these rhetorical strategies is to demonstrate that, regardless of what the statistical evidence says about their behavior, American physicians are not "racists" who require reformation or public exposure. Many self-exculpating formulations of this kind have appeared in the medical and public health literatures, including a recent proposal that "racially based clinical stereotypes" are merely "cognitive 'shortcut[s]' busy clinicians may use to help order their world."[83] Here again we see "time pressure" invoked as a mitigating factor in the event the doctor employs racial stereotyping. This is not to deny the real pressures that HMO-mandated assembly-line medicine inflicts on busy physicians. The problem is that the hectic schedule is invoked to deemphasize the racial stereotypes that may be affecting clinicians' judgment when they encounter black patients. The significance of this terminology lies in the discomfiting details it leaves out and in the alibis it presents to the reader: Physicians who practice racially biased medicine are not themselves racists, but are simply too busy to behave more carefully. They are distracted rather than negligent or hostile.

Racial bias is presented as an impersonal phenomenon for which doctors do not bear individual responsibility.

A major failing of the medical authors who have addressed the issue of medical racism in the medical literature is their lack of interest in the history of medical racism itself. Scientists' habit of relying on the most recently published work has come at the price of ignoring the history of medical thinking that has preceded and often influenced later thinking about race. Some physicians have thus acquired a naïve view of the history of race relations within the profession. Here, for example, we encounter the (white) physician who suggests in 1997 that African Americans' "lack of trust in the medical establishment may have originated with the disclosures about the Tuskegee syphilis study"—as if the racial misconduct of white physicians had somehow begun in 1972.[84] The overt racism displayed by American medical authors in *JAMA* and other medical journals up until the Second World War appears to be unknown to the great majority of medical authors. This historical ignorance has in turn had a profound effect on the capacity of physicians to even imagine that doctors might behave in racially biased ways for which they might be held accountable.

Another obstacle to acknowledging the role of race in medical practice is a disproportionate emphasis on the complexity of the origins of racial disparities and how much about them remains unknown. The truisms that result from this sort of agnosticism distract readers from what is or should be known about racial factors but was apparently unknown to the authors who profess ignorance. The coauthors of a study of racially unequal treatment for heart disease, for example, wrote in 1989 that "we need to understand more about the complex interaction between physician and patient" that leads to inequality of medical treatments.[85] In this case the tautological assertion that we need to understand more about what we don't understand obscures the more salient point, which is that critical analyses of "the complex interaction between physician and patient" had already appeared in the medical literature. In 1973 *JAMA* published David Satcher's observations on the racially insensitive conduct of many physicians and medical students he had watched interacting with black patients.[86] In 1979 the *Annals of Internal Medicine* published John Eisenberg's seminal article on "Sociologic Influences on Decision-Making by Clinicians."[87] In 1985 *Pediatrics* published David Levy's examination of "White Doctors and Black Patients: Influence of Race on the Doctor-Patient Relationship."[88] To be sure, these prescient essays and a few others were buried among thousands of other communications in the medical literature with which they competed for attention. (The African American–edited *Journal of the*

National Medical Association was then, and remains today, essentially ignored by the medical community and the news media.) The larger point is
that these publications demonstrated a keen awareness of what the medical
literature would eventually come to euphemize as "communication problems" between doctors and their patients. So it was, in fact, possible to
recognize and think systematically about these problems before the flood
of publications on racial health disparities began in the late 1980s.

What is most striking in retrospect is how impervious the medical literature has remained to the essential observations and recommendations
that appear in these "early" publications, all of which postdate the civil
rights era. The irony is that physicians' lack of interest in understanding their own professional behavior in its social context, which is one of
Eisenberg's basic points about how doctors see themselves, has played a
key role in keeping detailed and accurate accounts of black-white medical relationships and the effects of biomedical racial folklore out of the
medical and public health literatures. "Physicians often object," Eisenberg
notes, "to being asked questions relating to professional and social factors, especially religious affiliation and social class origin. This denial of
social influences is not limited to medical clinicians," since even clinical
psychologists tend to believe in their own invulnerability to social and
cultural factors.[89] Removing doctors from their social context offers the
additional benefit of preserving the privacy of professional conduct. The
absolute right to professional autonomy (and the authoritative judgments
this implies) thrives in isolation from challenges to physicians' conduct
toward patients who may or may not be satisfied with the doctors' manner or medical recommendations. Many years ago, David Satcher—who
would later became surgeon general of the United States—observed the
following: "Many white physicians with whom I trained preferred black
patients because they believed the black patient was less likely to be critical
and to express dissatisfaction or to question procedures. Most white physicians interpreted the master-servant relationship as a good doctor-patient
relationship. Their patients were 'happy.'"[90] Keeping the doctors "happy"
depended on their being unaware of how their ostensibly submissive black
patients might actually feel about them.

Socially progressive medical liberals also participate in the strategy of
denial through an inability or unwillingness to see medical race relations
in their historical context. Seeing the Tuskegee scandal as a unique and
temporary blemish on the honor of American medicine, they are likely
to have little or no idea of how their predecessors judged and treated "the
Negro patients" they encountered. Contemplating the possibility that

the racial health disparities they found so "disturbing" might be due to "racially discriminatory rationing by physicians and health care institutions," H. Jack Geiger commented: "We do not yet know enough to make that charge definitively."[91] In fact, Geiger's *New England Journal* editorial, titled "Race and Health Care—An American Dilemma?" (1996), is the prototype of the medical liberal response to racial health disparities. On the one hand, Geiger confronts the documented disparities and offers none of the conservative alibis that purport to explain them. But he simply cannot bring himself to believe "definitively" that his medical colleagues and the institutions to which they belong are capable of "racially discriminatory" professional behavior. Here, too, we see an important consequence of historical ignorance or naïveté. For either Geiger is unaware of the various forms of medical racism that were rampant in American medicine during the first half of the twentieth century, or he believes that racially motivated conduct on the part of American physicians was somehow abolished by civil rights legislation and the unofficial rules of political correctness that have been widely adopted since that time.

This sort of medical agnosticism has the advantage of incorporating a kind of intellectual modesty into its refusal to judge complex behavior. "We do not presume to know whether bias is truly at work in this setting," two medical authors state in their 1999 article on "Racial Disparity in Rates of Surgery for Lung Cancer." "Evidence that bias on the part of physicians (either overt prejudice or subconscious perceptions) influences access to optimal cancer care is disheartening," they comment, but it is too soon to tell whether even "subconscious perceptions" might be affecting the therapeutic relationship.[92] These authors, like Geiger, await "definitive" proof that would "truly" convince them. "Researchers," the *Chronicle of Higher Education* reported a year later, "want to investigate further whether minority patients are intimidated by white doctors, or whether doctors use medical terminology that some undereducated people, whatever their race, may have particular difficulty understanding."[93]

Even a passing familiarity with American social history would have assisted the researchers who were trying to figure out whether black patients might be intimidated by white doctors. Intimidation in every social venue was the social logic of Jim Crow racism, and the social universe of American medicine was no exception to this rule. The real question here is how medical researchers could be so unaware of the basic facts of life regarding race relations in the United States during the course of the twentieth century. This historical ignorance leads in turn to medical complacency toward the feelings of black patients whose personal histories lead back to the long era of Jim Crow medicine. Today's physicians seem to be unaware that the prejudices and practices of their predecessors traumatized generations of African Americans, for whom a distrust of white doctors became a cultural legacy that persists to this day on a scale few whites can imagine. Once again, the real mystery posed by these researchers is how they could have embraced the naïve assumption that black-white relations in medicine can be studied outside of the historical context that shaped them.

The agnostic approach to health disparities continues to predominate in the medical literature. The authors of a 2005 report on the management of heart disease in blacks and whites, which documents the persistence rather than the narrowing of racial health disparities, conclude the following: "Despite considerable debate, reasons for these differences are largely unknown. Potential explanations are sex and racial differences in eligibility for treatment, clinical contraindications, and confounding by other clinical factors." These authors propose that "persistent differences in treatments and procedures according to sex and race reflect some unmeasured characteristic of patients or a health care factor that has not changed over time."[94] The racist phase of American cardiology and its diagnostic legacy that are examined in Chapter 3 go unmentioned and, I suspect, unimagined by these authors. What is more, every explanatory term they use is obfuscating, misleading, or essentially meaningless. "Eligibility for treatment" usually refers to poverty; "clinical contraindications" can result from judgments by physicians that may express racial bias; "unmeasured characteristics" can include various aspects of an African American identity that may complicate diagnosis and treatment; a "health care factor that has not changed over time" could be virtually anything, including medical forms of racial bias. As we will see in greater detail, those medical authors who address racial issues in the professional literature employ a terminology and a rhetorical strategy that effectively eliminate the relevant historical factors as well as accurate descriptions of how race relations work in the world of American medicine today.

One issue that most medical authors evade is whether physicians have a responsibility to monitor their own unconscious motivations for the purpose of earning and retaining the trust of their patients. David Levy's 1985 paper on doctor-patient relationships introduces the basic distinction about conscious and unconscious behaviors. "The white physician," he points out, "need seldom contend with conscious prejudice in himself. However, he must be alert to the possibility of unconscious prejudice or negative counter-transference which impedes the doctor-patient relationship." For example, "unconscious prejudice may cause the white physician to over-identify with the black patient, i.e., lean over backwards and become overindulgent, paternalistic, and condescending."[95] But Levy's emphasis on the doctor's responsibility to monitor and adjust for his own state of mind—a well-known professional obligation of the psychiatrist—has not been taken up by the medical commentators who followed him.

Knowledge of the racial dimension of our medical history would also curb the temptation to excuse racially biased behaviors by distinguishing between "overt" and "subtle" misbehaviors. The physician's obligation to practice a degree of self-observation is noted by a few of the physicians who have touched on the interpersonal dynamics of race relations in medicine. "Many physicians would deny," John Z. Ayanian wrote in 1993, "that overt racism affects medical decisions, but few could overlook the subtle racial biases that can permeate reasoning and communication with patients and other physicians."[96] Here the distinction between *overt* and *subtle* is not invoked to excuse "subtle" physician behavior that might also be of "unconscious" origin. But the standard presentation of scenarios involving potential bias addresses the issues of motivation and self-awareness by establishing the racial innocence of the medical personnel whose behavior might be questioned. An early (1980) paper on measuring racial bias offers the following response to the discovery of possible bias: "Based on these measured treatment differences we conclude that there is some indication of racial bias. Our experience with the staff *indicates that this bias is not due to hostility or contempt for black patients but from subtle stereotyping* and greater familiarity with and preference for white patients. Feedback of the results of our data to the staff was met by an openness to consider racial bias as a possible explanation" [emphasis added].[97] The medical staff is given a clean bill of emotional health vis-à-vis race on the basis of the authors' "experience" with them. The preferred explanation of possible bias is, as is so often the case in these publications, "subtle stereotyping" for which no one is directly responsible. The "preference for white patients" that might be a sign of racist feelings about blacks is left unexplored.

Emphasizing the distinction between open racial hostility ("overt racism" or "overt prejudice") and ostensibly unconscious prejudice ("subtle racial biases" or "subconscious perceptions") is an essential feature of the rhetoric of exculpation that shapes most of these commentaries. "We're not talking about people who are overtly racist," a health disparities researcher said in 1998. "Physicians have very busy worlds. The encounters [with patients] are quick. These are things that increase stereotyping."[98] One problem with the frequently invoked distinction between the *overt* and the *subtle*, quite apart from the standard disconnect from historical experience, is the idea that objectionable racially motivated behaviors announce themselves in the form of overt prejudice. The rhetorical effect of this claim is to exonerate the silent majority whose feelings about race remain inconspicuous. To be sure, these people may be influenced by "subtle stereotyping," but this mental state is itself regarded as exonerating because the stereotyping is too subtle to be noticed by those who have fallen under its sway. The challenge of holding doctors accountable for their behavior remains deferred until that time when the entire situation will be better understood. A rationale for deferring the assigning of responsibility for racially unequal cardiac care appears in a 1993 *New England Journal* article:

> The extent to which subtle or overt racism underlies racial differences in the use of cardiac procedures is unclear. We believe that inadequate health education, differences in patients' preferences for invasive management, delivery systems that are unfriendly to members of certain cultures, and overt racism all may play a part. Allocating responsibility more precisely will require studies that control for angiographic data and directly examine interactions between patients and medical professionals.[99]

Deferred along with the allocating of responsibility is the question of why the medical profession has done so little to promote the studies of "interactions between patients and medical professionals" that might get physicians to recognize the ways in which medical relationships involving blacks and whites can and do go wrong.

This portrait of the physicians' vulnerability to "prejudice" effectively exonerates them of responsibility, since denigrating or hostile motives are presumed to be absent. Even though they are filled with "moral abhorrence" at racial prejudice, physicians "may not recognize manifestations of prejudice in their own behavior." Given this predicament, one might think that the authors would call for some sort of training to liberate doctors from their racial stereotypes. But they decline to do so, calling instead for more research, since the evidence linking stereotyping and prejudice to disparities in health care is merely "indirect."

The sheer obfuscation and confusion the agnostic approach to disparities can cause are particularly evident at the end of a *New England Journal* article that attracted wide publicity following its publication in 1999. The notoriety of "The Effect of Race and Sex on Physicians' Recommendations for Cardiac Catheterization" resulted from its misleading presentation of statistical evidence that exaggerated its findings of physician bias.[100] An unnoted irony of this media event was that a paper that infuriated some physicians by exaggerating findings of bias concluded with a version of the standard exoneration of physicians whose tangled jargon is in a class by itself:

> Our finding that the race and sex of the patient influence the recommendations of physicians independently of other factors may suggest bias on the part of the physicians. However, our study could not assess the form of bias. Bias may represent overt prejudice on the part of physicians or, more likely, could be the result of subconscious perceptions rather than deliberate actions or thoughts. Subconscious bias occurs when a patient's membership in a target group automatically activates a cultural stereotype in the physician's memory regardless of the level of prejudice the physician has.[101]

Following the familiar distinction between "overt prejudice" and "subconscious bias," the final sentence of this passage makes a point of dissociating physicians from their own racial bias. According to this psychology of prejudice, there is no relationship between the cultural stereotype that is "automatically activated" in physicians' memory and the "level of prejudice" they may harbor. Once again the minds of doctors are presented as playthings that are at the mercy of forces operating "automatically" outside them. Physicians "have" a "level of prejudice" in the same sense that they "have" other more innocuous traits for which they bear no responsibility. "Subconscious bias" serves as physicians' alibi not to be held responsible for their racially motivated behaviors.

Racially motivated feelings and behaviors on the part of physicians can also play a role in their decisions about whether medical treatments will be offered to patients, and whether those patients will feel inclined to accept treatments from medical personnel they may not trust. Black patients are frequently reported to be less willing to undergo "technologically intensive interventions" such as surgery. "Blacks with cerebro-vascular disease are more averse to the risks of surgery than whites and are more likely than whites to refuse coronary artery bypass surgery when it is offered. Similarly, blacks with end-stage renal disease are somewhat less likely than whites to want renal transplantation. . . . Black men with osteoarthritis perceived the risk of joint replacement to be higher, the rehabilitation longer and more painful, and the ultimate functional outcome less favorable than white men's perceptions. . . . Black patients appeared to fear perioperative risks of coronary artery bypass graft surgery more than whites did."[102] This reluctance to be operated on applies to a variety of procedures. "Blacks also report less confidence in the efficacy of knee or hip replacement, suggesting that lack of information about risks and benefits, compounded by a general distrust of the health care system, is a partial determinant of the observed lower operation rates."[103] Jeffrey N. Katz pointed out in 2001 that one source of these fears may be the fact that "the risks of mortality and complications following coronary artery bypass graft surgery are higher in blacks than in whites, even after adjustment for case severity. Referring physicians may communicate these local risk patterns to their patients." For example, black physicians tend to be somewhat more pessimistic about the benefits of joint replacement operations than their white colleagues.[104] White physicians may also doubt that kidney transplantation promotes the survival of blacks to the same degree as it does that of whites.[105]

The treatments black patients either prefer or avoid can have a great deal to do with beliefs or feelings of which white medical personnel may be unaware. Conspiracy theories and urban rumors about medical dangers have circulated in the black community for many years. Some African American patients have reported a widespread belief in the black community that being exposed to air during lung cancer surgery can make the tumor spread, causing some patients to refuse the surgery and to disbelieve physicians' assurances that this fear is unwarranted.[106] African American patients can also be influenced by racial stereotypes in ways that prevent them from acting on their preferences. One study, for example, found that "black women were uncomfortable talking to physicians about menopause, fearing that they would sound unintelligent or mentally impaired, and were dissatisfied with the discussions when they did raise the subject with their doctors."[107]

Many years passed before medical authors began to abandon the practice of invoking "patient preferences" as a convenient alibi for inferior medical care and to begin to talk candidly about the role that fear and distrust can play in these decisions. "Patient 'preference' for less intensive treatment," Katz noted, "may in fact represent resignation to the perceived status quo—that interventions are unavailable, unaffordable, ineffective, or unduly risky—even if those perceptions are not accurate."[108] But the greatest degree of candor about how preferences work appears, not in the medical literature, but in newspaper coverage of racial health disparities. It was *Newsday*, not the *New England Journal*, that in 1998 published the following commentary by Ed Hannan, a professor and chairman of the Department of Health Policy, Management and Behavior at the School of Public Health at the State University at Albany: "One of the things alleged by those who say that there are truly not racial differences [in treatment] is that blacks tend to turn down procedures that have been offered to them. But what we found, essentially, is that the physician did not recommend the surgery."[109] Dr. Robert Gaston, a transplant surgeon at the University of Alabama in Birmingham, the largest transplant center in the United States, told *Newsday* that doctors dealing with poor African Americans in particular "will come up to a person and say something like, 'You really don't want a transplant, do you?'"[110] A 1999 study concluded that: "Among the patients in our study who desired transplantation . . . black patients were less likely than white patients to have been evaluated and placed on a waiting list or given a transplant."[111] These black patients had expressed a preference for undergoing surgery. Their doctors, for whatever reasons, did not always prefer to accommodate their wishes.

These reports make clear the rhetorical significance of the term "patient preferences," which effectively removes physicians from the decision-making process, thereby exempting them from responsibility for whichever treatment choice is made. The other misleading function of this term is to endow black patients with an independence and a sense of security that not all of them are likely to feel in a modern hospital setting. A white physician who treats a black patient in 2012 may not realize that the patient's medical clock may be set at 1952 or 1922, depending on the legacy that medical racism has left in that person's family over many years. The patient's decision not to undergo surgery in the present may have been shaped by a traumatic past whose effects neither the doctor nor the patient understands. But the fact that the doctor does not grasp what is happening will not prevent the consequences of a misunderstanding.

The preceding analysis of medical rhetoric and vocabulary asserts that American medical authors have failed to produce an honest and accurate assessment of their own behaviors in the domain of race relations. The constant use of various euphemisms to gentrify race relations and envelope doctors' behaviors in a sanitizing jargon points to a deeply rooted resistance to self-scrutiny and real reform. The exceptions to this rule are few. M. Gregg Bloche calls the "overwhelming" evidence that "members of disadvantaged minority groups receive poorer health care than whites" a "bitter truth."[112] But this sharp acknowledgment of failure sounds a discordant note in a medical literature that has long been in denial about race matters. As three African American physicians pointed out in *JAMA* as far back as 1989, "the most likely reason for these inequalities is that physicians value black lives less than white lives." Commenting on a *JAMA* article on racial inequalities in treatments for heart disease, they go on to call this study an exercise in evasion, since "racism is considered only briefly, lastly, and politely as 'socio-cultural factors influencing physician and patient decision making.'" They cannot understand why the authors "stopped shy of implicating racism. Their own article carefully documents the evidence in the medical literature."[113] More than two decades later, the medical literature continues to practice this sort of denial. The verbal evidence of this stalemate is the persistence of stultifying jargon. The alienation of white doctors from black patients is a problem of "patient physician race concordance." Black patients may experience "less patient-centered" visits than white patients and hear a "less positive affective tone" when doctors address them.[114]

The medical literature thus remains in one sense an elaborate arrangement whereby white physicians are insulated from certain kinds of discomfiting information about the medical suffering of black people and from knowledge of how black patients or colleagues assess their professional behavior. The voices of black patients and physicians appear, infrequently, in newspapers.[115] Black people's analyses of how white physicians behave in interracial encounters play no significant role in American medicine's half-hearted attempts to deal with its half-acknowledged race problem.

The effect of these publications about doctor-patient relationships has not been to promote the reform of medical training or to negotiate a new relationship with the black population. The actual result has been more publications of the same kind. There are no studies of how doctors actually think about their black patients, no inventories of stereotypes, few inquiries into racially motivated diagnostic errors, and no analyses of the transmission of racial folklore from one medical generation to the next. Apart from an occasional reference to the Tuskegee Syphilis Experiment, references to the history of medical racism in the United States are almost entirely absent. Editorial gatekeepers ensure that potentially discomfiting penetrations of the physician's private sphere do not appear in the professional literature. American medicine thus persists in the mistaken belief that it has left the world of racially inspired medical folklore far behind.

Deciphering the racial complexes of physicians in the medical literature of the post–civil rights era is difficult due to the obscurantist jargon medical authors use to take the sting, the pungency, and the menace out of race relations as they are acted out in medical settings. Sanitizing race in this way also serves to protect the privacy of doctors whose racial beliefs are officially regarded as humane until there is dramatic evidence to suggest otherwise. The sanctity of the private sphere within which physicians' thoughts and feelings shape their decisions derives from their traditional sense of autonomy. Physicians who acknowledge that racially motivated judgments can affect medical practice may challenge doctors' assumed right to privacy by advocating some kind of therapeutic intervention. "If we recognize our own negative racial attitudes," David Levy wrote, "we should ask ourselves why we need them and then do something to effect personal growth and change. For psychiatrists who lack the empathy needed for work with all groups of people, psychoanalysis has been recommended to erase distorted perspectives concerning race or at least to enable them to become more aware of when their irrational attitudes might impede the treatment process."[116]

THE PHYSICIAN'S PRIVATE SPHERE

A generation after Levy wrote these words, prescribing psychotherapy for racially troubled physicians remains an improbable and even exotic proposal for reform. An alternative to the status quo would be the systematic detection and exposure of racially motivated conduct by doctors—an option the medical profession has never embraced. The legal scholar Dorothy Roberts, who has written on the medical racism that has been inflicted on black women, has challenged the pretense of medical autonomy and argued that "doctors' 'private' moral dilemmas involving their patients are actually interpreted and resolved according to relationships of power in the larger society." Highly trained and affluent physicians (or lawyers or professors) can, in fact, exercise illegitimate and unethical forms of power over their undereducated patients (or clients or students), white or black. Roberts's objective, therefore, is "to shatter the myth that the interaction between physician and patient is a private matter."[117]

Resistance to the shattering of this "myth" of privacy is embedded in the medical profession, and is directly related to physicians' sense that professional conduct is independent of the larger social forces (such as race relations) that operate in the wider world outside the office. Most doctors, according to the physician and health policy scholar Troyen Brennan, "think a patient is best treated if the physician follows her personal and ethical code in dealing with sensitive issues. . . . Nor do most of my colleagues think that medical ethics should define a public role for physicians, or that health law and policy should represent moral challenges for physicians."[118] The problem is that many (and probably a majority of) physicians have not developed "personal and ethical codes" that would enable them to deal successfully with "sensitive issues" like race in a comfortable and competent way. Where, indeed, would the physician's "personal and ethical code" for racial encounters come from? Our social institutions do little to prepare any of us for race matters, and medical education does little to remedy this deficit (see Chapter 5).

The result of laissez-faire race relations in the medical world is an unregulated environment in which patients in general, and black patients in particular, hold the weaker cards. The executive vice president for medical affairs at a Long Island, New York, hospital defended this limited view of a doctor's accountability (and his own) in 1998 in the following terms: "The issue for us is to accept patients without regard to race, creed, color, national origin or ability to pay. After that, how the cookie crumbles is something over which we have little or no control and, I think, little or no responsibility." This administrator had no plans to monitor the racial conduct of the physicians who practice medicine at his hospital, and he apparently saw no reason to do so. The consequences of this policy, according to Kathleen Gaffney, the Nassau County health commissioner, are predictable: "You get treated by what you look like. If you're black . . . the physician is less likely to take your symptoms as seriously, so you may not get the same response. There continue to be health care stereotypes in terms of minority patients being less compliant, they 'don't take their drugs,' and there is also a perception they are less motivated and less educated. It becomes a self-fulfilling prophecy because they're treated differently by health professionals."[119]

Physicians' sense of entitlement to privacy in their professional conduct is not limited to American practitioners. Most British physicians, too, expect to be left alone to manage race relations on their own terms. The following anecdote is instructive in this regard. After hearing a South Asian medical student speak on the needs of minority ethnic children in the National Health Service (NHS), the speaker's white peers "reacted negatively: 'He's off again!' some said. Others felt insulted that I could even consider that they would ever discriminate against anybody. Some groaned that they wanted a 'serious medical topic,' which to them this wasn't. Most saw it as a political statement, bearing no relationship to their future in medicine." And some white doctors extend the same racial privilege to white patients. A South Asian doctor in Birmingham "provoked outrage when he planned to screen his prospective patients for racist views."[120] Encounters with racist patients have long been part of being an African American physician.

The task of understanding how doctors think and feel about race is also made more difficult by the fact that the accumulated survey data about racial attitudes focuses on attitudes toward economic status, social policies, and other sociological topics. Opinion surveys of racial attitudes typically measure respondents' attitudes toward affirmative action, economic status, the state of race relations, voting rights, educational achievement, enforcement of civil rights laws, sources of inequality, the effects of interracial contact, or "the racial healing process." These data, too, present collective information about attitudes and pose few questions that are directly relevant to the medical setting. Questions focusing on racial stereotypes of laziness and intellectual inferiority would be relevant to studying the attitudes of doctors who may doubt the willingness of black patients to understand and follow their instructions. But doctors also deal with the intricacies, and the intimate aspects, of human bodies that do not figure in published survey data. The sociologists and political scientists who produce most of these studies do not include the questions about anatomical or physiological traits that could illuminate how medical students or doctors might think about their black patients.

In fact, it is unlikely that social scientists would see any reason to pose such questions, given the widespread and mistaken assumption that biological fantasies about racial difference are largely extinct. Second, many social scientists conducting research on race would feel uncomfortable about posing such questions. The days when whites refused to share the same swimming pool water with black bathers are gone, and modern people feel an understandable reluctance to revisit the primal fears that insisted on this sort of biological quarantine from racial aliens. Yet the biological level is precisely where we must go to explore the racial fantasies of medical personnel. There are even some survey data that can help us reassess the assumption that biological racism is a thing of the past. For example, a political scientist's 2004 study of support for the Mississippi state flag found that a biologically themed "old-fashioned" racism was far more prevalent among college students than he and others had expected it to be. "Old-fashioned" racism in early twenty-first-century Mississippi included the belief that "differences that exist between Blacks and Whites are attributed to God's divine plan"—implying a belief in the polygenist doctrine of separate creations—and that blacks and whites should not intermarry, thereby mingling their racially distinct genomes.[121] In fact, many years of social conditioning have made race biological thinking a fundamental aspect of how we continue to think about racial differences, even if understandable (and generally commendable) social pressures keep most of these ideas from circulating widely in our public media.

Social scientists' lack of interest in investigating biological fantasies about racial differences has been matched by a similar disinterest on the part of journalists, with a few exceptions. A *Washington Post*-ABC News poll reported in 1981, for example, that close to one-quarter of white adults still regarded blacks as inferior human beings, a judgment that suggests a belief in genetic inferiority.[122] A National Opinion Research Center study released in 1990 reported that 56 percent of whites believed blacks were "violence-prone," although the idea of a biological basis for this trait was not explored.[123] (A suspected biological trait *was* explored at the New York State

Psychiatric Institute during the period between 1993 and 1996, when 100
black and Hispanic younger brothers of juvenile delinquents were given the
subsequently banned diet drug fenfluramine "to test a theory that violent or
criminal behavior may be predicted by levels of certain brain chemicals."[124])
In October 1963, only months after Dr. Martin Luther King's March on
Washington, *Newsweek* reported that 71 percent of whites thought that
black people "smell different"[125]—a biological fantasy about black bodies that
can be traced back to the racist plantation physician Samuel Cartwright.[126]
Our problem is to relate such findings to how doctors think and behave.
For example, if about a quarter of white Americans believe black people are
somehow inferior, is there any reason to assume that about a quarter of
America's physicians are somehow immune to this sort of racial thinking?

PLAYING ANTHROPOLOGIST

An embarrassing and revealing episode involving racial misbehavior by a
physician was the 2000 scandal that engulfed Dr. William (Reyn) Archer III,
an obstetrician-gynecologist and the son of a powerful Republican congress-
man, who was appointed Texas health commissioner by Governor George
W. Bush in 1997. Over the next three years, Dr. Archer made a number of
eccentric and controversial statements, public and private, on such topics
as the emasculating effects of birth control and Hispanic attitudes toward
marriage. The end came when he told an African American doctor of internal medicine that she was "too smart in a way," and that using one's intel-
lect to get ahead was "what white people do." Then, playing anthropologist,
he observed that her light-colored skin placed her in an African American
"elite."[127] It turned out that Dr. Archer had once said "that he likes to look
at health and other problems with an anthropologist's eye, examining the
customs, behavioral issues and cultural values that might be contributing factors."[128] The racially eccentric conversations of the highest-ranking
physician in Texas were made public only because they were secretly tape-
recorded by the black female physician to whom he directed his remarks.
The medical profession did nothing to dissociate itself from this authoritar-
ian personality or his primitive racial fantasies. Dr. Archer's urgent need to
play racial anthropologist finally led to his resignation from public office in
late 2000, but the Texas chapter of the American Medical Association played
no role in removing him from public office.[129]

The ironic aspect of this awkward and protracted drama is that physicians should, in fact, take an "anthropological" interest in the backgrounds,
habits, and life circumstances of their patients for the purpose of giving

them well-informed care. But there is a crucial difference between the amateur cultural anthropology that acquaints the physician with the lives of his patients and the amateur racial anthropology that searches for racial essences and becomes fixated on apparent racial differences that can inspire both voyeuristic fascination and misleading fantasies in white observers.

What we may call "playing anthropologist" also occurs outside the doctor's office. Young African American women, for example, have told me of being approached in public places by white male strangers who proceeded to comment on the anatomy of their heads or bodies. The comments made by these men were not overtly lewd or hostile, but rather expressed an "anthropological" curiosity about black women. They also demonstrated a willingness to treat black women as if they were specimens on display, another ritual that was common in the nineteenth century. In this sense, "playing anthropologist" involves both a curiosity about the anatomy of the racial alien and a sense of entitlement that confers a right to examine her body for evidence of racial difference.

These inquiring approaches to black women are attempts to answer what the African American journalist Susan Richardson calls "black questions" from complete strangers. She found it frustrating that "after so many centuries in this country, my people were still a mystery to many whites. I have friends who belligerently refuse to answer questions about our curly hair, the variation in our skin color from chocolate to 'high yella' and our culture, especially when they are asked if we are related to the exotic peoples in *National Geographic*."[130] Troubling encounters with racially curious whites are among the emotional "micro-aggressions" many African Americans experience on a regular basis.[131] At the same time, these emotional stressors and their effects remain unknown to the great majority of whites, who assume that Americans of all skin colors share an essentially homogenous and egalitarian social environment in which everyone has an opportunity to thrive. Physicians who share this overly sanguine view of the black experience and who treat African American patients will eventually overlook signs or symptoms that are relevant to the proper diagnosis and treatment of people who are under more stress than the doctors perceive.

The behaviors of these amateur anthropologists are culturally aberrant only in their frank self-assertion. Most racial curiosity remains just that—an unexpressed interest in racial differences that might take the form of speculations about racial athletic aptitude or IQ scores or sexual prowess. Speculations of this kind originate in the traditional racial folklore that persists inside the heads of the vast majority of modern people, including the great majority of doctors, regardless of whether they are black or white.

The presence of discomfiting racial folklore inside the heads of modern people is continually on display in the awkward statements that prominent people have made in recent decades. In 2005, William J. Bennett, a former Republican secretary of education in the Reagan administration, ignited a national controversy when he fantasized on his radio program that "if you wanted to reduce crime, you could, if that were your sole purpose, you could abort every black baby in this country, and your crime rate would go down." He then added: "That would be an impossible, ridiculous, and morally reprehensible thing to do, but your crime rate would go down."[132] While Bennett defended his remarks as a "thought experiment about public policy," a black journalist at *The New York Times* called them "twisted fantasies."[133] Another African American commentator who was "shocked and angered" by these remarks noted that Bennett had "instantly connected crime and race."[134] Bennett countered that he could not grasp why a genocidal fantasy about a vulnerable racial minority descended from slaves might offend anyone. The Pulitzer Prize–winning syndicated columnist Charles Krauthammer, a graduate of Harvard Medical School, described "crack babies" in 1988 as a "biologic underclass whose biological inferiority is stamped at birth"[135]— a judgment that turned out to be as mistaken as it was heartless.

Another fantasy about racial biology appeared in a comment Senator Daniel Patrick Moynihan made in 1994 about the consequences of the out-of-wedlock births that occur at a higher rate among African Americans. "I mean, if you were a biologist, you could find yourself talking about speciation here," that is, the creation of a new species. "It has something to do [with] a changed condition in biological circumstances."[136] A year later the president of Rutgers University, a liberal affirmative-action proponent named Francis Lawrence, told a faculty meeting the following: "The average SAT (score) for African Americans is 750. Do we set standards in the future so we don't admit anybody? Or do we deal with a disadvantaged population that doesn't have that genetic, hereditary background to have a higher average?"[137] While none of the more than 30 faculty members who were present took exception to this assessment of African American intelligence, the release of a tape recording of the remark provoked a storm of publicity that almost cost Lawrence his job.[138]

None of these men belong to the racist fringe as it is traditionally defined; on the contrary, all of them have occupied leadership positions in mainstream American institutions: state or presidential cabinets, a flagship state university, syndicated journalism, the United States Senate. None of them were dismissed or demoted for endorsing or playing with race biological themes in controversial or offensive ways. Only the hapless and obsessive Reyn Archer, isolated in his Jim Crow world of uppity blacks and the specter of lynching, lacked the facile talent to talk his way out of trouble. The desperate Francis Lawrence, by way of contrast, claimed that, while he and his wife had refused on principle to read *The Bell Curve*, his preoccupation with its outrageous claims about racial intelligence had somehow reversed the ideological force field in his brain and prompted him to say the exact opposite of what he had meant.

These incidents offer useful evidence because they expose the private racial imaginations of modern people to public scrutiny. What they show is that race-biological ideas can still inform white thinking about blacks to a degree that goes unacknowledged in our episodic and fitful "dialogue on race" that promises so much and accomplishes so little. It should be obvious that physicians, given their intimate contact with patients' minds and bodies, participate in this process as much as or more than most other people. It is possible that physicians are exposed to more racial folklore than other professionals, precisely because they absorb the ideas that circulate in society at large as well as those that are generated within the medical culture and circulate by word of mouth.

One of the central claims of this book is that folkloric beliefs about racial differences have persisted over many generations and have kept an evolving racial anthropology alive both inside and outside the medical profession. American medical authors seem to be unaware of or uninterested in folkloric material of this kind. Reports of racially awkward incidents involving white doctors and black patients (or, for that matter, black doctors and white patients) almost never appear in print. An anesthesiologist who told a nonphysician I know that the spinal fluid of black patients is thicker than that of whites will never appear as a case study in a medical journal because editors do not regard reports of this kind as suitable for publication. Medical journals are more disposed to describing on occasion the folkloric beliefs of patients. A senior physician at a Veterans Administration hospital in New York told me: "In my experience, when the notion of folklore enters medical discourse it invariably concerns the patient's folklore about himself—a folk remedy, a 'primitive'/uneducated/unscientific/old country notion they have about their body. That doctors have a 'folklore' about their patients, let alone that they operate on the basis of folklore, is hardly ever recognized, talked about or acknowledged. The flip side of course is that the patients have their own folkloric concepts of their doctors (e.g., 'you just want to experiment')".[139] It is not surprising that doctors can think of themselves as immune to folkloric thinking while ascribing such beliefs to their unsophisticated patients. This is, however, an illusion that is encouraged and maintained by the absence of appropriate instruction about racial folklore in medical school curricula and continuing education.

Medically significant racial folklore is known among African Americans and some doctors as the "silent curriculum" or, as the VA hospital physician reported to me, as the "hidden curriculum."[140] "Are you aware of the term 'hidden curriculum' as it applies to medical student education?" the VA doctor asked me:

> The term is very much in vogue in med-ed [medical education] circles. It refers to precisely what you're referencing . . . the under-the-radar shaping of attitudes and behaviors that can lead to a lifetime of bad habits, a parallel education picked up despite the best efforts of formal lectures and rounds. So much of medical education is informal, anecdotal, on the fly, and unsupervised. Residents are largely educated by other residents. It's all very intense, imitative, personal, hierarchical and riddled with "dependency issues." An off-hand remark in a midnight I.C.U. to a sleep deprived intern can make an impression disproportionate to its accuracy.[141]

This insider's account of how medical habits are acquired focuses on the role of oral tradition—the private transmission of concepts and information, whether accurate, inaccurate, or innocuous—beyond the purview of formal instruction or supervision. Dr. Judith Gwaltmey, a professor of medicine and physiology at Boston University, puts it as follows: "There are lots of little stories that physicians believe that are neither scientifically based nor proven. That's the problem."[142] As the VA doctor points out, the oral transmission of these "little stories" can have a profound influence on how medical personnel interpret a patient and his or her symptoms:

> Are you aware that the in-hospital case presentations frequently begin something like: Mr. Jones is a 70-year-old African-American/white/Hispanic (choose one) male with a chief complaint of x-y-z? The racial identifier has a privileged status, up front, implying that everything that follows is potentially colored (no pun intended) by that fact as importantly as the facts of sex or age. The alternative in the case presentation format is to put that piece of information into what is called the social history or physical exam, assuming it even merits inclusion as a pivotal fact. Case presentations are delicate organisms, and the activation of bias early in the hearing can be deadly.[143]

This account of how the racial presentation of a patient occurs in clinical medicine corresponds perfectly to a description that appeared in the *Annals of Internal Medicine* in 1996. The problem with giving patients racial identities in this manner is that "a physician's assumptions about a patient's race that result in the elimination of possible diseases or the narrowing of focus to one disease in the differential diagnosis may have serious negative consequences." This author points to the case of a European boy (coded "white") who presented with abdominal pain and anemia and whose surgery was abruptly canceled when his previously undiagnosed sickle-cell anemia came to light. A second case, concerning a young man coded "black," ended in his death after he was treated for a sickle-cell crisis his doctors inferred on the basis of his presumed "race" and the patient's remark that he had once been told he had "sickle cell."[144] "What surgeon has not been embarrassed," a white physician asked in 1960, "by operating for acute appendicitis, only to find a normal appendix because he failed to remember sickle cell disease in the differential diagnosis."[145] The fact that this physician, Dr. John Scudder, registers embarrassment rather than alarm reflects the casual approach to diagnosing black patients we have already seen in a number of cases from previous decades. A year earlier, a paper on blood transfusions by Dr. Scudder had produced a front-page story in *The New York Times* titled "Blood Expert Says Transfusion Between Races May Be Perilous." "This may sound wrong sociologically," he commented, "but it is scientifically correct."[146] In May 1960 the African American–edited *Journal of the National Medical Association* noted that, following the news coverage of Dr. Scudder's paper, "several states have enacted laws or implemented old measures stipulating that Negro blood be separated."[147] What *had* alarmed Scudder was the immune response of "a white war veteran" to a blood transfusion from a "Negro donor" whose blood did not contain an atypical antibody matching that of the white patient. Scudder proceeded to recommend, on the basis of the differing racial distributions of blood groups and antibodies, the racial segregation of blood to avoid dangerous incompatibilities.

Case studies of medical folklore and how these ideas are transmitted from one generation to the next are never analyzed in the mainstream medical literature. An interesting example of this sort of analysis appeared several decades ago in the black-edited *Journal of the National Medical Association*, at a time when the civil rights movement was encouraging black self-assertion in every social venue, including medicine. In his article on "Racial Contrasts in Obstetrics and Gynecology," the white obstetrician William F. Mengert announced that his purpose was "to examine objectively each racial contrast in obstetrics and gynecology and place it in one of two categories: folklore or real difference. When this is done it becomes obvious that many racial contrasts depend upon social factors such as custom, social and financial station, rather than race." Over the previous century, as we will see later on in this book, many medical authors had made little or no effort to distinguish between the folkloric beliefs that circulated among doctors and real scientific information.

The white physician who confesses in print to having mistakenly believed in "Negro" traits or disorders has been an absolutely exceptional contributor to the medical literature. White physicians commented occasionally during the Jim Crow era on their colleagues' inaccurate ideas about racial differences, even as pseudoscientific racial interpretations of the human organism and its diseases continued to predominate over this sort of caution. Some physicians understood, for example, that the stereotype of the venereal disease-ridden Negro was likely to produce some medical misjudgments. "In approaching the subject of syphilis in the negro," a Charleston, South Carolina, doctor writes in 1915, "there is especial need to guard ourselves against preconceived notions. It is the prevailing opinion that practically every negro who has reached middle life is syphilitic, an opinion which finds support in the exceedingly lax moral standards of the race. This opinion may be true, but I have not been able to find any definite and exact data upon which it is based."[148] "I am . . . prepared to admit, in the light of recent investigations," another Charleston doctor wrote two years later, "that in all probability some [eye] affections which were attributed to syphilis may have been tuberculosis. . . . It behooves us to jack up, as it were, our diagnostic machinery to meet the times."[149]

The medical men of this period were willing to concede that physicians were vulnerable to some other mistaken ideas about black patients in addition to the constant harping on the perils of the syphilitic Negro. It is not true, a professor at the Atlanta Medical College asserts in 1915, that the Negro race "is not afflicted with adenoids in the nasopharynx," even if local variations in the disorder have created this impression.[150] In 1925, a *JAMA* editorial on "Rectal Pathology in the Negro" warned against making "sweeping generalizations" about Negro tissues on the premise that the black man is an evolutionary ("atavistic") throwback.[151] It is now clear, a New Orleans doctor wrote in 1932, "that in spite of a rather widely held opinion to the contrary, the negro race is quite as susceptible to this terrible disease [cancer] as is any other race and people."[152] (*Newsweek* told its readers in 1963 that "Negroes are far less prone to cancer than whites."[153]) A Columbia University psychologist who in 1939 compared blacks to apes cautiously noted that the medical literature "has carried with it many superstitions in regard to predisposition of the colored race for certain types of mental disturbances or a relative infrequency for others."[154] If doctors think infectious mononucleosis is relatively rare among "the colored," two physicians from Richmond, Virginia wrote in 1944, it is probably because they have not bothered to examine the blood smears of their black patients.[155] A counterpart to the Southern physician, the British colonial physician, could make his own mistakes. A doctor who had assumed that "reticulocytes were larger in Africans than in Europeans" confessed his "misapprehension" in 1952.[156]

These confessions of error in the medical literature show that the pseudoscientific consequences of racially motivated medical thinking—"preconceived notions," "sweeping generalizations," and "superstitions" among them—were making themselves apparent to the more open-minded sort of medical man even during the era of Jim Crow segregation. The other major theme that runs through these observations about diagnosing blacks is the careless and mistaken assumption that these people enjoyed various degrees of immunity to a variety of disorders: adenoids, cancer, mononucleosis, and many more. In addition, these doctors sometimes concede that such careless and mistaken diagnoses were the direct result of medical negligence on the part of white practitioners who did not take the trouble to examine their black patients with sufficient care. As one physician noted in 1920, in the case of suspected exophthalmic goiter, blacks "are often less minutely examined than white patients."[157] If the Negro infant death rate for congenital malformations is half that of white infants, another doctor surmises in 1932, "This difference is probably due, in part, to less careful observation of Negroes."[158] A 1946 *JAMA* commentary on "Maternal Care and the Negro" concluded that "errors in judgment and technic as well as neglect on the part of the physician were 50 per cent more frequent in the care of colored mothers."[159] The impact such observations might have had on the doctors who made them would surely have been buffered by the profound racial paternalism that characterized the medical profession at this time. In the words of the commentator on obstetrical neglect: "The educational and intellectual deficiencies of the Negro favor poor obstetric results." It is for this reason that these comments should be read as confessions of error rather than as a recognition of ethical deficiencies.

Apart from this climate of prejudice, there is another way to understand why physicians might avoid careful examination of black patients in some cases. In some Southern towns, black patients could wait from four to six hours just to be seen, and some were not asked to remove their clothes for physical examinations.[160] There is no one way to explain physician behavior of this kind; some practitioners must have made a conscious decision to give black people short shrift, while others may have been reacting to phobias rooted in apprehensions about racial differences, whether these were cultural or biological. The psychoanalyst and anthropologist George Devereux has offered some explanations of such behaviors based on what he observed while instructing fourth-year students at the Temple University School of Medicine in the 1960s. His assignment was to show the medical students the "psychiatric clues" that emerge during physical examinations. "The assumption that the racially alien patient must look 'different,'" he says, "leads to diagnostic oversights quite as often [as] does an unawareness of genuine racial differences." Uncertainty about the thin calves of a South African tribesman or the scanty pubic hair of Indian patients could lead to false diagnoses. He points to a syndrome he calls the "'tactful' reluctance to examine closely the most distinctive portions of a racially alien patient's body." The small healed scars on an elderly black patient elicited no inquiries from "an exceptionally able" white doctor. Similarly, Devereux noticed that the medical students generally avoided "the characteristically prognathous lower half" of black people's faces. This may have been due to a phobic response to a frequently (and viciously) caricatured aspect of "black" physiognomy racists have traditionally associated with the great apes. One doctor did not examine an abdominal scar resulting from an appendectomy because he assumed, in accordance with the stereotype of the knife-wielding black criminal, that it was a razor slash. "I never saw a doctor *routinely* examine a Negro male's inguinal rings," Devereux reports, "perhaps because of the myth that a large penis is a racial characteristic of the Negro."[161]

More recent evidence described in the following suggests that the hidden (and occasionally overt) complexes and phobias that white doctors brought to the interpretation of the black body in the 1960s continue to affect the behavior of a significant number of doctors today. The tightening of politically correct rules governing racial discourse that has taken place since that era should not be mistaken for a purging of racial folklore from the minds of modern people. Few doctors, David Levy noted in *Pediatrics* many years ago, "are free of unconscious fantasies about imagined racial characteristics." His analysis of how the white doctor–black patient relationship can go wrong is still a rarity in the medical literature. Unlike the numerous commentators on racial health disparities who employ terms like "unconscious prejudice" and take the analysis no further, Levy describes specific scenarios that can result from this syndrome. He thereby enters that private domain medical editors have long treated as inviolable. There is, for example, the doctor who overcompensates for his racial feelings by becoming "overindulgent, paternalistic, and condescending."

Then there is the doctor who enters into "a conspiracy of silence" about the race issue with his black patient, in that both "share the view that [ostensible racial] differences are signs of minority group inferiority and to discuss them would be tantamount to discussing a missing limb with an amputee." Physicians can also be naïve about what counts as maladaptive behavior in the context of the African American experience; for example, suspiciousness that might strike whites as pathological may be justified given the emotional stressors many black people have to deal with.[162] The conventions that have determined what can be published in mainstream medical journals have effectively prevented the mapping of this terrain.

African American physicians' observations of how their white counterparts treat black patients have occasionally appeared in medical publications. "It may not be in bad taste," a black gynecologist wrote in the *JNMA* in 1920,

> to call attention to the young doctor of the dominant race who must get his first practical experience at the risk of our women. All of us who reside in the larger cities are aware of his activities. It is only necessary to say in regards to his efforts that more organs of female reproduction are laid upon his altar, a sacrifice to his ignorance and for the benefit of his training than perhaps ever was sacrificed, as to function, by the ignorant mid-wife or the criminal abortionist.[163]

Half a century later the future Surgeon General David Satcher described a less destructive, but similarly exploitative, arrangement that put black women's reproductive organs at the disposal of white doctors-in-training. Black patients, he wrote in *JAMA*, "are frequently exploited for teaching sessions. One black woman related to me that she had had nine pelvic examinations by physicians and students and had never been told whether her pelvis was normal or abnormal."[164]

The official publication of the Urban League, which was founded in 1910 as the Committee on Urban Conditions among Negroes, noted in 1924 that in many American localities there was "a prevalent idea among white medical men that all Negroes, especially if they cannot make another diagnosis, have syphilis. This idea is so well grounded that they will often treat as syphilis a case that shows repeated negative blood tests, absolutely lack all clinical symptoms and with an entirely negative history." Here are the careless diagnostic habits noted earlier by white physicians who mention (but do not quite deplore) this sort of racially motivated neglect. This black author also emphasizes the importance of "the Negro physician and nurse," since "those of the white race in quite a number of cases look upon Negroes as mere subjects for observation."[165] Here is an early reference to the African American anxieties about being mistreated as experimental material that haunt the black community to this day. The power of the syphilis theme to shape medical thinking was evident the same year in Mississippi; there, medical men were speculating about why they had been unable to find any blind newborns among the black population. "Some doctors say that the Negroes, through generations of contact with venereal diseases, have developed a kind of immunity which protects the new-born baby's eye from the ever-present sources of infection."[166] As was often the case, the imagined racial trait was a protective effect—"a kind of immunity"—that implied black people required less medical attention than less hardy types. As Gunnar Myrdal pointed out most of a century ago in *An American Dilemma*, "Diseases which are not frequently a cause of death are reported so badly or reported for such inadequate samples that it is almost inevitable that Negroes would appear to be immune to them even if they were not really so."[167]

Careless diagnostic habits can still occur when black patients seek treatment. Racial misinformation about blacks and heart disease causes some physicians to regard high blood pressure as "normal" in African American patients. (There are doctors in Europe who regard hypertrophic cardiomyopathy [an enlarged heart] as "absolutely normal" in Africans.[168]) Disputed assumptions about racial physiology and drugs causes some doctors to believe that certain blood pressure medications do not benefit black patients—a claim that black cardiologists have contested. There are physicians who assume that most black patients are diabetic. Others assume that the painful symptoms of sickle-cell disease are signs of drug withdrawal and refuse these patients the narcotic-grade drugs that can relieve their pain. Antiquated ideas about blacks' immunity to pain manifest themselves in the failure to provide adequate doses of analgesic drugs in hospitals and emergency rooms; the refusal to provide pain relief may also originate in ideas about blacks as drug-seeking or especially prone to addiction. Many gynecologists have automatically diagnosed a black woman with symptoms of endometriosis as having pelvic inflammatory disease (PID), based on the assumption that black women are sexually promiscuous. This diagnosis can lead in turn to the sterilization of the affected woman. "Physicians have been known to diagnose, manage, and make recommendations based on perceptions they acquire from the literature. They have, for example, failed to order appropriate tests to detect macrosomia or intrauterine growth retardation because 'black women are less apt to know they are pregnant early in pregnancy than white women'."[169] Today, it is indefensible to offer medical advice based on folkloric assumptions about what African Americans know or don't know about their health. This practice continues on account of the sheer momentum of traditional racial folklore. We will now examine how the assigning of racial essences to human traits originates and is perpetuated both outside and inside the world of medicine.

FROM RACIAL FOLKLORE TO RACIAL MEDICINE

When modern physicians offer racially motivated diagnoses and treatments, they are participating in a living tradition of which they are unaware, and medical school curricula do little to enlighten them. The fundamental tenet of Western racism is that blacks and whites are opposite racial types, and the most important correlate of this principle is that black human beings are less complex organisms than white human beings. These two ideas, operating together, have created a racially differentiated human biology that has suffused the tissues, fluids, bones, nerves, and organ systems of the human body with racial meanings that over the last century have influenced medical thinking in significant ways. Most of the major human organs and organ systems have their own racial histories, depending on how they have been interpreted in their social and historical contexts. In a similar fashion, many diseases and disorders have been effectively coded "white" or "black," depending on whether they are associated with modernity ("white") or socially backward ("black") ways of life. The various forms of black medical "hardiness"—dermatological, neurological, surgical, venereal, cardiac, reproductive, and more—all presume a more primitive (and less complex) human type that is biologically different from the civilized white man. This racial doctrine of biological (and medical) difference is the ideological dimension of the "colonial medicine" described at length in a later section of this book.

The racial anthropology of the nineteenth century and the colonial medicine to which it gave birth are the prototypes of the modern-day racial medicine described previously in capsule form. The racial anthropology of this era was also an evolutionary doctrine that posited a developmental hierarchy predicated on a polarity between racially inferior blacks and racially superior whites. A representative text of this genre is "On the Negro's Place in Nature," published in 1864 by James Hunt, PhD, president of the Anthropological Society of London. "The Negro race, in some of its characters, is the lowest of existing races," he writes, "while in others it approaches the highest type of European; and this is the case with other savage races. We find the same thing in the Anthropoid Apes, where some species resemble man in one character, and some in another."[170] This Victorian Age theme of differential human evolution and its related analogy between the "lower" races and the great apes or other animals persisted for many years in the thinking of Euro-American anthropologists and medical men.

This evolutionary theory of human racial differences also appears in later medical publications on race. In 1925, *The Journal of the Michigan State Medical Society* published an article endorsing the view that "the female negro pelvis is similar in many respects to the pelvis of the female gorilla," arguing that "it seems but logical to conclude that the negro pelvis shows a reversion toward the type found in the lower animals."[171] The 1929 volume of the *Transactions of the American Gynecological Society* includes a casual endorsement of the idea that "the negro lies nearer to the common stem than does the European and so is nearer to the childhood of the race."[172] In 1939, the flagship journal of American psychiatry allowed a Columbia University psychologist to propose in its pages "that in the negro there are characteristics approaching the apes with a greater variability of form and structure."[173]

Simpleminded pseudo-Darwinian reasoning also equated black human beings with darker kinds of animals. Researchers at the University of Oklahoma in 1925 conducted a pharmacological experiment on the premise "that black feathers in chickens were the genetic equivalent of African heritage in humans."[174] Readers of the 1928 volume of the *American Journal of Physical Anthropology* were told that, "It is natural to associate the low death rate of negroes from skin diseases and skin cancer with the presence of large amounts of pigment. Among animals there are many cases in which darker varieties are relatively immune to various diseases."[175] Two contributors to the 1930 volume of *JAMA* compared black and white babies with black and white rats on the premise that skin color corresponds to a deeper biological analogy.[176] Other publications suggested that "evolutionary changes in teeth" had left black dental development at a primitive stage.[177]

That such primitive pseudoscientific fantasies about racial differences passed editorial review at flagship journals like *JAMA* and *Psychiatry* during this period is a commentary on how influential some of the categories of Victorian racial anthropology remained well into the twentieth century. Nor should we assume that this influence was extinguished on account of the racial watershed marked by the Second World War. The racial integration of professional sports and the military services were landmark social and political events that were catalyzed by the drafting of African

American men into the racially segregated armed services. But these and other social reforms such as school integration (1954) and voting rights (1964) did not remove the racial folklore inside people's heads.

The ignorance that results from this information vacuum helps to account for the shock and surprise that attend the scandals caused by prominent people who finally succumb to the power of racial fantasies that would have been better left unspoken. It is significant that these awkward events entangle liberals as well as right-wing ideologues like William Bennett and Patrick Buchanan, who once wrote that black crime "is, like sickle cell anemia, a ghetto sickness"—as vicious an example of racist medical defamation as our society has heard since the days of Jim Crow.[178] When presidential candidate Jimmy Carter suddenly endorsed the "ethnic purity" of American neighborhoods in April 1976, he showed—as the case of Francis Lawrence did twenty years later—the fine emotional line that can separate professed racial enlightenment from the unreformed thought habits that lurk within.[179] It is a measure of our racial civility that the threshold of socially acceptable discourse is seldom breached in public life. But not all violations of this standard result from heretical impulses that break through the ideological self-discipline of those who profess racial equality. We must distinguish between those whose principled self-restraint has been breached by the sudden urge to express a socially forbidden racial thought, and others who ignore or disdain the social rules that govern public talk about racial differences. These are the commentators who can slip into a nineteenth-century racial idiom and wonder what all the fuss is about.

The influential official or policy maker of this kind who appears oblivious to the unofficial rules of racial discourse is useful for our purposes, because he allows us to see how racial folklore can still shape the thinking that goes into medical policy making. A notorious case of this kind erupted in February 1992 when Dr. Frederick K. Goodwin, then administrator of the Alcohol, Drug Abuse, and Mental Health Administration, commented on the so-called Violence Initiative that was being sponsored by the Department of Health and Human Services. The goal of this program was to develop pharmacological or other therapeutic interventions against male violence that was implicitly identified as violent behavior by young blacks. Dr. Goodwin's remarks made it seem as though he had traveled back in time and embraced the mentality of a racial "ethnologist" like James Hunt. According to Goodwin's evolutionary model, the male violence of the black American ghetto was a reversion to the chaos of the primeval African jungle and its primitive inhabitants. Male monkeys, he said, are violent and hypersexual, suggesting "some interesting evolutionary implications." The progeny produced by their frequent copulations will "offset the fact that half of them are dying." He then proposed an analogy with "inner city areas" and "the loss of some of the civilizing evolutionary things that we have built up. . . . Maybe it isn't just the careless use of the word when people call certain areas of certain cities, jungles."[180] The medical and social implications of the Violence Initiative were clear. As the African American political scientist Ronald Walters put it: "If there is a reason for this kind of research, the aim is to find a drug. And if you begin using drugs to pacify young black males, as is often done with Ritalin for hyperactivity, you're creating a regime of social control."[181] Goodwin's grossly stereotyping and speculative sociobiology provoked both support for the project and a bitter backlash.[182] This controversy made it clear that the evolutionary racism of the late nineteenth century could still play a role in late twentieth-century thinking about race among influential psychiatrists.

Late nineteenth-century racial anthropologists aimed at creating a comprehensive inventory of the anatomical, physiological, psychological, and cultural traits of the racial alien. Hunt's original and borrowed observations included physiognomy ("absence of expression in the features"), muscularity ("the shoulders are less powerful"), the skeleton ("the bones larger and thicker"), the calf ("usually weak"), the skull ("very hard and unusually thick"), the nerves ("larger than in the European"), the skin ("much thicker"), the voice ("peculiar"), precocity, cranial capacity, convolutions of the brain ("less numerous and more massive"), eyes, teeth, and pain threshold ("physical pain never provokes them").[183] This inventory belongs to the European colonial project that assessed native human material for the practical purpose of politically controlling and economically exploiting what black Africans had to offer to colonial regimes.

Colonial medical science thus combined intellectual curiosity with the ambition to control the natives and to change them in ways that were advantageous to Europeans. Combining intellectual curiosity with racial anthropology produced the phenomenon we may call *racialization*, the imposing of a variety of racial meanings onto anatomical, physiological, and psychological traits. Racialization floods the body and everyday life with racial meaning by generating folkloric interpretations of apparent racial traits and oppositions: what blacks eat, how well they sleep, how fast they run, how musical they are, how often they have sex, how they age, how their children gestate and grow, and so forth. The racial interpretation of black bodies and behaviors, whether on a Southern plantation, in an African colony, or at a medical clinic in an American city, is a form of surveillance that expresses motivations that may be benign or malign, depending on social and historical context. What is more, the racial folkloric themes that have come to be associated with these black lives have encouraged whites to interpret black food habits, sleep patterns, sexual activity, musical aptitude, athleticism, the aging process and other capacities, experiences, and behaviors in various ways that have influenced how doctors think about their black patients.

3. Medical Consequences of Racializing the Human Organism

Introduction

The racializing of medical thinking is the process that translates the racial folklore circulating in the larger society into a medical doctrine of perceived (and usually imaginary) racial differences. The racializing of the human organism has a logic that conforms to the fundamental principles of Western racial doctrine referred to previously. The first of these principles posits the complexity of the civilized versus the simplicity of the primitive. The second (and related) principle posits the *hardiness* of the primitive versus the *delicacy* of the civilized. Medical distinctions between "white" and "black" disorders developed over time as scientists and physicians made distinctions between the greater and lesser biological and psychological complexity of whites and blacks, respectively. These opposing racial images present a sharp contrast between diametrically different racial types, between civilized and sensitive whites who differ profoundly from primitive and hardy blacks. Invidious distinctions between these racial types provided the basic axioms of the racist anthropology of the nineteenth century. It is striking that some of these distinctions have persisted to the end of the twentieth century and beyond.

Racial Interpretations of Black Infants and Children

Traditional images of black infants and children are a form of racial folklore that generates contrasting images of either their robust health or special infirmities. These images have played a role in shaping how doctors diagnose and treat black children, including at times the negligent strategy of not treating them at all. Here the process of racialization has generated a system of extreme (and often opposing, or "bipolar") stereotypes that effectively deny normal human status to the racial type that is portrayed in this way. In the case of black children, contrasting bipolar images of supernormal health on the one hand and abject medical distress on the other can turn these children into exotics, aliens, or little monsters.

Conforming to this dramatic and at times bizarre folk history of black children and their traumas, the standard public health–style narrative presents the familiar recitation of disquieting statistics and warnings. Black children suffer from higher rates of infant mortality, low birth weight, deadly infections, injuries, episodes of sudden infant death syndrome (SIDS), drownings, burns, suffocations, and deaths from choking, poisoning, homicide, and AIDS. Vastly elevated lead levels in black children's blood may lead to the hyperactivity and attention deficit disorders that become disciplinary issues in school. Hyperexposure to cockroach antigen leads to childhood asthma and its deleterious consequences.[1] Public health data of this kind confirm the stark reality of a permanent medical emergency that will require a profound social transformation if it is ever to be alleviated. Understanding how medical personnel have reacted to this crisis over the past century requires us to see how Western societies and their doctors have imagined black children. We will find a surprising and troubling history of ideas about black children that has consistently cast them in abnormal roles—as superhealthy or medically doomed, blessed or cursed by nature, as adorable cherubim or damaged creatures that are beyond medical salvation.

The idealized or demonized biology of the black infant can begin in utero when it is a fetus. The demonizing variant of this biology stigmatizes most dramatically the legendary creature known as the "crack baby" that is supposedly devastated by "the unique effects of intrauterine cocaine exposure."[2] We will analyze the medical and political hysteria over "crack babies" during the 1980s and 1990s later in this chapter. Let us begin, however, with a history of ideas about black infants and children that has emphasized their preternatural health and vitality rather than their pathology.

The Afro-Caribbean psychiatrist Frantz Fanon satirized the stereotype of the hardy and supervital black child half a century ago. "The Negro symbolizes the biological," he writes in Black Skin, White Masks. "First of all, he enters puberty at the age of nine and is a father at the age of ten; he is hot-blooded, and his blood is strong; he is tough. As a white man remarked to me not long ago, with a certain bitterness: 'You all have strong constitutions.'"[3] Fanon's wariness regarding this "positive" image of black juvenile biology was entirely warranted. In fact, the image of the healthy and even adorable black child has been favored by a series of commentators we may charitably call racial paternalists. Black school children, Frederick L. Hoffman wrote in his *Race Traits and Tendencies of the American Negro*, present "a better physical type than do the children of the whites."[4] "The negro boy," Ales Hrdlicka wrote in 1898, "is generally well built, lean, and muscular."[5] In addition to superior physique, there is a special innocent vitality. The Negro child, one cardiologist writes in 1932, "laughs easily, dances, sings, plays, and that usually in rags and wretchedness," thereby transcending the misery of his social condition.[6] (This physician also believed that blacks possessed "less highly organized" nervous systems than whites.) Nor is this the only example of racial folklore about the singing and dancing Negro that has found its way into the medical literature. The happy-go-lucky Negro personality was, in fact, a staple of American psychiatric commentary for decades. Imagining a Negro gift for carefree living and relaxation served to diminish white society's responsibility for African American suffering. Physicians also embraced this opportunity to find emotional relief along with others who intuited the cruelties of Jim Crow racism.

Idealized visions of black infancy could also take on a utopian quality. "Consider our colored countrymen," the famous psychoanalyst Erik H. Erikson wrote in 1959. "Their babies often receive sensual satisfactions of oral and sensory surplus, adequate for a lifetime. It is preserved in the way in which they move, laugh, talk, sing. Their forced symbiosis with the feudal South capitalized on his oral-sensory treasure to build up a slave's identity: mild, submissive, dependent, somewhat querulous, but always ready to serve, and with occasional empathy and childlike wisdom."[7] This was the year that saw the publication of Stanley Elkins's *Slavery* and its controversial theory of the submissive slave personality represented by the figure of "Sambo." It was left to Erikson to trace this syndrome back to the special satisfactions of black infant sensuality that whites could only imagine. And, once again, the compensatory role of these fantasized satisfactions is evident; for whatever the travails of adult black life, these unfortunates would have known perfect happiness as infants in their mothers' arms. Two years later, *JAMA* published a comparable fantasy about the African newborn who "enters a world where every need is anticipated and met by his mother." The anxieties that characterize the African adult are seen as rooted "in the fact that his own early emotional relationships within the family seem to have been so undisturbed, indulgent, and satisfying that he believes this utopian simplicity should continue forever."[8] Promoting a myth of idyllic African infancy in the flagship journal of American medicine was business as usual for a medical establishment that had been absorbing medically themed racial folklore for decades.

The utopian infancy that will eventually cripple the black adult can be seen as a variation on the theme of black precocity that dates from the most denigrating racial anthropologists of the Victorian Age. As James Hunt phrases it, "Young Negro children are nearly as intelligent as European children; but the older they grow the less intelligent they become. They exhibit, when young, an animal liveliness for play and tricks far surpassing the European child."[9] Here is the "hyperactive" black schoolboy a century before the social workers diagnosed him. By the 1960s, the term *precocity* had come to refer to early physical more than mental vitality[10], yet here too it could be appropriated by those harboring doubts about the equality of the races. The possibility that "the [developmental] precocity of Black infants may be related to 'optimal intrauterine and perinatal' conditions" was endorsed by Arthur C. Jensen, the author of "How Much Can We Boost I.Q. and Scholastic Achievement?," a paper on race and intelligence that provoked a firestorm of controversy in 1969.[11] Jensen's interest in "differences in intrauterine pressure" can be seen in relation to the traditional racist theory that black precocity is inevitably followed by a decline in intelligence as adolescence sets in. In summary, one lesson of the precocity myth is that a romantic human biology that extols sheer vitality does not always flatter the people it describes, even if they are children. The same caveat also applies to the romanticizing of what appears to be precocious intelligence. "Everybody knows that pickaninnies can be smart as paint," *Time* commented in 1940, employing a racist term for black children that is now extinct, "but many a white doubts the innate intelligence of Negroes."[12]

The image of the healthy black child was encouraged by African Americans who wanted to emphasize progress in public health within the black community. For example, the 1934 National Negro Health Week celebration included "cups and medals for the best teeth, the healthiest boy or girl, etc."[13] At the 1941 Memphis Tri-State Negro Fair, black doctor-judges assessed "54 wonderful black babies [who] were competing in a healthiest-baby contest."[14] Such events were African American variations on the "scientific" Better Babies Contests of the early decades of the twentieth century that were inspired in part by the eugenics movement.[15] Morris Steggerda, an associate of C.B. Davenport, conducted a eugenic competition involving "50 nigger babies" in Kingston, Jamaica, in 1926.[16] U.B. Phillips, the prominent historian of the Old South whose work tended to sympathize with the slaveholders, included "winsome pickaninnies" in his portrait of an idyllic antebellum world of benevolent plantation masters and contented slaves—an imaginary realm from which the disastrous health problems and premature deaths of these black children were conspicuously absent.[17] Racial paternalists promoted the image of the healthy black child while ignoring their diseases and shortened lives.

The romantic biology applied to black children has also invoked "the survival of the fittest" theme as evidence of their hardiness. "Undoubtedly," an *Archives of Pediatrics* article states, "'survival of the fittest' plays some part in eliminating the physically unfit before the school age."[18] It is likely that many observers of black life, both white and black, have found this idea attractive. To whites it offers the spectacle of a primal competition that confirms their view of blacks as primitives; to blacks it offers the prospect of a dignity that is earned by persisting in the struggle to survive against formidable odds. A medically informed and more realistic view of this sort of struggle for survival appeared in the *American Journal of Public Health* in 1938:

> One might expect that the unnecessarily high death rates among the young children, due to the operation of "survival of the fittest," would eliminate the weak and leave only the strong. In many sections of the lowlands, if only the physical stature of the young adult is considered, the expectation is confirmed to some extent. If, on the other hand, one considers the whole individual: his physical and mental attributes, and his personality, together with their interrelationship, the wholesome, positive qualities are few.[19]

The fantasy of Darwinian fitness debunked by this author depends on imagining the black child as a purely physical creature. "The Negro symbolizes the biological," Fanon wrote, and this is the operative principle here. Simply reciting a slogan like the "survival of the fittest" begs the question of which kinds of fitness might confer long-term advantages on black children. The skeptical author wisely looks beyond physical survival to the eventual fate of the physically sturdy black boy whose "mental attributes" are left in a state of underdevelopment.

This debunking of the myth of black juvenile hardiness and vitality is an appropriate introduction to the more prominent of the "bipolar" images of black children that has predominated both inside and outside the world of medicine. Here we encounter the traumatized black child who is diseased, frightened, and abandoned, a pathetic little figure who incarnates the dark-skinned wretched of the earth in their collective misery. The African version of this child-victim will be familiar to Westerners everywhere—the hollow-eyed, swollen-bellied, fly-tormented waif who stares out at the affluent white readers or viewers whose donations represent the last chance to save him. The traditional racist versions of this forlorn child take the form of caricatures that appeared during the era of racial segregation. One racist variation that aimed at comedy made these children "all teeth and bug eyes and hair sticking up all over their heads as they dug into slices of watermelon."[20] There is "the figure of the nostalgically forlorn [black] child" evoked in the Mammy songs of long ago.[21] One of LeRoi Jones's apocalyptic essays of the 1960s speaks of "the children's eyes deep in their black skin."[22] Here, too, are the imperiled children of Alice Walker's novel *The Color Purple* (1982) with their "strong white teef [teeth]."[23] These victims are the abused and neglected descendants of malnourished and sickly slave children who had gone through much worse.[24]

There have been many medical versions of the traumatized black child. The dirt-eating Negro ragamuffin and his distended "pot-belly" combine poverty and hunger in a uniquely disturbing image.[25] "Here, children are filthy: sleep in filthy houses, eat filthy food and your attention is called to the mortality of children under ten years of age," the *American Journal of Public Health* reports in 1915.[26] There are the "venereal infections, innocently acquired" that the *Southern Medical Journal* reports a year later "in children of both sexes."[27] Rickets and pneumonia take their disproportionate toll among black children in particular.[28] The "babies are starved even though their bellies be full," the *Southern Medical Journal* reports in 1923.[29] The black child can also be the medical victim of parental incompetence and neglect: "He was one of eight children. The mother was lazy and indifferent. This child was responsive and eager to gain but both parents delayed giving permission for the tonsillectomy."[30]

The problems of medically victimized black children originate in poverty, prejudice, and troubled families. The black child is burdened with "all the handicaps resulting from fears, low ideals, and primitive notions," the *American Journal of Psychiatry* states in 1921, and only good fortune can "prevent him from making a complete wreck of his physical and mental life."[31] According to the *Archives of Pediatrics*, "Negro children in cities are victims of communal neglect or indifference and their behavior responses are more understandable in the light of their lack of intelligent outlets for emotional development and social control." Almost half of the children in jails and workhouses in 1923 were black.[32] It is even worse for those "negro defective children" who "suffer from feelings of inferiority in relation to their conspicuously-shaped heads." Children of normal appearance could suffer their own special kinds of heartbreak: "Lonely, homeless children, usually negro boys who had vague memories of their mothers, hallucinated their mother's voice reassuring them, telling them to be good and promising to come back to them or to see that they got a good home."[33]

And there are terrible accidents: "Small colored children," according to the *Tri-State Medical Journal*, "frequently receive severe burns from falling over or into pails of boiling water."[34]

Black children are also subject to special emotional traumas. In 1956 the *American Journal of Psychiatry* reports the following: "It is all too clear that Negro children not yet five can sense that they are marked and grow uneasy. They can like enormously what they see across the color line, and find it hard to like what they see on their side. In this there is scant comfort or security, and in it are the dynamics for rending personality asunder."[35] In 1963 *JAMA* sounded what would become a familiar warning about the damage caused by the dysfunctional black family: "The Negro child is thus exposed to emotional deprivation and appears to suffer from problems stemming from culture conflicts, caste restrictions, and minority status, mediated in part through the family structure. . . ."[36] Over the past half century, the haunted faces of these children, and those of the many who have followed them, came to symbolize a racial crisis that will not be resolved in the foreseeable future.

These images of African American children have been intensified by the traumatizing images of the emotionally unbearable, virtually unthinkable millions of infants with AIDS and orphans in Africa whose needs exceed even those of the urban ghetto and its victims. In fact, the image of the medically doomed African child long antedates the plague of HIV/AIDS. "Africa," the *British Medical Journal* declared in 1952, "is littered with the graves of babies the cause of whose death can never be guessed at."[37] Five years later the *BMJ* notes "a fatalistic acceptance of death in childhood" in Africa that discourages visits to whatever doctor might have been found out in the wild.[38] Medical disasters in Africa have shaped our images of black people and their seemingly intractable medical problems for many years. The secular sainthood granted Albert Schweitzer for his humanitarian work in French Equatorial Africa was rooted in the urgent and unmet needs of the Africans who flocked to Lambaréné to be cured by the great man. In this sense, black disease and white medicine have long been locked into a symbiotic relationship of which the AIDS catastrophe is the most recent, and most horrifying, example.

Bipolar images of preternaturally healthy or traumatically afflicted black children have proliferated in the medical literature as well as in the larger world outside the clinic. This brief history of such images demonstrates the interdependence of the medical realm and the society it serves. During the first half of the twentieth century, racial folklore about black children passed easily into the medical journals where it was endowed with professional authority by medical authors. During the second half of the twentieth century, the problem of the black family became a racial and political preoccupation in the United States; consequently, social workers, sociologists, and journalists have produced the most familiar medical images of black children. The medical literature of our era no longer dramatizes their medical problems in vernacular terms, with a single exception—the pathology-ridden "crack baby" who was conjured out of the cocaine epidemic that took off in the mid-1980s. The point here is that fascination and horror can take on a life of their own; and in so doing, they distort medical reality and create in its place an appalling drama, either heartbreaking or repellent, that captivates spectators who gradually become voyeurs.

The "crack baby" panic that erupted during the late 1980s was an event of this kind, living on for years before physicians finally concluded that it had been an artificial crisis. The crisis mood was sustained by a peculiar form of medical hysteria that was fed in turn by deeply rooted societal views about black people, their weaknesses, and their behavioral problems. The medical report that launched the media's promotion of the "crack baby" issue, "Cocaine Use in Pregnancy," appeared in the *New England Journal of Medicine* in September 1985. Dr. Ira J. Chasnoff and his coauthors reported "findings of depressed interactive abilities and significant impairments in organizational abilities in infants exposed to cocaine as compared with control infants or with infants whose mothers used methadone." Their study had enrolled only 23 women who had also variously used alcohol, marijuana, and cigarettes, thereby complicating the task of isolating the possible effects of intrauterine cocaine from those of the other drugs.[39] On September 11, 1985, the *CBS Evening News* broadcast a story on a "crack baby" allegedly suffering from a cocaine "withdrawal" syndrome that does not, in fact, exist:[40]

> Yet the myth of the "crack baby" grew ever larger. Syndicated columnist Charles Krauthammer dismissed "crack babies" in 1988 as a "biologic underclass whose biological inferiority is stamped at birth." Boston University president John Silber criticized "spending immense amounts on crack babies who won't ever achieve the intellectual development to have consciousness of God." The *New York Times* declared "crack babies" unable to "make friends, know right from wrong, control their impulses, gain insight, concentrate on tasks, and feel and return love." Even *Rolling Stone* condemned "crack babies" as "like no others, brain damaged in ways yet unknown, oblivious to any affection."[41]

It would be difficult to assemble a better collection of proxy images for the animating themes of antiblack racism. In this narrative the "crack baby" simultaneously symbolizes genetic inferiority, intellectual deficiency, juvenile delinquency, and the conscienceless males known as psychopaths.

By 1992 *JAMA* was reporting "an apparent rush to judgment about the extent and permanency of specific effects of intrauterine cocaine exposure on newborns. Predictions of an adverse developmental outcome for these children are being made despite a lack of supportive scientific evidence." These authors objected to media representations of these children "as severely or even irrevocably brain damaged" and to the influence these images were having on the ability of doctors to make clinical decisions unbiased by sensationalism.[42] A year later two authors confirmed the hysterical basis of the "crack baby" phenomenon: "We think it is clear now, from a multitude of studies, that the effect of prenatal cocaine exposure is minimal at birth and is probably limited to minor growth deficits." By this time, however, the damage had been done. As Dorothy Roberts pointed out in 1997: "The image of the crack baby—trembling in a tiny hospital bed, permanently brain-damaged, and on his way to becoming a parasitic criminal—is indelibly etched in the American psyche. It will be hard to convince most Americans that the caricature of the crack baby rests on flimsy, exaggerated data."[43] By 2001 and 2002, *JAMA* was describing the prenatal cocaine issue as an example of "how sociopolitical forces shape discrepant interpretations of similar scientific data" and how the "popular perception of the 'crack kid'" had "undoubtedly shaped physicians' attitudes and public policies."[44] "The term 'crack baby,'" another expert stated in 2004, "is an urban legend masquerading as a medical diagnosis. It is a label that stigmatizes, marginalizes and endangers children and their mothers who are desperately in need of care. Born from the combination of an ongoing crisis in urban health care and draconian zero-tolerance drug policies, the crack-baby myth thrives even though it has no basis in science."[45] Two decades after this myth had been launched, it was still affecting how doctors thought about black children.

"Why," *JAMA* asked in 1992, "is there today such an urgency to label prenatally cocaine-exposed children as irremediably damaged?"[46] Answering this question requires us to situate this emotional "urgency" in its historical context, for the purpose of examining comparable campaigns in which physicians stigmatized or predicted doom for black children or the black "race" in general. The extinction theory that flourished around the turn of the twentieth century predicted the eventual disappearance of a tubercular and venereal disease–ridden black population that was doomed to succumb in the racial "competition" with stronger whites. This prognosis also expressed an unmistakable *wish* for black extinction shared by the many whites who saw post-emancipation blacks as a failing and degenerate population of racial inferiors that was, as Frederick Hoffman put it, "unsuited for the battle of life."[47] The Detroit doctor who recommended in 1903 that white society "help along the process of extinction" expressed a view that reflected an impatience with blacks and their problems that was typical of the medical profession at the time.[48] This sort of thinking also helped to prepare the ground for the conspiracy theories about white medical authorities that continue to flourish in African American communities to this day. The point of this comparison is to suggest that a misguided and "urgent" campaign to find irreparable medical damage in "crack babies" may originate less in therapeutic motives than in racially motivated impulses that echo the wish for black extinction being expressed a century ago in the United States. The familiar fixation on black fertility that provokes resentment of "welfare mothers" seems to represent another example of unconscious white ambivalence toward the desirability of black survival. Those who wish to protest such speculations will have to demonstrate that the hostile and destructive feelings directed at black people that some physicians were expressing openly a century ago have actually become extinct.

The sudden demand for mandatory sickle-cell testing of black infants, children, and adults that erupted even before the passage of the National Sickle Cell Anemia Control Act on May 16, 1972, represented another collective response to an invented "black" medical emergency on the part of a white-dominated lobby that included several Southern state legislatures. The question "Why is this limited to Negroes?" was already being heard in 1970.[49] The mandatory testing campaign was both medically unjustified and substantially harmful to its target population. As the African American physician Charles F. Whitten explained in 1973, mandatory testing inspired fears of genocide through population control, misrepresented the disease, created unwarranted anxiety in those tested, failed to provide counseling, encouraged misdiagnoses, destabilized families, eliminated informed consent, and targeted children for no valid medical purpose.[50] African Americans, *The Black Scholar* declared in 1974, "have a right to ask whether they want the government to wage war on the fetus and black children with the aim of *controlling* sickle cell for their benefit"—an impossible objective, in any case.[51] In its euphemistic way, *JAMA* recognized the emotional burden that testing inflicted on its black victims, but this was a one-sided contest between a medical establishment carrying out a political mandate and a resentful black population that had grown accustomed to medical neglect and abuse.

The extinction theory, the "crack baby" diagnosis, and the sickle-cell crusade were all temporarily persuasive and pseudo-scientific delusions that took for granted the reality of something like "racial" disease. These diagnoses also incorporate a pessimism about the fates of medically afflicted blacks that commands our attention. And once again we confront the question of where pessimistic diagnosis ends and hostile wish fulfillment begins. What are the motives that prompt whites to fantasize repeatedly about the medical hopelessness of blacks? Is it compassion or schadenfreude or a combination of both?

The "crack baby" is the most ominous representative of what one reporter called "a new *'bio-underclass'* of infants who are disadvantaged almost from the moment of conception."[52] The idea of a "bio-underclass" suggests a perfect fusion of biopathology and sociopathology that transforms the "crack baby" into the violent and psychologically deformed criminal of the future. Two years after Daniel Patrick Moynihan speculated about "speciation" in the ghetto, the academic criminologist John J. DiIulio, Jr. was talking of young black males as "juvenile super-predators" who "seem not merely unrecognizable but alien."[53] In the case of the "crack baby," the coding of deviant intrauterine development as "black" precedes the coding of predatory male crime as "black," so that medical personnel wind up colluding in the criminalization of the black child. Ascribing the alleged deformation of these children to the cigarettes or alcohol that their mothers have smoked or ingested was seen as too anticlimactic to report. This lack of interest in noncatastrophic outcomes regarding fetal exposure to cocaine was actually reported in *The Lancet* in 1989; the evidence showed that medical editors overwhelmingly preferred studies that indicated cocaine-induced fetal damage over superior studies that indicated otherwise. "The subconscious message may be that if a study did not detect an adverse effect of cocaine when the common knowledge is that this is a 'bad' drug, then the study must be flawed."[54] This is a prime example of how racially coded "common knowledge" can dictate a medical diagnosis.

Racial Interpretations of the Black Elderly

The racial interpretation of the aging process in elderly blacks resembles the racial interpretation of black children in two major respects. Here, too, one observes an oscillation between folklore and science, along with the contrasting ("bipolar") extremes of hardiness and vulnerability. The important difference between racial interpretations of children and the aged is that, while black children have been hypervisible as presumed victims and sociopaths, the black elderly have tended to be socially invisible because they are not associated with pathological behaviors. There is, consequently, no "common knowledge" about the "black" aging process comparable to the "crack baby" mythology, because there is no ideologically motivated demand for pathological images of the black elderly.

The absence of such a stigma does not exempt aging blacks from racial interpretations of their bodies and symptoms. Quite apart from how their doctors may think about their "racial" traits, the black elderly construct ideologically motivated interpretations of themselves. As the African American psychiatrist James H. Carter has pointed out, "Senior black Americans take great pride in having lived through varying degrees of deprivation and racism, leaving behind a legacy that reinforces the notion that 'only the strong survive' and negates suicide." The African American value system includes the claim "that survival of aged black men and women is testimony to individual emotional and physical ruggedness."[55] For many of these people an ideology rooted in the demand to survive is a principal source of dignity, and this demand can have medical consequences. For example, toward the end of life, black patients want more life-sustaining treatments than their white counterparts, and white physicians should understand why this is the case.[56]

The African American commitment to survival points to a contrasting pair of themes that present the "black" aging process in opposing ways. On the one hand, medical authors have speculated repeatedly that a kind of natural selection promoting "the survival of the fittest" among the black elderly has produced a superlongevity phenomenon among the oldest blacks: "It seems premature to discount the idea that very old blacks constitute a group with 'extra-special hardiness'—the physical and psychological survivors."[57] This phenomenon became known as the "crossover effect," although its origins remain unclear. The observed superlongevity could be due to a more rigorous natural selection of old blacks, an underreporting of black deaths, or inaccurate reporting of ages.[58] The temptation to explain the alleged black advantage as the result of an unusually severe process of natural selection will be strong among both blacks and whites.

The black superlongevity phenomenon coexists with stronger evidence of a contrary trait, namely, accelerated aging among blacks: "Certainly, early aging among blacks is evident in several physical and social areas. Blacks, for example, experience earlier sexual maturity, onset of certain diseases, functional limitation, and mortality than whites. And socially, the timing of certain critical life events is accelerated: the birth and loss of first child, the loss of spouse, and the earlier ending of work lives."[59] Here is a sobering counterpoint to the alleged "crossover effect" that contrasts so starkly with the African American longevity deficit of six fewer years in relation to whites. This premature aging process appears to also include much higher African American vulnerability to dementia, including Alzheimer's disease.[60]

Contrasting ideas about the "black" aging process can disorient diagnosis on account of how the black elderly can see themselves. The "hardiness" doctrine is evident in the folklore about black skin that is expressed in the African American adage: "When women get old, black don't crack."[61] A more scientific rendering of this folk wisdom appeared in *JAMA* in 1962: "Because Negro skin has natural protection in its high melanin content, elderly Negroes often appear deceptively young."[62] On the other hand, older African Americans have been reported to regard their mental health and cognitive functioning as being more impaired than is the case in whites despite the absence of more objective corroborating data.[63] Listening too credulously to these patients or looking at their skin could mislead unwary physicians.

Physicians who are unaware of racially inflected medical folklore may assume that black skin is endowed with a natural protection against skin cancers, that the black elderly are not at risk for suicide, that certain symptoms are due to the "accelerated" aging of black patients rather than disease processes, that black women do not experience the symptoms of menopause, and that black patients are unusually susceptible to dementia. Given a tradition of racist thinking about black intelligence, it is not surprising that false positive rates for dementia have been found to be higher in the black elderly.[64] In these cases, a doctor might incorrectly diagnose a black patient who may have underestimated his or her own cognitive functioning and thus misled the doctor. It is, therefore, important to keep in mind that the "common knowledge" about racial differences that can skew a physician's judgment may come from patients themselves.

Racial Interpretations of the Black Athlete

The influence of black athletic achievement on twentieth-century physiological and medical thinking appears as early as 1940 in the *Journal of Biological Chemistry*. Four years after Jesse Owens won four gold medals in sprinting and long jumping at the 1936 Berlin Olympic Games, a team of physiologists interpreted the growing prominence of black athletic stars in the following terms:

> The existence of physiological differences between Negroes and Whites other than those dependent on pigmentation and external anatomical features is suggested by the superior records of Negroes in track and

field athletics and by the commonly expressed opinion that they have greater resistance to high temperatures. So far, however, no one has demonstrated unique physiological characteristics of the Negro that might be related to the capacity for energy transformation.[65]

The racial physiology they derived in part from athletic performance also included a psychiatric evaluation of blacks as well as the composition of their blood. "Negroes," they write, "are reputed to have a different emotional make-up than Whites and it is true that emotional make-up can be reflected in the properties of blood obtained by puncturing an artery, or even a finger." As for the properties of their blood, "It appears to be a racial characteristic of Negroes to have thin blood in the sense of low hemoglobin [8 per cent less than in White subjects]. . . ."[66]

Here is more evidence that the penetration of the scientific literature by racial folklore can have diagnostic consequences. In this case, the folklore acquires credibility through the charisma of the celebrity athlete and is received uncritically by scientists who might be expected to respond with greater skepticism. The fact that "no one has demonstrated unique physiological characteristics of the Negro" is less persuasive than what is "suggested" by spectacular athletic performances. That Negroes "are reputed to have a different emotional make-up than Whites" is granted scientific status on the fanciful proposition that emotional make-up can be read in a blood profile. The ease with which some scientists are overwhelmed by athletic "evidence" appeared again in 1984 when Dr. George E. Graham, a professor of international health and pediatrics at Johns Hopkins University and a member of President Reagan's Task Force on Food Assistance, asserted that black children were probably "the best-nourished group in the United States," his evidence being the proliferation of African American sports stars.[67]

During the 1960s many athletic trainers and football coaches regarded black football players as virtually indestructible and thus immune to injury.[68] The same idea about Africans appeared in *The Lancet* in 1945.[69] Almost half a century later, this racial folklore entered the life of an African American female athlete who was taking my course on "Race and Sport in African-American Life" at the University of Texas. At the end of the semester she wrote:

> This class has already helped me understand my white coaches better. . . . [When] I tore my ACL and MCL and chipped my femur in a basketball game my coaches kept talking about how [the African-American professional football star] Jerry Rice had come back after only 5 1/2 weeks and how I could still have a great season if I wanted it. A few days after my

injury one of my white teammates tore a muscle in her thumb; all the coaches freaked and she sat out two weeks of practice and was constantly being checked on and pampered. I on the other hand was ignored once it was discovered that I could not play this season. The coaches could not have cared less how I was doing. This class helped me not be so angry about all of that. I realize now that they genuinely thought that because Jerry Rice came back in record [time] I should as well, because we are both black.[70]

This informant was a more than competent and uncomplaining student who came to class on crutches; her constant companion was a white teammate. Several African American male athletes later told her they had had similar experiences.

Another version of the medical "hardiness" doctrine applied to African American athletes can also affect black athletes outside the United States. After the Cameroon soccer star Marc-Vivien Foe collapsed and died during an international match in France in 2003, it was learned that he had been allowed to continue playing despite the detection of his enlarged heart, because this condition (hypertrophic cardiomyopathy) was considered "normal" for his race. The manager of his former British team commented that, "when we sent him to one specialist, they told us that Foe's condition is absolutely normal and common among African athletes, and that because of that we could proceed with the signing of the contract."[71]

The medical irony of all this is that ideas about black athletic aptitude promote positive images of black health and hardiness that contradict African American (and African) medical realities, such as Dr. Graham's misguided assumption that elite black athletes must have been well-fed children. More than any other social venue or institution, the sports world creates and disseminates apparent evidence of racial differences that include pseudo-indices of superior black health.[72] The ubiquity of these images of black supervitality makes them a potential threat to the health of black patients around the world.

Racial Interpretations of Black Musical Aptitude

While medical interpretations of African American musicality and musical aptitude have appeared occasionally in the medical literature, this particular variation on the medical "racializing" of blacks appears to be an archaism in a way that the medical interpretation of athleticism is not. During the early decades of the twentieth century, scientific speculation about blacks' special affinity for musical expression was stimulated by the growing influence of "black" musical forms such as jazz and the blues. American psychologists published studies of racial musical aptitude in children during the 1920s and 1930s, often finding that black children possessed a superior sense of rhythm. Given the pervasive racial dichotomies of the Jim Crow era, it is not surprising to hear one researcher announce in 1933 that "we have found distinct racial differences in musical ability."[73] This kind of research could also produce findings that appeared to have some medical or anthropological significance. A University of Pennsylvania psychologist thus claimed in 1928 that the musical aptitude of black children amounted to "a verification of the oft-stated idea that the Negro child matures more rapidly than the white child"—a reiteration of the "precocity" theory that attributes arrested mental development to black adolescents and adults. The black child's alleged "superior vocal ability" signified "an anatomical difference between the races in the organs of vocalization,"[74] a finding that could only confirm the contemporary belief that blacks and whites were different racial types. Such investigations transcended the realm of music and promoted popular ideas about blacks and their special temperament.

The idea that African Americans and Africans possess a special aptitude for music was embraced on both sides of the color line. "No one," we read in W. E. B. DuBois's anthology *The Health and Physique of the Negro American* (1906), "will question this gift of music in the Negro."[75] In "The Poor White Musician" (1915), the black man of letters James Weldon Johnson credits his race with a "natural musical ability" whites must labor mightily to equal.[76] At the same time, medical and other scientific racists were only too happy to endorse the inherent musicality of blacks. "Motion, music, and excitement, or a combination of these make up much of the life of the colored people," a psychiatrist at St. Elisabeth's Hospital in Washington, DC, wrote in the *American Journal of Psychiatry* in 1921. "Their natural musical ability of a peculiar type, and their sense of rhythm, are too well known to make comment necessary."[77] "As a group," the racist psychologist J. C. Carothers wrote in 1951, "Africans also excel in musical ability," a faculty that "must leave the frontal lobes in relative idleness" and thereby doom the African to the limitations of his primitive state.[78]

What doctors believed about the role of music in black life could help them make sense of racial temperament and thus of human diversity as they understood it in the era of Jim Crow segregation. A cardiologist writing in 1931 about "Nervous and Mental Influences in Angina Pectoris" connects racial temperament to chest pain in the following way: "The psychology of stress, strain and struggle in the white races is in sharp contrast to the humorous carelessness of the musical negro or the placid acceptance of the gentle Chinaman."[79] As improbable as it may seem today, racial caricatures of this kind played a significant role in the medical thinking of that era. As late as 1963, a report in *JAMA* on Negro schizophrenics cites "the Negro's reaction to religion and music" as a cause of his allegedly greater susceptibility to hallucinations.[80] These episodes are instructive because they show how easily folkloric material can be absorbed into physicians' worldviews and then into their diagnoses. They demonstrate that a fanciful logic of racial difference can operate by taking up residence in as familiar a venue as popular music and then serving as an interpretive resource. It would be naïve to assume that today's physicians are immune to the racial "logic" that inheres in our ideas about African American affinities to certain musical styles. In fact, modern people are fully capable of regarding musical temperament and other cultural markers as racial traits. This was confirmed in a 1995 opinion survey that reported "blacks were roughly 10 times more likely than whites to be seen as superior in athletic ability or rhythmic ability."[81]

Racial Interpretations of Losing Consciousness

Multiple references in the medical literature to the special hallucinatory potential of blacks raise the question of whether various types of consciousness and unconsciousness might be seen as subject to racial variation. The answer, of course, is that such fundamental categories of human experience could not have escaped racial interpretation over the past century. "Some American psychiatrists," one sociologist wrote in 1967, "have asserted that Negroes are less able to distinguish between 'objective existence' and hallucinations, that is, objective or everyday existence for the Negro can be closer to what the hallucinatory state is for a member of another group."[82] This view of black mental functioning can be understood as one of various ways in which whites have sought to infantilize or pathologize blacks as a group. Denying a "racial" population the capacity to engage in the reality-testing and empirical reasoning we associate with "objectivity" means condemning them to a primitive level of mental functioning. Commentaries by physicians and others on the ease with which blacks lose consciousness in various ways thus belong to the same racial psychology that has long assigned blacks the lowest status in the racial hierarchy.

Observations on the capacity of black people to lose consciousness have played a significant role in the medical literature of the twentieth century. Loss of consciousness can take the form of falling asleep, falling into a hypnotic state, or yielding to the techniques of anesthesia. These reports have always attributed to blacks an enhanced capacity to achieve these unconscious states. This special gift for achieving mental oblivion finds its place in a doctrine of black inferiority that emphasizes a primitive mentality, general passivity, and the stigma of laziness that was long a part of both colonial and Southern racist lore.

An early racial interpretation of the capacity to fall asleep appears in Thomas Jefferson's *Notes on the State of Virginia* (1781). The racial anthropology that informs Jefferson's views on the anatomical and psychological traits of the Negro would reappear intact most of a century later in the pseudoscientific doctrine of the plantation physician Samuel Cartwright. Blacks, Jefferson says, are more prone to "sensation than reflection," and this imbalance accounts for "their disposition to sleep when abstracted from their diversions. . . ." Consequently: "An animal whose body is at rest, and who does not reflect, must be disposed to sleep. . . ."[83] "Left to pursue their natural inclinations," Cartwright declared in 1851, "they devote a greater portion of their time to sleep."[84] Cartwright's physiological theories were intended to explain the practical necessity of slavery, and the portrait of naturally sleepy slaves who required the guidance of white masters served this objective well. A Viennese physician who went to Uganda in 1911 asserts "beyond any doubt" that Africans sleep more deeply than whites, and that they manage to do so on hard wooden benches on which Europeans could not catch a moment's sleep.[85]

The idea of a somnolent Negro race was well known to the African American intelligentsia during the early twentieth century. W. E. B. DuBois wrote that the black race from "the dawn of creation has slept, but half awakening in the dark forests of its African fatherland."[86] A racially condescending white character in Langston Hughes's story "Slave on the Block" (1934) decides to paint a picture of her black gardener called "The Sleeping Negro": "Dear, natural childlike people, they would sleep anywhere they wanted to."[87] This image of the naturally sleepy Negro eventually played various roles in the medical literature. The *Southern Medical Journal* reported in 1913, for example, that Negro patients responded especially well to "nerve sedatives and hypnotic" drugs and suffered only infrequently from insomnia. And they were very receptive when they were awake. "Psychotherapy among the Afro-Americans," says Dr. Niles, "is almost like planting good seed in virgin soil," a happy consequence of their "primitively developed mentalities."[88] (This optimistic assessment of the value of psychotherapy for blacks would eventually prove to be an anomalous viewpoint in American psychiatry.) A report on "Behavior Problems in Negro Children" that appeared in *Psychiatry* in 1939 describes as a "characteristic of the race . . . the capacity for so-called laziness" that is the same as "the ability to go to sleep. . . ." "Frequently," according to this psychologist, "children are brought to us because of sleeping attacks or so-called narcolepsy. These have invariably been negro boys of early adolescent or pre-adolescent age." The author appears to assume that this special vulnerability to "sleeping attacks" has a biological rather than a social basis, since she speculates, not about the stressful living conditions these children might have been dealing with, but rather about "specific brain impulse tendencies."[89] In this case, the ability to fall asleep is not a normal but rather an abnormal trait associated with an indolent temperament and the social irresponsibility it implies.

The capacity to lose consciousness includes being anesthetized, and the black response to anesthesia, like the propensity to sleep, could be linked to passivity and low intelligence. "The average negro," a News Orleans doctor commented in 1932, "because of his duller perceptions, is an excellent subject for any sort of anesthesia, and perhaps his traditional confidence in the white man gives him a feeling of security which the more highly organized white patient sometimes lacks."[90] The African American pathologist Julian H. Lewis, author of *The Biology of the Negro* (1942), claimed that "the first person to be completely anesthetized was a Negro."[91] Submitting to anesthesia in a segregated society where blacks often feared white doctors must have been an ordeal for many black people. The New Orleans doctor's misplaced faith in the black man's "traditional confidence in the white man" contrasted sharply at this time with the somber views of more perceptive white colleagues who recognized racial estrangement when they saw it. There is no suggestion in his account that he was aware of black patients' anxiety about anesthesia. And there was plenty to be anxious about, given that anesthetized blacks were dying in far greater numbers than their white counterparts.[92]

The capacity to sleep was also seen in relation to mood and the mood pathology known as depression. In 1932, for example, the *American Heart Journal* presented a paraphrased dialogue sent in by a cardiologist who had asked "a very sensible negro" about "suicide in his race." This black man confirmed for the doctor the folkloric image of the happy-go-lucky Negro and his presumed immunity to depression. He then said that "when he sat down he went to sleep so easily that the worry passed away."[93] Such vignettes suggest that the apparent somnolence of patients could mislead physicians who missed (or were deliberately misled about) various clues that could have given them a better grasp of doctor-patient relationships across the race barrier. How many physicians of this era were aware of what was going on when they were being taken in by the African American technique of "putting on the white man"? How many physicians of our own era are aware that they might be subjected to ruses of this kind that might result in mistaken diagnoses?

The ability to fall asleep easily is widely regarded as an enviable trait that suggests relaxation and the sound mental health the absence of stress promotes. In retrospect, we can understand the sleepy Negro syndrome as a variation on the theme of the physiologically noble savage whose effortless adaptation to Nature stands in stark contrast to the anxiety-inducing stresses and complexities of white lives. Responsiveness to hypnosis was yet another version of this doctrine. "The native," a South African physician reports in 1939, "is very susceptible to hypnotic influence, and it was comparatively easy to hypnotise him, and one made many interesting experiments in this field."[94] The various reports of diminished consciousness in blacks reassured whites by confirming that blacks were passive by nature and receptive to white influence; there is, after all, no greater imbalance of power than that which separates the conscious from the unconscious, regardless of whether the state of oblivion results from sleepiness, anesthesia, or hypnosis.

The evidence bearing on African American sleep is diametrically opposed to the medical myth of the sleepy Negro and his contented state of mind. In 1975, the African American psychiatrist Chester M. Pierce stated the obvious: that there was every reason to believe that "ghetto sleep" was inferior to the sleep patterns of those who did not have to live crammed into thin-walled apartments and constantly exposed to the violence and bedlam of inner-city streets.[95] It is even possible that a belief in the deep sleep enjoyed by ghetto dwellers and other black people living under stress is a compensatory response to repressed knowledge of, and discomfort about, living conditions that would keep most of us up at night. Why traits are ascribed to African Americans as a group should be scrutinized every time such claims are made.

The evidence reported in recent years shows that blacks are at greater risk for obstructive sleep apnea (OSA), a disorder that can also promote hypertension and obesity.[96] Sleep disordered breathing (SDB) is reported to be twice as common in young blacks as in young whites. The higher rate of SDB may also be related to the fact that black children are only half as likely to have had their tonsils and adenoids removed as their white peers. Non-Caucasian adults report a rate of insomnia twice that of whites.[97] African Americans have also been shown to have a higher rate of isolated sleep paralysis.[98] This terrifying condition is known in the African American vernacular as "being ridden by the witch."[99]

Given these reports of disproportionately severe sleep disorders among African Americans, it is at first surprising to learn that "African Americans appear to have fewer chronic sleep complaints than Caucasians." Their rate of waking up in the middle of the night is said to be only 60 percent that of whites.[100] Snoring is a symptom of obstructive sleep apnea, yet black spouses report leaving the bedroom for this reason only half as often as their white counterparts; almost twice as many blacks as whites regard snoring as "normal." "From this study," commented Dr. Kelvin Lee, director of the division of general otolaryngology and sleep surgery at the New York University Medical Center, "it appears that in the black community there isn't a perception of snoring being a problem. That's a big opportunity for outreach and education."[101]

This physician's plan to educate African Americans about the medically harmful consequences of OSA involves a therapeutic option that is somewhat more complicated than it looks. On the one hand, OSA has been linked to the obesity and cardiovascular diseases (CVDs) that exact a terrible toll among African Americans. This would argue for making people aware that snoring is a symptom of a disorder that requires treatment. At the same time, the relative absence of concern among blacks about OSA and some other disorders should be understood in its historical context. During and after slavery, African Americans were conditioned by the medical racism of their times to respond late (or not at all) to a variety of disease states and medical discomforts. In this sense, lack of concern about an ostensibly minor symptom like snoring is an adaptive response that has an experiential logic and, perhaps, a value of its own. People simply did not rank it very high on the list of threats to their health. We have already seen that a kind of stoicism about medical problems remains embedded in the African American experience.

The racial interpretation of entire categories of human experience in terms of "black" and "white" variants, such as aging, childhood, athleticism, and sleep, has made it difficult for physicians to remain unaffected by these folkloric ideas; it is hard to resist the temptation to find or invent racially differential traits when a preoccupation with such traits has established itself as a social convention. The importance of racial folklore about musical and athletic aptitude came about because racist restrictions on employment and education that operated for most of the twentieth century caused African Americans to invest a disproportionate amount of effort and talent in becoming entertainers. "Black dominance" of certain musical idioms and high-profile sports has, consequently, promoted a belief in racial aptitudes and essences as effectively

as media coverage of black SAT scores and crime rates; and medical professionals are exposed to this lore like everyone else.

Racial Interpretations of the Nervous System

The nervous system can be thought of as the organic site of human identity and temperament. It is the anatomical basis of important social performances, including the faculties of intelligence, empathy, and self-control.
Its disorders are often both conspicuous and dramatic, as in the case of
various mental illnesses or a lack of physical coordination. The nineteenth-
century racial anthropological model of racially distinct nervous systems
thus led doctors over many years to make profound and invidious distinctions between black and white human beings. Today, as we shall see, there
is abundant evidence suggesting that the racial neurology of this earlier
period lives on in two ways. First, it has promoted an unfair distribution of
analgesic medications along racial lines; and, second, its crude anatomical
hypotheses have evolved into more sophisticated theories of racially differential nervous reactivity that currently occupy a place in modern medical science. Between the age of Victorian racial anthropology and this late
twentieth-century medical research, racial themes in neurology influenced
how doctors thought about a variety of medical topics.

The crude, anatomically based neurology of Samuel Cartwright asserted that "the nerves going from the brain, as also the ganglionic system
of nerves" in blacks were larger than those of whites, thereby accounting for their mental inferiority and immaturity.[102] James Hunt's "On the
Negro's Place in Nature" (1864) repeated this idea that black nerves were
thicker, and therefore less sensitive, than those of whites.[103] American scientists and physicians of the first half of the twentieth century abandoned
the emphasis on gross neural anatomy in favor of a focus on nervous
"organization" that called into question the fitness of blacks to be members
of a modern society. "Is the pure-blood negro so stabilized in his nervous
organization," *Science* asked in 1929, "in racial habits, as to be limited to
fewer lines of thought and work and cooperation in civilized life, or does
no such restricting influence exist in his constitution?"[104] "Certainly," the
American Heart Journal said in 1932, "there is a profound dissimilarity in
the psyche and sensorium in the two races under consideration. Therefore,
it seems logical to assume that [there is] an inherent difference in the sensitivity of the nervous system in the two races."[105]

This doctrine served the ideological needs of societies that practiced racial apartheid; so that while the *Southern Medical Journal* spoke of the
black's "less highly organized nervous system,"[106] the *South African*

Medical Journal asserted in a similar fashion that the black person's "central nervous system is in a lowly stage of development."[107] Racially differential nervous systems could also be seen as a cause of differential crime rates. "Another fact supporting the differences in nervous system and psychic development," the *American Journal of Physical Anthropology* noted in 1937, "is the frequency of homicides among the Colored."[108] The idea of racial intelligence also played a role in this discussion. *JAMA's* 1939 editorial on "Angina Pectoris in the Negro" observed the following: "While a disturbed emotional state can precipitate an anginal attack, a more than moronic intelligence is required to describe that attack. A difference in nervous system sensitivity seems a plausible explanation for why blacks were not reporting angina attacks."[109] Such assessments of black intelligence in the medical literature were in no way controversial at a time when the prevailing racial etiquette required few concessions to black dignity; indeed, some journals did not even bother to capitalize the word "Negro" as late as the 1930s.

The bipolar stereotypes associated with the "black" nervous system are stoicism at one end of the spectrum and excitability at the other. Neurological stoicism has long included the idea that blacks are not as sensitive to pain as whites—a stereotype that is one of the fundamental tenets of Western racial folklore.[110] Medical discussions of racial pain sensitivity have often focused on the chest pains known as angina. At least a few medical authors, however, argued that, while many doctors accepted the idea of racially differential pain, this purported racial difference was an illusion that originated in the differential social conditioning of whites and blacks:

> Angina pectoris, as one sees it in the Caucasian, hardly occurs in the negro, and it is because the term angina pectoris is purely symptomatic fear. The fear that is so prominent a symptom in the white person does not occur in the negro, but I will venture to say that the pains are just the same. The negro does not complain of them, although he has felt them. That which the white man speaks of in a striking, graphic manner, the negro refers to as "misery in the stomach" or "misery in the chest."[111]

This passage from 1927 contains some essential themes: the white patient's need or willingness to express fear, the black patient's refusal to complain about physical discomfort, and the language barrier that could make it difficult or impossible for white physicians to "read" their black patients. The assumption that blacks did not experience angina went hand in hand with a belief in the black man's immunity to heart attacks that lingers on to this day. "I am unable to find in the literature a description of the clinical picture of myocardial infarction in the Negro," a cardiologist writes in 1946. "The diagnosis is rarely made clinically." And this practitioner offered a different explanation for the observed absence of angina in black patients; the pain is absent in blacks because the early onset of hypertension has dilated their blood vessels. While he is aware that the rarity of reported angina in blacks "is commonly ascribed to lack of stress or to inability of the Negro to feel or express pain," he refuses to believe in racially differential pain thresholds.[112]

The other bipolar extreme of the "black" nervous system is an alleged nervous excitability that has taken various forms, from the "vociferous lamentations" of the hyperemotional "Negro patient" of the early twentieth century to the modern theory of racially differential neurohormonal reactivity.[113] "The negro," the New Orleans doctor writes in 1929, "is an excellent subject for local anesthesia and he bears general anesthesia equally well unless his emotional nature has been aroused, in which case the excitement stage may be extreme." A British colonial physician writes in 1945 of the African patient's "hysterical and functional disabilities."[114] Terms such as "psyche," "emotional nature," "excitement stage," and "hysterical disabilities" convey impressions of racial temperament rather than anything resembling scientific speculations about the state of the nervous system.

This stage of racial neurology appeared later during the 1950s in conjunction with speculations about racial differences and neurohormones. In the meantime, a crude "gland theory" that derived racial differences from "the functioning of the endocrine glands" appeared in the *American Journal of Sociology* in 1927. Six years later, a prominent American endocrinologist expressed his skepticism about the idea that racial traits resulted from hormone deficiencies or excesses. "The evidence," he wrote, "is thus ambiguous."[115] In 1937 a comment about "racial peculiarities" and "endocrine products" appeared in the *American Journal of Physical Anthropology.*[116] But naïve speculations of this kind were already dated and could not survive scientific scrutiny.

The early neurohormonal doctrine of the 1950s combined speculation about hormone deficiencies in Africans and African Americans with other speculations about their vulnerability to hypertension and the neurological stress of surgery and anesthesia. In 1955 a lecturer in anesthesia at the University College Hospital of the West Indies, in Saint Andrew, Jamaica, told his audience at the World Federation of Anesthesiologists in Holland that "patients in tropical countries" were far more endangered by the stress of surgery than whites:

> There is a quantitative difference in the blood pressure reaction to a
> standard vasomotor stimulus (cold pressor test), the Negro reacting
> more sharply than the European. This reaction is usually regarded as

a sign that the person concerned is liable to develop essential hypertension. Excessive autonomic reactions to surgical procedures are certainly very common in Jamaica and appear to be due to an excessive action of the sympathetic nervous system as shown by the following reactions. . . .[117]

The terminology this author employs emphasizes pathological (black) deviations from presumably white norms: There are "excessive autonomic reactions to surgical procedures," an "excessive action of the sympathetic nervous system," and "an overactive sympathetic nervous system" that produces an "excessive rise in the blood glucose levels."[118] Higher levels of hypertension and higher death rates among blacks suggested that the observed ("excessive") state of the nervous system was, in fact, both deviant and potentially lethal to black patients. The potential problem with such speculative claims is that they may be rooted in a deeper paradigm of a pathological "black" biology that belongs to the Western racial imagination rather than to biological science. This conundrum was recognized in 1952 by the unusually perceptive authors of a letter to *The Lancet.* "Is the African reaction to stress abnormal," they ask, "or is it normal and the European reaction abnormal?"[119] This was a surprisingly open-minded perspective for that era, and it raises an important question about comparisons involving human beings and their varying cultural norms, such as a society's conception of and attitude toward stress. For the pathological effects of stress mean that a society's definition of stress will influence its definition of pathology, along with the medical judgments that employ that definition as a clinical norm.

Robert A. Hingson of the Departments of Obstetrics, Surgery, and Anesthesia, University Hospitals of Cleveland and Western Reserve School of Medicine, in Cleveland, Ohio, adopted the pathological model of the black nervous system. Writing in the African American medical journal, Dr. Hingson declared that the long ordeal of forced transport from Africa and forced adaptation to North America had "resulted in *a racial melancholia,* associated with suprarenal hypertension, cardiovascular crises, and eclamptogenic toxemia with convulsions, that have greatly increased rates of morbidity and mortality in the Negro race" [emphasis added]. The explicit reference to a neurohormonal factor appears in the author's advice to medical personnel everywhere: "Develop in the environment of hospitals and clinics an atmosphere of friendliness, tranquility and fraternity designed to overcome his inherent fear and initial hypertension and *epinephrine arousal storms* which multiply his hazards during these emergencies" [emphasis added].[120] This text is notable for its use of a colorfully folkloric term like "racial melancholia" at the same time that it offers a reasonable scientific hypothesis regarding the stress hormone (catecholamine) epinephrine, which is known to have deleterious effects on cardiovascular functioning, such as the accumulation of plaque in arteries (atherosclerosis) and the disruption of the electrical rhythm of the heart.

Medical research on racial physiological differences in sympathetic nervous system reactivity over the last half century has focused on the causes of hypertension and heart disease.[121] The modern neurohormonal theory, involving hormones that are secreted by or act on the nervous system, holds that "heart failure develops and progresses because endogenous neurohormonal systems that are activated by the initial injury to the heart exert a deleterious effect" on the cardiovascular system.[122] This is why drugs known as neurohormonal antagonists, the most important being beta-blockers and angiotensin-converting enzyme (ACE) inhibitors, are widely used to mitigate the effects of heart disease. Reports that these drugs work less well in African Americans than they do in whites have caused controversy, and especially among black cardiologists, because they are so effective in most patients. This controversy and the story of the "race-specific" antihypertensive drug BiDil (isosorbide dinitrate and hydralazine) are analyzed later in this book.

The racial dimension of heart disease and its treatment by neurohormonal antagonists provoked some controversy in 1999 in the pages of *The New England Journal of Medicine*, when a team of authors used the neuroendocrine theory to account for the poorer prognoses of black patients with left ventricular systolic dysfunction whose treatments had been the same as those of comparable white patients. Blacks, these authors suggested, "may have a greater degree of activation of neuroendocrine compensatory mechanisms than whites with a similar degree of left ventricular systolic impairment." In this case the authors' speculative theory actually recommended, rather than discouraged, the use of beta-antagonistic drugs: ". . . if black patients with left ventricular systolic dysfunction, as compared with white patients with similar degrees of left ventricular dysfunction, have an exaggerated neuroendocrine compensatory response, they may be ideal candidates for the early use of third-generation beta-blockers. . . ."[123] It is important to recognize that, given earlier accusations that black patients had been denied potentially beneficial beta-blockers, this was a political as well as a clinical statement.

The idea that a genetically regulated physiological difference between blacks and whites was exacerbating heart disease in the former group provoked objections from scientists who doubted the adequacy of the statistics, the ability to control for relevant environmental or behavioral factors, and the reliance on the presumed genetic homogeneity of the white and black populations in the United States. The authors' reply pointed to their intention "to illustrate the importance of self-reported [as opposed to genetically defined] race with respect to outcome." Moreover, they continued, "the blood pressure response to angiotensin-converting-enzyme inhibition and neuroendocrine activation in heart failure differ between black Americans and white Americans, providing a plausible mechanistic explanation for our observations."[124] This model of racially differential physiologies elaborated on the molecular level would suggest that the racial physiology being proposed may have a rational basis and does not necessarily express a racial fantasy.

What changed after the 1950s was the image of the black man whose nervous system had always been open for racial interpretation. Over the course of the decade that followed Hingson's expressed concern about "the Negro's need for special attention," bloody racial uprisings in the inner cities and the ideal of Black Power in racial politics transformed American society's idea of what black people wanted and what they were capable of doing to get it. In the course of this political transformation, an abnormal capacity for violence became associated with black male identity, and social scientists as well as psychiatrists responded accordingly. With African American prisoners today occupying just over half of all prison cells in the United States, the conjoining of black identity, psychopathology, and psychopathy has become a standard theme of American racial folklore. If the racial meaning of a "black" nervous system is emotional instability, then the idea of the unstable neurological apparatus will constantly be fed by social imagery that derives from the "black" misbehaviors that appear in the mass media.

Racial Interpretations of Pain Sensitivity

A less publicized consequence of racial interpretation of the nervous system is the denial of equitable pain relief to black patients. This scenario can be complicated by acquired cultural attitudes toward pain that include the stoic coping strategy many African Americans have chosen as a matter of practicality and self-respect. As one public health researcher points out, some blacks' discounting of pain as a remediable condition "may be a vestige of past circumstances in which only the most disabling conditions could serve as justification for interruption of one's duties in order to seek care. This habit may persist today even for individuals who have more resources and autonomy over their personal lives."[125] Traditional

stoicism of this kind can only exacerbate the undertreating of pain (oli-
goanalgesia) that has been observed in the treatment of both black and
Hispanic patients.[126] These scenarios, which often play out in emergency
rooms, can be a form of racial theater in which medical personnel assign
predetermined roles to nonwhite patients seeking relief from pain. As one
African American physician puts it: "Do some patients express pain in a
way that is more convincing that they need medication? Do some patients
present in a way that they are viewed as overly dramatic, drug seeking,
or for some societal reason not deserving of pain medication?"[127] Exacerbating this situation is the fact that pharmacies in predominantly African
American neighborhoods usually do not stock enough analgesic drugs to
meet the needs of black patients.[128] And even if they did, as another African American physician notes, "Some doctors are afraid of being profiled
by the DEA, regulatory agencies, or pharmacies, so they may be hesitant
to prescribe medicines to a profiled set of patients."[129] Given the distorted
view of blacks and their drug-consuming habits promoted by the war on
drugs, many of the profiled patients will be black.[130]

   A racially motivated physician who denies pain relief to black patients
does not rationalize his actions by imagining thicker nerve fibers or
slower conduction of nerve impulses—the naïve racial physiology of his
nineteenth-century predecessors. Imagining black humanity's immunity
to pain today is not an individual decision; it is rather a conditioned response
or set of responses to the sheer volume and spectacle of black suffering in
the ghetto or in poor societies in Africa that are experiencing mass death
from AIDS. Contemplating this suffering is likely to be an overwhelming
experience for many whites, whose coping strategies will include numbing
and dissociation from black pain with which they can empathize on some
level. Turning off the empathetic response in this situation enables individuals to preserve their emotional equilibrium and keep on functioning
unimpeded by altruistic impulses to help those in pain.

Racial Interpretations of Heart Disease

Over the past century, the medical discussion of heart disease in African
Americans has demonstrated a prodigious capacity to absorb racial folklore and reformulate these ideas as medical doctrine. The familiar bipolar
model that features opposing images of supernormal fitness and racial pathology is much in evidence here. The idea that blacks enjoyed a relative
immunity to heart disease—in effect, cardiac hardiness, except for their
special vulnerability to syphilitic infection—was an important cardiologi-
cal dogma throughout most of the twentieth century and one that persists

in the thinking of some physicians even today. At the same time, we must recognize that the idea of black cardiac hardiness exists in two versions. On the one hand, there is a racially motivated and pseudoscientific doctrine of black immunity that originated in a failure to properly observe the natural history of the disease in blacks. More scientifically grounded speculations about "protective factors" that prevent African Americans from experiencing more heart disease than they actually endure have been appearing in the medical literature since the early 1980s and require further evaluation. Finally, medical discussions of heart disease in blacks have often included assessments of alleged racial character traits that supposedly affect blacks' ability to compete and survive in a modern society.

The bipolar model of black cardiac functioning has generated the usual stereotypes of special immunity and special vulnerability to disease. The prominence of physical labor in the lives of so many black men and women during most of the twentieth century prompted cardiologists to speculate about the relevance of overexertion to heart disease in blacks. While the hardiness stereotype led to one interpretation, doctors' doubts about the maturity of their black patients pointed in another direction. "Hard work on the docks is an infrequent cause of heart disease among blacks," *JAMA* reported in 1915, "the natural cardiac strength of the negro enabling him to continue work at very hard labor."[131] Here we encounter a traditional hardiness stereotype, reminiscent of plantation medicine, that rationalized putting blacks to work for long hours in hot temperatures. The idea that there might be a downside to black men's being engaged in "very hard manual labor" was invoked in 1927 to confirm once again the role of venereal disease in black lives. It is overwork and syphilis that account for "the high rate of syphilitic heart disease among them," and this observation also implies an organic racial difference: "Apparently, then, the cardiovascular apparatus of the negro is more susceptible to syphilitic infection than that of his white brother."[132] A year later the *Southern Medical Journal* lamented how difficult it was to persuade heedless black patients to avoid "over-exertion" and thus avoid congestive heart failure.[133] In short, discussing the medical aspects of the everyday lives of their black patients provided cardiologists with opportunities to comment on their ignorance, their irresponsibility, and the innate racial differences that separated them from their "white brothers."

The pathologizing interpretation of black cardiac functioning reproduced the image of a sickly and degenerate black "race" that, by the 1890s, had become a familiar rationalization for the American racial hierarchy. While the standard doctrine of this era claimed that blacks were more *resistant* than whites to "the diseases of civilization" and its complexities, this version made blacks more *vulnerable* to the complications of modern life, thereby emphasizing their biological unfitness and their inability to compete against the better adapted whites. One version of the unfitness doctrine that lasted well into the twentieth century held that "blacks had worse survival after coronary bypass surgery than whites."[134] But regardless of which version doctors applied to their black patients, the fundamental point was that both variants played upon ideas about black disabilities. On one level or another, medical commentary always served a racial agenda that favored whites.

The contest between these two ideas—black cardiac hardiness versus blacks' "defective cardiovascular apparatus"—was resolved in favor of the hardiness stereotype, since for many years doctors believed in the rarity of coronary heart disease (CHD) in African Americans. Two kinds of medical racism caused this diagnostic asymmetry. First, negligent observation of black patients accounted for the many underestimates of disease prevalence in blacks during most of the twentieth century; people who were worth less than whites simply did not warrant proper medical attention. The other racist premise originated in the socially sanctioned theory that blacks and whites were biologically different organisms; the idea of their racially differentiated pain thresholds appeared often in discussions of angina pectoris. The pioneering paper that found black heart patients presenting "clinical and pathologic features in every way similar to the Caucasians" appeared in the *American Heart Journal* in 1948. Having established the biological parity of blacks and whites, these authors also took the trouble to point to the medical neglect of black patients, in that "Negroes with coronary artery occlusion are rarely hospitalized in civil life, if one is to judge from the literature."[135] This failure to hospitalize black patients resulted, as we have seen, from a dysfunctional collaboration between doctor-avoiding (and pain-tolerating) blacks with heart problems and the white physicians who chose not to diagnose them as carefully as whites with similar symptoms.

The myth of black immunity to heart disease was noted and deplored in the medical literature for decades after the 1948 paper that refuted the claim that the symptoms of coronary artery occlusion differed in blacks and whites.[136] "The doctor's patient-admitting behavior," the African American cardiologist Richard Allen Williams wrote in 1975, "is conditioned by his personal prejudices, by anecdotal experience passed on by colleagues (e.g., 'Black people just don't have heart attacks') and by basic ignorance of those conditions which primarily affect Blacks."[137] As another cardiologist pointed out in 1982, with no more than an estimated 30 black cardiovascular surgeons and 200 black cardiologists in the United States at that time, the care of black heart patients was "largely in the hands of white physicians, many of whom subscribe to the misconceptions about the rarity of occurrence of CHD in blacks purveyed in the 1950s and 1960s and to some extent even today."[138] The influence of such "misconceptions" was not always evident to physicians. One author wondered in 1984 "whether a 'traditional' diagnostic belief exists that blacks simply do not develop myocardial infarction."[139] In fact, the persistence of such a tradition was still being noted during the early 1990s.[140] Yet survey data on the extent of this sort of medical ignorance do not appear in the medical literature.

Medical speculation about "protective factors" that might prevent higher levels of heart disease in African Americans has been appearing in medical journals over the past half century.[141] This medical mystery has also shown up in the popular press. "Why, if it has been clearly proved that hypertension increases the risk of heart disease, don't Negro men (who have a higher hypertension rate) suffer more heart attacks than white men? Heart specialists are still stumped by this puzzler," the popular African American magazine *Ebony* commented in 1962.[142] Twenty years later, an expert on heart disease in African Americans reiterated this observation in the *American Heart Journal*, even as he deplored the standard mythology about black cardiac hardiness: "The only validity to the 'immunity' concept is that, given their high risk factor levels vis-à-vis whites, it is surprising that United States blacks do not have much higher CHD mortality and morbidity than whites," wrote Richard F. Gillum.[143]

The paradoxical coexistence of high (yet, in relation to healthier whites, relatively low) black mortality from coronary heart disease on the one hand, and greatly elevated black rates of CHD risk factors such as hypertension, diabetes mellitus, female obesity, and low socioeconomic status on the other, has presented Gillum and other researchers with a medical riddle. Twenty-five years ago, Gillum offered a biological hypothesis that other medical authors later adopted in various forms:

> Recent findings of higher HDL cholesterol in blacks may be one explanation. The HDL differences are probably genetically determined, being apparent in childhood although not at birth. . . . Lower triglyceride levels, higher alcohol intake, greater fibronolytic activity, lower type A behavior pattern prevalence, and some unexplained genetically determined resistance to coronary arteriosclerosis are all hypotheses awaiting data to substantiate or refute them.[144]

The early 1980s saw much discussion of the "protective factors" hypothesis. One commentator argued that environmental factors would be likely to overwhelm genetic effects, "given the overwhelming evidence about social disadvantage of U.S. blacks," since "ten variables that represent an additional social burden to blacks are likely to be detected for every one variable that may act in a protective fashion."[145] Yet this response to the genetic hypothesis evades the challenge of accounting for the improbably low prevalence of heart disease that requires an explanation in the first place.

Since that time, the idea of genetically regulated protective factors in blacks has persisted in the medical literature while remaining unresolved. One group of investigators presented some elements of this theory in 1984:

> It thus seems likely that whereas environment has a substantial effect on HDL cholesterol levels in both blacks and whites, there must be a "genetic" vector accounting for higher HDL levels in blacks. It is known, for example, that HDLs facilitate the macrophage immobilization of *Trypanosoma brucei*, the spirochetal factor vector for sleeping sickness, which is endemic in equatorial Africa. Many American blacks came from such geographic areas. One might then speculate that the relative protection offered by HDLs against sleeping sickness would have led to a natural selection of African blacks with higher HDL levels, a genetic selection now still expressed after generations of American life.[146]

In fact, it has been confirmed that HDL ("good cholesterol") does protect human beings against certain parasites, including the *Trypanosoma brucei brucei* organism that causes sleeping sickness.[147] Yet we must also ask whether casting high "black" HDL levels in an evolutionary drama about sleeping sickness may owe something to a tradition of racial thinking that has long associated the process of natural selection with Africa, black people, and the "hardiness" that evolutionary pressures have been assumed to confer on people of African origin. Ascribing any form of medical hardiness to a racial or ethnic group is potentially consequential, because it can imply that such people will require less medical attention and treatment than others.

In the meantime, the "protective factors" conundrum remains alive and well. As one cardiologist, Dr. Edward Havranek, told me in 2006:

> The subject of "protection" of black men from cardiovascular disease came up at our research group meeting today. Someone suggested that the origin of the concept probably lies in the observation that cardiovascular mortality is lower in black men than white men, but that the concept is fallacious because of competing mortality—black men have a lower percent mortality from CVD because they have higher mortality from suicide, violence, prostate cancer, etc. If they didn't have these causes of death related to low [socioeconomic status] and racial disparities in health care their CVD mortality rate would be the same as whites.[148]

Comprehensive thinking of this kind about "racial" differences in mortality rates is a necessary counterweight to assumptions about "protective factors" that may derive, at least in part, from the twentieth-century assumptions about cardiac hardiness among blacks that can still influence physicians' thinking today. What is more, there are other ideas about black people that, having originated outside of the medical subculture, have been absorbed by the medical literature about race and heart disease.

Cardiologists' assessments of black personality have sometimes addressed the question of how black people deal with a modern way of life that is associated with white values and achievements. For example, what high technology means to African Americans is an important dimension of their medical experience. Think, for example, of those black male patients, described in a 1955 medical article as "tense individuals," who admitted to "a profound fear of the electrocardiograph which could not be resolved by repeated reassurance."[149] We have already seen that black patient responses to sophisticated medical technology continue to be relevant to the problem of racially differential diagnosis and treatment and, in particular, "patient preferences" about whether to undergo surgical procedures. But the most significant issue of "racial character" that cardiologists raise, quite unintentionally, pertains to whether or not African Americans demonstrate the "type A" personality associated with ambition, achievement, and the stressful lives that so often produce social and professional advancement.

The classic 1960 formulation of the type A personality had nothing to say about race. The point of this report was to define an "overt behavior pattern A" that demonstrated seven times as much coronary heart disease as the converse personality designated "overt behavior pattern B." Type A behavior was "characterized by excessive competitive drive, a persistent desire for recognition and advancement, a persistent involvement in multiple functions subject to 'deadlines,' and a habitual propensity to accelerate their pace of living and working. . . ." The singular significance of this personality trait became apparent when both type A and type B individuals were found to have comparable "dietary, drinking, smoking, exercise and other living habits."[150] The crucial difference between type A and type B personalities is that the type As appear to be better prepared for the competitions that produce social, professional, and financial success in a modern society.

The latent racial dimension of the type A/type B dichotomy becomes evident as soon as we recall that whites, but not blacks, have been regarded as especially vulnerable to diseases that are supposedly caused by fast and stressful modern lives, accounting for the 1929 observation in *Science* that "cardiovascular diseases are correlated with civilized life, a reaction to nervous strain."[151] For most of the twentieth century many physicians embraced the idea that blacks possessed a "natural immunity to the so-called diseases of civilization,"[152] making the type A personality the opposite of what a "black" personality should be. In particular, the observation that type A individuals exhibit "a severe sense of time urgency" puts these high achievers completely at odds with a familiar stereotype about African Americans and their relationship to time.

The idea that black people lack "a chronic sense of time urgency"—the ability to set and adhere to deadlines—is a well-known example of racial folklore that inhabits an uncertain twilight zone between accepted fact and racial defamation. Judgments about their punctuality have been made about both Africans and African Americans. Half a century ago a British colonial physician in Uganda described his patients' relationship to time as follows: "Questions must be leading, and answers often vague, especially as to time. The recognized intervals, days, weeks, and months, deeply impressed on the English mind, become a continuous blur in that of the African, who seldom thinks back more than a few weeks. Ages are rarely known."[153] Such accounts of cultural ("racial") differences that seem to produce dysfunctional behaviors always raise questions about the competence and motives of observers. In the case of time urgency, however, there are corroborating observations from black commentators who point to life experiences that have made some black lives less time-fixated than others. LeRoi Jones once commented that "given his constant position at the bottom of the American social hierarchy, there was not one reason for any Negro, ever, to hurry."[154] The African American psychiatrist James H. Carter portrayed the time conundrum with both candor and clarity:

> Perhaps too much has been made of the disregard for time in the lives of black people, although it may be true that for many educationally and economically deprived blacks, watches are for pawning and not for telling time. However, the realities of transportation, health and economics must not be forgotten. To "be on time" can be meaningless for those blacks for whom the lack of transportation or other inconveniences are at issue. Therefore, in working with black patients, especially those from extremely low socioeconomic groups, the professional must be aware of differences in values regarding time. The inappropriate interpretation that the client is acting out because he is late for an appointment may simply have no usefulness.[155]

Young blacks may regard "being on time" as an undesirable example of "acting white."[156] Among African Americans, "Colored People's Time" has long been a vernacular term signifying a lack of interest in fixed schedules and appointments. Nevertheless, it should be obvious that African Americans could not have survived, let alone advanced to the degree that they have, had the rank and file of black Americans indulged in the luxury of living in accordance with a "Colored People's Time" that was out of synch with the time standards of white society.

The sheer implausibility of the idea that African American laborers and professionals have managed to escape the temporal requirements of modern life prompted the African American epidemiologist Sherman A. James to challenge the tacit assumption in the medical literature that the type A personality did not occur among blacks. James pointed to "the *coping styles* that the poor and the nearly poor commonly use to deal with recurring behavioral stressors in their lives. Type A behavior represents one such coping style, and although this behavior pattern may be more widespread among the middle and upper-middle classes, it could also be fairly common among certain subgroups of the working poor." For example, "It is conceivable that the multiple responsibilities faced by working women who are also single parents may predispose many to become time-urgent, hard-driving, and impatient (i.e., "type A") persons in an effort to make ends meet."[157] Similarly, "Many of the jobs that industrial black workers hold involve repetitive, routine, time-paced work."[158] Having grasped the disturbing implications of dividing whites and blacks into time-responsive and time-indifferent "racial" groups, James resolved to resist this sort of segregation and to demonstrate that "the conceptual properties of type A behavior must be the same for blacks and whites."[159]

To provide blacks with a category of stressful experience comparable to that of whites, James described a coping style he called "John Henryism":

This psychosocial construct refers to a strong personality predisposition to cope actively with behavioral stressors in one's environment. The concept is based, in part, on the legend of John Henry, the famous black steel driver who defeated a mechanical steam drill in an epic battle of "man against machine" but fell dead from exhaustion immediately thereafter. In addition to its folkloric origins, the "John Henryism" concept is also based on results from controlled laboratory experiments by investigators interested in characterizing patterns of cardiovascular reactivity to behavioral stressors.[160]

James's theory held that high levels of "John Henryism" combined with low levels of formal education in black subjects would produce higher blood pressures and higher levels of cardiac stress.

A generation elapsed between the classic formulation of the type A personality (1960, and coded white) and the formulation of "John Henryism" (1984, and coded black). Today, another generation later, "John Henryism" is regarded as "a coping style that has a clear genetic basis in African Americans and reflects clear personality traits." These traits include extroversion, conscientiousness, striving for achievement, self-discipline, and assertiveness. It now appeared that black Americans had finally achieved psychological parity with their hard-working white fellow citizens.

The cruel irony, researchers maintain, is that these achievement-promoting traits can also impair the emotional and physical health of the black people in whom they occur. According to Christopher L. Edwards, a psychiatrist at Duke University Medical Center, these "intensely success-oriented and goal-directed" people "are likely to fail because their lack of resources will catch up to them. Add to that the African American situation, which, for many, includes an expectation that failure is inevitable, and you find yourself in a most destructive situation. They end up compromising their health, with higher rates of cardiovascular disease and death as compared to any other population in the world. We also see evidence of this self-destructive behavior in African Americans with breast cancer, osteoarthritis, and, of course, sickle-cell disease."[161] The stresses that are built into the African American predicament are pathogenic in ways we still do not understand.

RACIAL INTERPRETATIONS OF
HUMAN ORGANS AND DISORDERS

The infiltration of racial folklore into medical thinking about anatomical, physiological, and psychological differences between blacks and whites has been a profoundly influential and largely unacknowledged aspect of modern medicine. Every human organ system has presented an opportunity for doctors to formulate claims about biological differences between the black and white "races," and many doctors over the past century and a half have promoted the racial interpretation of human organs. In the following section we will examine how medical thinking about eyes, skin, and teeth has conformed to a unified doctrine of racial difference that is evident from the end of the nineteenth century until the middle decades of the twentieth century and beyond.

Racial interpretations of organ systems have both biological and social dimensions. The biological argument promotes ideas about racial differences that are rooted in the nineteenth-century racial anthropology that stigmatized black Africans as biologically deviant or deficient. The social dimension of racial folklore involves the conversion of anatomical characteristics into a widely circulated racial folklore that serves to stereotype, stigmatize, and ridicule blacks, or draws attention to their real or alleged disabilities. In this way, physical traits attributed to the eyes, skin, and teeth of black people are absorbed into familiar racist narratives about the nature and quality of black lives.

The racial interpretation of human organ systems employs a standard repertory of related themes. The first step in this process is to identify anatomical or physiological forms of racial difference. The next step is to conjoin this anatomical or physiological deviation from a white norm with the evolutionary retardation of black human beings. A natural corollary of the evolutionary argument is ascribing "hardiness" to various aspects of the purportedly less evolved black organism. All of these biological themes can be translated into invidious comparisons and judgments about black health and character.

Racial Interpretations of the Eyes

Reports of racial differences in vision and the structure of the eye appear in the medical literature around the turn of the twentieth century. Ophthalmologists commented on blacks' apparent immunities to a broad spectrum of eye diseases: trachoma, myopia, conjunctivitis, and color blindness among them.[162] In 1924 it was reported that black babies appeared to be immune to blindness at birth (opthalamia neonatorum): "Some doctors say that the Negroes, through generations of contact with venereal diseases, have developed a kind of immunity which protects the new-born baby's eye from the ever-present sources of infection. Others scoff at that, and insist that it could not be so."[163] (The claim presented in this 1914 report appeared again in 1944.[164]) The white ophthalmologist H. Phillip Venable's essay on "Glaucoma in the Negro" appeared in the African American medical journal in 1952 and raised uncomfortable questions about black pain sensitivity and the usefulness of glaucoma surgery in the black patient, thereby suggesting biological differences between the races. At the same, he was careful not to make bolder claims about racial differences. "Some writers maintain that the eye of the Negro is anatomically and physiologically different from that of other races," he writes, but the differences he sees are more subtle than apparent. "We question seriously whether his eye is different physiologically," he concludes.[165]

Venable's "white" perspective on glaucoma in the Negro, its courteous tone notwithstanding, drew a withering response from six black ophthalmologists several months later in the same journal. At a time when overt black challenges to white authority were difficult, the dramatic exchange that occurred in the pages of the *Journal of the National Medical Association* gave vent to the pent-up outrage of black physicians, who used this "Negro" venue to expose the naïveté of white practitioners whose social imagination was shaped by confident assumptions about black people's bodies and habits. Employing an ironic professional courtesy of their own, these black doctors attempted to debunk Venable's claim that glaucoma pain was racial in origin, that Negro patients were irresponsible procrastinators, that there was any evidence whatsoever of racial differences between white and black eyes, that glaucoma surgery in black patients was futile, and that the white surgeons who attempted it knew what they were doing. "It is difficult to say what an American Negro is," writes Dr. Malcolm Proctor, "let alone find him an anatomical or physiologic variant."[166] Dr. Venable's thinking, wrote Dr. Theodore R. George, remained trapped within the racist premises of American society as a whole. Appearing in the black medical journal that white physicians did not and still do not read, this unsparing assessment of what white physicians took for granted about their black patients went unheard by Dr. Venable, who thanked his critics for their "very gratifying" comments, and by the medical profession as a whole.

Medical commentary about the eyes of black people over the past century demonstrates how easily ophthalmological diagnosis could feed the racial stereotypes of the Jim Crow South. The allegedly pathological consequences of emancipation were confirmed by one doctor's claim in 1893 that "the eye of the negro had deteriorated since he became free."[167] The assertion that "syphilis is a potent cause of eye affections among the negroes" was only one of the ways medical authors linked venereal disease to other Negro disorders, thereby reinforcing popular ideas about Negro sexual promiscuity.[168] The reported absence of myopia in blacks placed them outside the sphere of social progress in that "myopia is a concomitant of civilized life." Perhaps blacks did not suffer from myopia because "the great majority of negroes whom I have treated were uneducated and, in many instances, unable to read and had never used their eyes for work of a trying nature."[169] Eye injuries suffered by Negroes that were reported from hospital emergency rooms opened a window onto the violent side of black life and the dangerous recreations of alcohol-fueled Saturday nights.[170]

More than a half century after Dr. Venable encountered his black critics, racially differential treatment for glaucoma has become an accepted, yet sometimes problematic, standard of care. It is known that glaucoma exacts a heavier toll on the African American population than on whites, and in 1998 the National Institutes of Health endorsed different surgical glaucoma treatments for white and black patients. According to a 2000 report, "Blacks and whites respond differently to certain surgical procedures, so some physicians may view differences in treatment as medically justified." The problem is that some physicians may simply assume that racially differential treatments are warranted when they are not, thereby leading to inadequate treatment of black patients.[171]

Racial Interpretations of Black Skin

Dark skin has been the most prominent anatomical signifier of black racial identity. This important symbolic role has imposed on black skin medical significance of two kinds. First, the conspicuous role of black skin has encouraged white doctors and others to focus attention on the surface of the black body to emphasize its differences from white skin; in addition, the sheer visibility of skin has made some black people painfully self-conscious about dermatological traits and disorders in racially specific ways that do not affect whites because they do not deal with the experience of being black.

The predominant "racial" characteristic of black skin has always been its hardiness and presumed resistance to heat, chemicals, and penetration by insects or ultraviolet rays. "The epidermis of most Afro-Americans is rather thick," a physician wrote in 1913, "while the terminal sensory nerves do not appear to be normally impressionable, as a general rule."[172] The eugenicist Charles B. Davenport attributed to black skin an impressive resistance to "venomous bites and stings" as well as skin cancer.[173] As late as 1985, a contributor to the African American *Journal of the National Medical Association* speculated: "Possibly, the thicker, darker skin of the Negro may decrease the number, or penetration, of mosquito bites."[174] It would appear that a full century of medical speculation about the properties of black skin had failed to resolve basic questions about whether dermatological hardiness was grounded in science or folklore. In fact, all of the alleged characteristics of black skin, whether real or imagined, have symbolic meanings that extend their significance beyond the realm of clinical medicine. The uncertainty about what is real and what is imagined is itself an important factor, since it raises questions about whether race is a medically significant category of analysis.

Like black people's eyes, their dark skin has played public roles that project the alien qualities of blackness far beyond the medical clinic and its concerns about the identification and healing of disease. We have already encountered the potentially harmful effects of dermatological hardiness, which can create a willingness among whites to expose black workers to a variety of physical traumas, including the extreme heat of a cotton field or a blast furnace, industrial chemicals, or exposure to invasive insects. But the recognition of dermatological hardiness is also a symbolic form of racial segregation. "Due to anatomical differences," the *Southern Medical Journal* reported in 1939, "the full-blooded negro is seldom affected by skin diseases common to the white man."[175] In this and in other ways, blacks and whites led medically separate lives, in that "black" and "white" diseases were treated in racially segregated facilities. Body odor was another skin-related physiological variable with its own social significance. In 1940, *JAMA* endorsed the notion that "there are some differences in the odor of sweat of Negroes and of white persons" due to "the fatty acids and oils present."[176] It is not surprising that the racial dimension of American life at that time made body odor a social as well as a physiological phenomenon. Like super-tough skin, "black" fatty acids and oils helped to make social segregation seem like a natural and appropriate arrangement.

Racial Interpretations of Human Teeth

During the first half of the twentieth century the medical and dental literatures contained numerous reports of the superiority of black people's teeth. These accounts of black dental hardiness were preceded by much earlier accounts of splendid African teeth. The "Kaffirs or Hottentots," says one European observer in 1668, are equipped "with teeth beautifully clean and white, like ivory, and hard, so that the bite is firm."[177] Other such reports of "beautifully white" African teeth appeared for many years afterward and eventually began to appear in Western scientific journals. "The negro teeth," the eugenicist C. B. Davenport wrote in 1919, "are naturally resistant to the organism of tooth caries."[178] But the image of healthier Negro teeth alternated with contrary reports of conspicuous tooth decay and other dental problems, including two *JAMA* articles that appeared in 1941. One report on pregnant Negro women attributed their miscarriages, not to their syphilis, but to their infected teeth: "The teeth of practically all of these women were uniformly bad, the good ones being the exception and could easily account for the number of miscarriages seen."[179] The study of Negro sharecroppers noted that, "in spite of the excellent appearance of the teeth, purulent matter could be pressed out easily from the gingival margins, which bled readily on slight pressure."[180] Appearances could be deceiving. As a third *JAMA* author noted: "The impression has prevailed that Negroes are blessed with unusually good teeth, but dental authorities state that this is another exploded tradition. Their teeth look white in comparison with their black skin."[181] While it is possible that this simple trompe l'oeil had played a role in promoting a myth of dental hardiness, an equally plausible (and less innocent) source of this myth was a white society's disinterest in offering dental services to poor blacks. It was far more convenient to assume that dentally robust blacks did not require this sort of medical attention at all.

In accordance with the pervasive racial interpretation of human organ systems, dental hardiness was integrated into the traditional racial biology that favored genetic mechanisms as *the* explanation for observed racial differences. Thus a physical anthropologist writes in 1937: "The dentin and cementin of the teeth, being really a part of the osseous system, show, as a rule, in the Negro a very good development, *seemingly a dominant gene in this race* [emphasis added], thus accounting for their beautiful sets of teeth."[182] More sophisticated scientific commentaries on racial differences in dentition, regarding genetics and dental development, appeared in 1969 and 1976.[183]

The theme of the exceptional whiteness of black people's teeth described previously eventually took on a life of its own as an instantly recognizable and denigrating form of racial folklore. Racist caricatures turned gleaming white teeth into a public spectacle that often took the form of *the grin*. As Frantz Fanon noted in *Black Skin, White Masks* (1952): "The smile of the black man, the *grin* [in English in the original], seems to have captured the interest of a number of writers. Here is what Bernard Wolfe says about it: 'It pleases us to portray the Negro showing us all his teeth in a smile made for us. And his smile as we see it—as we make it—always means a *gift*'...."[184] The gift referred to here was the invitation to whites to enjoy the giddy mindlessness of the grinning "happy Negro" and his flashing teeth. In 1965 the black psychologist Kenneth B. Clark identified "shiny teeth" as a standard feature of the "stereotyped Negro you see in the movies or on TV."[185] Sparkling white teeth conveyed a comically dazzling image of dental health that obscured the actual conditions in which black people lived and tried (or did not try) to maintain their teeth. As one observer noted in 1941: "Broad grins may have displayed glistening white teeth but physicians complained that there were 'few negroes not subject to toothache.'"[186]

The health status of black people's teeth also became a theme within their own community. Booker T. Washington himself made the use of the toothbrush a kind of obsession at the Tuskegee Institute. Students who failed to use them were expelled, and Washington commented on "the effect that the use of the tooth-brush has had in bringing about a higher degree of civilization among the students."[187] During the 1930s the National Negro Health Week celebration featured the awarding of "cups and medals for the best teeth."[188] Alice Walker's famous novel *The Color Purple* (1982) refers several times to the impressively white teeth of Negro children and Africans, whose teeth "remind me of horses' teeth, they are so fully formed, straight and strong."[189] Today, however, the once ubiquitous folkloric theme of dazzling African teeth has given way to the less entertaining news that poor children of all colors suffer from "shockingly bad" dental health.[190]

Racial Interpretations of "White" and "Black" Disorders

Racially differential images of diseases are rooted in social and economic disparities that create insignia of advanced development and stigmata of retarded development. Medical disorders have usually been identified with higher rather than lower social and economic status. Few medical disorders have been specifically associated with lower-class people; the medical costs imposed on the hearts of manual laborers were once an example of such medical damage. In the same vein, a 1936 medical report noted that it was generally accepted that Addison's disease was "prone to occur more frequently in members of the laboring class." In fact, these authors had expected to find more cases among Negroes, given "the heavy manual labor by which many of them earn their livelihood."[191] This is one of the many reports appearing in the medical literature of the twentieth century that refer to an apparent and inexplicable resistance to disease among blacks.

The "diseases of civilization" have always been associated with higher social and cultural classes. It was once easy to believe that myopia occurred primarily in people who were educated enough to strain their eyes by reading. Myopia was, then, "a concomitant of civilized life."[192] Dyspepsia, according to the plantation physician Samuel Cartwright, "is, *par excellence*, a disease of the Anglo-Saxon race. I have never seen a well-marked case of dyspepsia among the blacks. It is a disease that selects its victims from the most intellectual of mankind, passing by the ignorant and unreflecting."[193] The *Southern Medical Journal* noted in 1913 that "digestive discomforts" afflicted "those higher in the social and financial scale."[194] The *British Medical Journal* predicted in 1960 that black Africans too would eventually develop peptic ulcers once they had assumed "the burdens and responsibilities of administration and management in business and politics."[195] Physiological delicacy is presented as a direct concomitant of the kinds of stress that result from the challenges of modernity and its complications.

Nor was this idea limited to white medical personnel. The black physician Charles H. Garvin predicted in 1924 that the rising social status of black Americans would make them more vulnerable to various diseases: "It is not a direct race question but a question of civilization and its 'hustle and bustle' and 'burning the candle at both ends'," he observed.[196]

Diabetes mellitus, the *Southern Medical Journal* commented in 1921, "is notoriously a disease of the well-to-do." "Nervous strain, intense application to business, mental shock and worry have frequently seemed to play an important role, at least in precipitating the phenomena of the disease or aggravating it."[197] This is the cultural syndrome that also produced a term such as "nervous indigestion" to make the connection between a physiological disorder and an out-of-kilter nervous system. "Cancer is a disease of civilization," a Dallas proctologist declared in 1925, though he did not offer a rationale for his claim. More interesting is his claim that "primitive races" are almost entirely immune to hemorrhoids, "as are the lower mammals."[198] The implication is that whites have evolved to the point where they have become vulnerable to a skin problem to which "primitives" are immune.

Hypertension offers a rare example of a disorder whose racial image has reversed itself over the past century. Today it is well known that hypertension occurs at a much higher rate among African Americans than among white Americans. At the same time, it is not surprising that a disorder associated with nervous stress was once seen as a "disease of civilization," since premodern peoples were assumed to live in a state of tranquility, untroubled by the complications of modern life. "Primitive communities from four continents have been found to be almost completely free from hypertension," the *British Medical Journal* commented in 1953.[199] Not long afterwards an American doctor was pointing out that hypertension had become "popularly associated with executives" and the medical price they paid for their high-powered roles in the business world.[200]

Heart disease, in particular, became identified with mankind's forward march into a dynamic and technologically sophisticated modern age. "Civilization as we know it," an American cardiologist wrote in 1932, "in Western Europe and America, the ambition, effort and community state of mind of these areas, the increasing responsibilities that come with age, and an aging circulation, apparently are the foundations for the increasing prevalence of angina." Small wonder, he continues, that this form of chest pain "occurs usually in the sensitive, nervous type, as the Jew, or in the tense, efficient American, rather than in the dull, happy negro or the calm, accepting Chinaman."[201]

The quintessential "white" disorders are those that become identified with white women, because they afflict the physiologically and psychologically unstable "weaker" sex of the "civilized" race. The delicacy and sensitivity of white women have long been symbolic correlates of their medical vulnerability, and their weaknesses have been understood in relation to hardier women of color. In her study of female "hardiness" a century ago, Laura Briggs points out that "it was simply an article of unshakable faith that black women did not suffer from 'nerves,' nor have difficult labors." In his *American Nervousness* (1881), George Beard presents this racial dichotomy as follows: "Woman in the savage state is not delicate, sensitive, or weak, [but] strong, well-developed, and muscular, with capacity for enduring toil. As well as childbearing."[202] The ultimate claim about white female physiological delicacy appeared in 1925 in the form of an assertion by a white gynecologist in Dallas that the vaginal tissues of black women were less sensitive than those of their white sisters.[203]

It is not difficult to understand why a white gynecologist of this era would have adopted this belief about the sexual physiology of black women. First, as we have seen, black women were denied the traits of delicacy and sensitivity as a matter of principle. A correlate of this principle was the belief among many doctors that almost all black women (and girls) were sexually promiscuous by nature. These doctors may have regarded undiscriminating behavior of this kind as antithetical to real sexual passion. (I have never seen a report of a black nymphomaniac in the medical literature, perhaps because black women have been collectively stereotyped as oversexed and promiscuous rather than presented as individual case studies.)

"White" female disorders continue to be conceptualized in relation to their perceived absence in black women. This habit of thought is so powerful that the *Journal of the American Medical Association* saw fit to publish the following admonition in 2003: "If a researcher finds a higher prevalence of a given medical condition among individuals identified as white than among individuals assigned to other racial/ethnic groups, it should not be assumed, in the absence of evidence, that white people have some quality or characteristic that makes them more susceptible to the particular condition."[204]

If the quintessential "white" disorders are female complaints, then the quintessential female disorders are those of the reproductive organs. How doctors think about endometriosis, for example, offers an opportunity to watch race-based thinking about female biology express itself as an oral tradition. For example, in 1966 the white obstetrician-gynecologist William Mengert confessed to the African American readership of the *Journal of the National Medical Association* that, up to about 1950, "I did not believe that endometriosis as recognized in the Caucasian ever appeared in the Negro." Subsequent experience had taught him that this disorder was a consequence of upward social mobility rather than any organic racial factor.[205] Forty years later, a female physician in Texas told one of my students that she too had been taught in medical school that endometriosis was a "white woman's problem." Experience as a practitioner had shown her that this disorder appeared in women irrespective of race or ethnicity.[206] And here, too, white fantasies about black sex lives appear to have played a role in the racial construction of disease, since "gynecologists would almost automatically diagnose a black woman with symptoms of endometriosis as having pelvic inflammatory disease (PID). The underlying reason was an assumption that black women were sexually promiscuous (which is a known factor in contracting gonorrhea and PID)."[207]

Other racially differential diagnoses of "female" disorders are further evidence of how influential the paradigm of "white" female delicacy and medical vulnerability has been. One feminist scholar found herself wondering why public discourse on menopause has omitted black women from this narrative of female suffering. Perhaps, she suggests, the marginalization of black women is so complete that they simply take menopause less seriously than more privileged white women.[208] Reports suggest this interpretation of older black women's views of menopause is at least partly correct. Far from enjoying immunity to menopause, African American women suffer many of the familiar symptoms such as hot flashes, night sweats, and mood changes. At the same time, it may be that black women do accept menopause as "a natural life transition" to a greater degree than white women do and are less inclined to begin hormone replacement therapy (HRT).[209] At the same time, we must recognize that black women's apparently voluntary acceptance of medical suffering raises once again the meaning of "patient preferences" when medical stoicism is rooted in social disadvantage rather than a genuine freedom to choose. Black people have sometimes accepted medical suffering because they have become habituated to discomfort and do not see any prospect of obtaining relief. Similarly, black women's reported aversion to hormone replacement therapy, while apparently voluntary, may also be a consequence of black distrust of white doctors and the medications they prescribe. In this sense, a disorder may be regarded as "white" in part because many blacks do not identify with the diagnosis, or do not regard the disorder as serious enough to accept the prescribed treatment.

Eating disorders among young women, and especially anorexia nervosa, have long been seen as a "white" disorder of the privileged classes.

"Conspicuous is the absence of Negro patients," a psychiatrist wrote in 1966. Given the affluence of this young clientele, the absence of black children was hardly surprising: "They had been well cared-for children for whom things were done and who had been offered all advantages and privileges of modern child care. They had been exposed to many stimulating influences, in education, in the arts, athletics, and the like." Small wonder these patients included a disproportionate number of New York Jewish children.[210] Two decades later, when a visiting physician gave a talk at the Adolescent Rounds of the Department of Pediatrics at Howard University Hospital in 1984, "the vast majority of the audience considered eating disorders an esoteric disease that they would probably never encounter in their practice" at this African American institution. The purpose of the presentation was to alert the medical staff that "talented, affluent, and gifted" black teenagers were developing anorexia nervosa, and that they should be prepared to deal with this ostensibly new phenomenon.[211] By 2005, awareness of eating disorders among African American teenagers was growing, but the old stereotypes were still firmly in place. Anorexia and bulimia were still seen as affecting affluent white teenage girls. "Minority women are not getting treated," said Dr. Ruth Striegel-Moore, a Wesleyan University psychologist. "It's very clear from my studies that black American women do experience eating disorders, but doctors and therapists still operate under the assumption that they don't; therefore they aren't prepared to deal with them clinically."[212]

The eating disorders conundrum offers another opportunity to look at the relationship between a medical disorder and African American women's relationship to the norms of a white society whose media bombard everyone with idealized images of young women who are overwhelmingly thin. A common explanation for the lower reported rates of eating disorders among black women has been a greater acceptance of plump or obese women who do not experience the same compulsion to lose weight that is so common among young white women. The reality, however, is that black women's relationship to the idealized female body is conflicted. It is well known that African American women have an obesity rate of around 50 percent, which is significantly higher than that of white women. An argument rooted in one type of multicultural relativism has claimed that African Americans' alleged acceptance of "full-figured" women is actually a healthy sign of independence from the dieting compulsions that drive so many white women to try to lose weight. While such claims have an understandable appeal for advocates of a "Black is Beautiful" aesthetic, they are undermined by black women's ambivalence about whether being "overweight" is a lifestyle or a disorder that is now on the nation's health-promotional agenda. In fact, the greater the awareness of black women's vulnerability to eating disorders, the more "delicate" and "sensitive" they will appear to be. Given the emotional costs of the "strong black woman" stereotype that are borne by many African American women, giving them a less "hardy" image would serve as a corrective to the popular image of their supposedly superhuman stoicism and durability.

Fibromyalgia (FMS) and chronic fatigue syndrome (CFS) are two poorly understood disorders that have been conspicuously coded as affluent white women's diseases. Fibromyalgia is a chronic condition, nine times more common in women than in men, that produces fatigue, widespread pain in muscles, ligaments, and tendons, and many tender points on the body that produce pain when touched. Chronic fatigue syndrome is characterized by extreme fatigue, experienced over many months, which is not relieved by rest. It occurs twice as often in women as in men. The fact that the causes of these conditions are unknown has caused great uncertainty about symptoms and possible treatments, and has conferred upon them a quasi-mythic aura that has produced some imaginative ideas about the people who contract them.

While syndromes that involve chronic suffering can afflict both rich women and poor women, it is not surprising that pharmaceutical companies eventually decided to sponsor advertising that presents FMS patients as confident and high-status people with options, rather than as people who are imprisoned, emotionally and socially, inside their disease. Pfizer's first ad for its FMS drug Lyrica featured a "suffering, sighing woman" of about fifty. "Then there was the 'battered-woman' fibromyalgia disease awareness ad that attempted to portray how sufferers felt by showing bruised images of a woman who says something like 'maybe if people saw me this way, they will believe that fibromyalgia is a real medical condition.'" While the class affiliation of the (young) woman portrayed in the second ad is not clear, the older woman in the first ad, presenting an anxious facial expression and straining neck tendons, is upscale and well-groomed, complete with tasteful, dangling earrings. In a third Lyrica ad, "an older, but attractive woman obviously enjoying her vacation" strolls through an urban passageway with a distinguished-looking and barrel-chested gentleman who looks like a well-preserved male model.[213] This Lyrica ad begins as follows: "We open on a middle-aged woman with silvery-white hair (beautifully coiffed, I might add) sitting at a table. She tells us how fibromyalgia limited her life and how she suffered with the pain. But no more, she tells us as the camera begins to pan out and the music swells. Lyrica has changed her life. We see she's sitting in a café in a very 'old Europe' style setting—perhaps Venice or Rome, with the music we hear. A good-looking man who is supposed to be her age (but to me looks younger) walks up. She gets up and they walk away, conversing."[214] Other female activities in Lyrica advertisements include writing in a diary and gardening.

These advertisements are coded "white" in several ways. Attractive grooming suggests privileged (white) status and access to high-class cosmetic services. "Old Europe" identifies this satisfied patient with symbolic European whiteness and its fabled sophistications. Blacks till cotton fields, whites cultivate English gardens. It is introspective whites, who enjoy the luxury of quiet contemplation, who keep diaries, while blacks toil to keep body and soul together. Small wonder a British psychiatrist referred in 1960 to "the Nigerian's apparent lack of need to engage in the elaborate introspections and soul searchings in the way the European does."[215] It would not occur to a Nigerian to keep a diary, because he has nothing to say about his inner life, such as it is. Here is one more way the designation "European" codes race: White means complexity, while black signifies truncated consciousness and a diminished capacity to deal with the complications of human existence.

The alleged association of chronic fatigue syndrome with "white" and privileged people has been evident since the 1980s, when it became known as "yuppie flu," defined as "a psychosomatic illness restricted to members of the young middle and upper classes."[216] Over time the class privilege theme stayed constant even as the disorder came to include older people: "One of the common stereotypes [in 2006] is that this is a bunch of hysterical upper-class, professional white women who are seeing physicians and have a mass hysteria."[217] When Jerome Groopman attended an educational meeting for fibromyalgia patients outside of Boston in the spring of 2000, here is what he found: "The meeting was free, its costs underwritten by pharmaceutical companies, which had set up marketing booths in the entryway. Nearly all the participants were white women between the ages of twenty and sixty. Some walked with canes that had a four-point base, others wore braces on their wrists or ankles, and many limped. The cavernous hotel ballroom, which seats more than seven hundred and fifty people, was filled beyond capacity."[218] This spectacle of infirmity, featuring an army of disabled white women with disposable time, begs for an explanation of their homogeneity.

But the identification of FMS and CFS with high social status has been discredited. It is likely that sampling bias prompted researchers to go looking for FMS and CFS in the more affluent communities where they expected to find disorders of this kind.[219] In fact, chronic fatigue syndrome occurs throughout the social classes.[220] One report claims that CFS is actually more common in African Americans than in whites.[221]

The persisting fantasy that these disorders afflict privileged victims suggests that a kind of compensatory schadenfreude may be involved. Privileged lives provoke a combination of envy and vicarious enjoyment. The ensuing resentment may produce a feeling that these spoiled people "deserve" the mysterious ailment that seems to descend on them like a curse. Interestingly, the fantasy of high-status disorders has been strong enough to prevail against other factors that assign to these disorders a distinctly *lower* social status. For example, patients with FMS or CFS have frequently been regarded as hypochondriacs, and doctors resent, as Jerome Groopman puts it, "constant complaining about imagined issues." Small wonder that a survey of Norwegian doctors and medical students found that fibromyalgia was ranked at the very bottom of a prestige hierarchy of various diseases. Indeed, the fact that some diseases are more prestigious than others makes it "likely that considerations other than strictly medical ones tacitly influence medical decisions."[222] A medical world that assigns different measures of prestige to different diseases is also a medical world that can identify diseases as "black" or "white," or identify blacks and whites as more or less likely to complain about imaginary symptoms. This is the medical world in which FMS and CFS have been coded "white" and that has long excluded blacks from the domain of imagined illnesses.

Black people make implausible hypochondriacs because we know (or assume) their infirmities are all too real. In reality, black Americans *do* feel sicker than whites, because they *are* sicker than whites. But the implausibility of black hypochondria is not just something we infer from black people's actual health status. It is also an illusion promoted by blacks' exclusion from the domain of human complexity, where FMS and CFS are coded "white" because of their psychological complications. The assumed "hardiness" of black people would appear to eliminate any interest they might have in persuading themselves that they are ill. Hypochondria itself is coded "white" because it is a compulsive and perverse kind of *introspection*. So whites get credit for being sensitive, cultured, and complicated, while blacks may well suffer disproportionately from psychologically complicated disorders like FMS and CFS, which are still associated with privileged white lifestyles.

Given how thoroughly racial identity and social class can overlap, it is only natural that hypochondria has been coded "middle-class" as well as "white." Lee Rainwater, a prominent sociologist and a prolific white interpreter of the African American experience during the 1960s and 1970s, makes this argument in a 1968 essay on how lower-class and middle-class people supposedly feel about their illnesses. Middle-class people, according to Rainwater, are simply more sensitive than members of the lower class. Middle-class people believe in "the intrinsic value and worth of the self and of the body" and in "the sacredness of their persons." Every symptom is perceived as potentially incapacitating, because symptoms of illness threaten the "more perfect person the middle-class individual likes to think of himself as being."[223]

Lower-class feelings, according to Rainwater, are duller and less differentiated than those of their more prosperous neighbors. Lower-class people possess a "very primitive level of existential comprehension" and "learn to live with illness." That is why lower-class people seldom "organize their lives around being ill, as in hypochondriasis."[224] Their general incuriosity about illness prevents the sort of exaggerated interest in symptoms that can turn into hypochondria.

This account of the mental world of the lower classes closely resembles American psychiatry's portrait of the African American personality throughout the twentieth century. Blacks have always been regarded as possessing truncated mental lives and duller feelings than those of more sensitive whites. Rainwater also points out that middle-class professionals, such as doctors, are often hostile toward such "problem" people and may have little interest in learning how to serve them. American medicine's long struggle to understand "the Negro patient" has been one aspect of the larger struggle to establish therapeutic relationships between the uneducated masses and the learned professionals who are supposed to serve them.

The same racial dichotomy that has brought into being "white" diseases has also produced a comprehensive doctrine of black "hardiness." These conceptualizations of racially segregated medical phenomena are, of course, two ways of naming and identifying a single dichotomy that has long distinguished between the alleged anatomical, physiological, and psychological characteristics of whites and blacks. According to the medical folklore we have been examining, blacks have often been regarded as being too "hardy" (or too "primitive") to contract "white" disorders. We have also seen that cultural as well as biological factors have been invoked to account for purported racial "hardiness" or "immunity." Indeed, the most conspicuous differences between whites and blacks in the United States, apart from skin color, have everything to do with social and economic status and the deprivations and opportunities a person's status makes possible or, in some cases, inevitable.

Black "Hardiness"

The idea of black hardiness and vitality is a system of interrelated themes, all of which presume a more primitive human type that is biologically different from civilized man. A fundamental dogma of this dichotomous racial biology has been the idea that blacks possess a relative immunity to various disorders that renders them less sensitive to physical discomfort than whites. This racial myth represents a hardiness paradigm that was more conspicuous during the period when the claims of overtly racist anthropologists were published and discussed in the medical community without shame or embarrassment.

Physical Hardiness

White racist judgments about the character and intelligence of black people have long coexisted with positive and even admiring assessments of blacks viewed as physical organisms. For example, the racist biologist and eugenicist Charles B. Davenport made this case in 1919, not in an obscure tract, but in the *Proceedings of the National Academy of Sciences*: "But the uninfected negro is highly resistant to diseases of the skin, mouth and throat. He seems to have more stable nerves, has better eyes and metabolizes better. Thus, in many respects the uninfected colored troops show themselves to be constitutionally better physiological machines than the white men."[225] "Nature," an Arkansas physician wrote in 1926, "endows the negro with strong passions, strong muscles and a vigorous constitution."[226] In a similar vein, in 1928 the flagship *American Journal of Physical Anthropology* credited blacks with "a power of vital resistance both to infection and to malignant growths."[227] A year later a Dallas gynecologist credited blacks with "naturally higher resistance to trauma and to infection."[228] The evolutionary subtext that framed these endorsements of black vitality is evident in the Arkansas doctor's observation that "the negro is only a few generations removed from savagery. We should expect very little of a person whose great-grandfather was a cannibal."[229]

It should be noted that the white consensus on black physiological superiority was never complete. For one thing, some racists found no pleasure in extolling the organic superiority of an inferior race. "I fancy that a great deal of nonsense has been written about the vigorous health of the savage," a Victorian racist wrote in 1864, and he was right as *The Lancet's* declaration in 1936 that: "The rude [robust] health of the savage is as imaginary as the rude health of our own forefathers."[230] Neither the disparaging racist nor the realistic physician saw any point in promoting a myth of the physiologically noble savage. An influential disparager of black health during the 1890s, Frederick L. Hoffman, argued that "the smaller lung capacity of the colored race is itself proof of an inferior physical organism, and this assertion is proved by the greater mortality of the race as compared with the white."[231] Yet his book also contains medical testimony asserting the physical superiority of the black male of the Civil War era. Hoffman's book served the great medical racist argument of the latter part of the nineteenth century, namely, that emancipation had ruined Negro health. This, he argued, was demonstrated by the contrast between the physically robust slave and his degenerate offspring whose health had been subverted by freedom. Both claims about the black organism—its inherent vitality or its inherent pathology—could serve racist ends. While the disparagers stigmatized blacks as unfit for modern society, the promoters of the black "hardiness" doctrine provided white doctors with a convenient alibi for the medical neglect of an impoverished black population. The lasting effects of the hardiness doctrine on the medical treatment of later generations of African Americans are described throughout this book.

It is important to understand that white commentators have not exercised a monopoly on romantic and pseudoscientific claims about the superior vitality of the black organism. White racist interpretations of black vitality have coexisted with African American claims about black "hardiness" that promote the theme of black survival. African American doctors have articulated their own interpretations of black physiological normality or superiority to refute the image of a Negro race that was fatally afflicted by tuberculosis and syphilis. Organizing a National Negro Health Week and Negro Health days in the 1920s was one way of expressing Black America's determination to join the larger world of "sanitary science and preventive medicine," but more pointed declarations were required. Dr. Charles H. Garvin, writing in 1924 in the organ of the National Urban League, cited a white public health expert to argue that the Negro *did* possess "biologic fitness." Despite a "lack of racial immunity" to the white man's diseases, the black man "will respond to the treatment for pulmonary tuberculosis, and if that treatment is begun early he will continue [to do] well."[232] (Appeals for the recognition of black people as normal human beings remain a part of the black experience to this day.) Half a century later, W. Montague Cobb, MD, PhD, physician, anthropologist, and a prominent African American of the intellectual class, was making more aggressive claims about the biological qualities of the black race in nakedly Darwinian terms. Cobb asserted that "the American Negro was *the most highly selected biological element* in the American population" [emphasis added]. The horrors of the various stages of the Middle Passage meant that "every African who landed on these shores had undergone *a more rigid biological selection than any group in the history of mankind.* Moreover, over 250 years of hard labor, long hours, and meager food, clothing and shelter are not calculated to promote the survival of the unfit" [emphasis added].[233] It should be emphasized that this melodramatic narrative had already appeared in African American doctors' commentaries on their survival as a people. A black physician named N. O. Calloway had made the same melodramatic claims in a speech at the 1962 meeting of the (black) National Medical Association. "Slavery began," he said, "with the trip to America, during which all of the weak ones were killed or thrown overboard or allowed to die. This was followed by the slave block, further selection and sales as desirable animals. From this point on, artificially controlled mating occurred." He also asserted that inherited diseases such as Friedreich's ataxia, Sydenham's chorea, and progressive spinal atrophy had "entered the Negro race through the inheritance of their white blood."[234] The black Harvard psychiatrist Chester M. Pierce found in 1969 a measure of compensation for the shortened lives of black people in their physical hardiness: "It is my contention that despite harrowing and grisly environmental onslaught our bodies withstand and prevail to an amazing degree. We have strength to do the heaviest labors. We have coordination to succeed in any athletic contests." The shortened life span, he says, is due to "the fact that the energy requirements to be black are of a vastly greater order of magnitude than those used by a white man."[235]

This "hardiness" doctrine, which can also be a form of racial chauvinism, has not been limited to highly educated African Americans such as physicians. On the contrary, the black survival-of-the-fittest story is a folk belief established in the minds of the black rank and file and "trickled up" to a black professional class that shares certain emotional needs of the less educated that derives from the shared ordeal of being black in a white society. Indeed, the traditional narrative of black suffering has largely suppressed a counternarrative of black racial superiority that appeared even before emancipation. The abolitionist Martin Delany declared in a 1852 pamphlet that: "We are a *superior race*, being endowed with properties fitting us for all parts of the earth, while they are only adapted to *certain parts*."[236] In 1927, the black writer George S. Schuyler wrote : "The rigid training and discipline that the Negro has received since his arrival on these sacred shores has left him *with a lower percentage of weaklings and incompetents* than is shown by any other group" [emphasis added]. According to Schuyler, "in America conditions have made the average Negro more alert, more resourceful, more intelligent, and hence more interesting than the average Nordic."[237] Here the black intellectual invokes black survival as a tremendous achievement that turns racial inferiority doctrine on its head. The "folk" equivalent of this inspirational racial biology appears repeatedly in *Drylongso: A Self-Portrait of Black America* (1980), an extraordinary anthology of grassroots African American opinion about racial matters large and small. "Most black people think that they are mentally and physically better than white people," says Ellen Turner Surry, "and I think that they are physically superior to white people. I think it goes back to slavery-time. I think that only the strongest of us were able to survive, so that gave us better stock to start with."[238] Many of the black people of modest means interviewed for this book offer their own variations on the theme of black physical and psychological superiority over white people. But the primal theme of this doctrine has always been the Middle Passage drama, recited here yet again by the daring and later degenerate leader of the Black Panther Party, Huey P. Newton: "Well, think about it. They came over here in boats as slaves, and the ones who were weak died. Only the strong ones could survive the boat ride. Then they became slaves and they lived in these places with no heat, no plumbing, nothing. They didn't get any medical care. There were rats and all kinds of diseases, and we're still alive."[239]

The medical consequences of the "hardiness" doctrine have been profound in two ways. First, the historical record as presented in the medical literature makes it clear that white (and, undoubtedly, some black) doctors have overestimated black resistance and "immunity" to disease to the detriment of many black patients. The pseudoscientific or self-deluding rationales that made these misperceptions possible are described in detail throughout this book. Here we see how often doctors' racial interpretations of various human organ systems have assumed that black "hardiness" is an inherent aspect of human biology. "There is good evidence that Negroes have extraordinary power to survive both wounds and major surgical operations and that, once convalescent, they are less liable to the reactions of fever and other complications."[240] The potential medical consequences of such a hardiness doctrine can easily be imagined.

Second, the "hardiness" doctrine has over many years caused many black patients to discount or disregard their own symptoms by endowing them with the belief that they are tough or resilient enough to manage without medical care—a kind of medically dysfunctional black pride that may also draw on religious beliefs to reject medical assistance. This doctor-avoiding syndrome is also related to how African Americans deal with pain as a medical symptom, a response that may involve social factors medical personnel should be prepared to recognize. As we saw earlier, Dr. Jean Bonhomme, president of the National Black Men's Health Network in Atlanta, calls this stubborn refusal to seek help "pathological stoicism."[241]

The medical stoicism of black people belongs to the larger drama of black life that has often been portrayed, by blacks and whites alike, as an ordeal requiring "hardiness" to survive its destructive effects. The archetypal Negro engaged in hard labor thus found his way into the medical literature, where the black "hardiness" doctrine proliferated even if it did not always prevail. The *American Journal of Public Health,* for example, commented in 1932 that, given the enormous number of physical defects found in Negro industrial workers, "we wonder how these men can endure [the] moderate to great amounts of physical effort exacted of them. As a matter of fact, many do not long endure; they suffer physical breakdown relatively early in life."[242] It appeared there was less to black hardiness than many white physicians believed. But as the black psychiatrist Alyce C. Gullattee noted in 1969, whites had long promulgated a myth that portrayed blacks as "capable of hard physical labor with little need for rest or relaxation," thereby enabling white exploiters to "utilize Negroes for hard labor and menial tasks."[243] At the same time, many blacks embraced the idea of their own hardiness as an emblem of racial pride.

Emotional Hardiness

The idea that black Americans are psychologically stable and durable to a greater degree than whites is an important consequence of the racist myth of black mental simplicity. In the absence of complication, stability reigns because a disorder requires an ordered system of some complexity that is vulnerable to disruption. Conversely, the less complex the mind, the fewer ways in which it can go awry. For this reason, the prominent black psychiatrist Carl C. Bell wrote in 1980, blacks receive "unsophisticated medical care because of the misconception that as an unsophisticated people we have a limited number of diagnostic categories."[244] How and why American psychiatry limited the number of diagnostic categories that have been applied to African Americans is described in detail later in this book. At this point we may simply note that the psychiatric profession has promulgated its own version of black emotional hardiness over the past century by defining blacks as resistant or immune to depression, manic-depressive illness, and obsessive-compulsive neuroses, among other psychiatric disorders. What is more, each and every claim that blacks enjoy resistance or immunity to a specific disorder can be explained by examining a social logic that incorporates the notion that black human beings are less complex, and therefore less suited for modern life, than whites are.

The idea that blacks enjoy immunity to depression grew out of the old racial stereotype of the "happy-go-lucky" Negro. The social logic (or rationale) of this caricature is rooted in the emotional needs of whites, who require relief from the emotional burden of observing, or simply intuiting, black suffering about which they do little or nothing. It is, therefore, not surprising that the heyday of "happy-go-lucky" imagery, which included black smiles the size of watermelon slices, was the era of Jim Crow racism during which black suffering was much more visible than it is today. The black psychiatrist James H. Carter commented in 1974: "The pervasive myth that blacks are happy-go-lucky must no longer be accepted. A gross error was made in the past by characterizing depression first as an English malady and subsequently as the 'white man's malady' in the United States."[245] A decade after the passage of the Civil Rights Act, Dr. Carter still found it necessary to campaign against racial folklore in American psychiatry and the color-coding of a major psychiatric disorder.

Understanding black emotional hardiness requires us to recognize its effects on black people as well as depression's illusory role as "a white man's malady." Acknowledging the real and the illusory aspects of emotional hardiness means acknowledging the reality of "pathological stoicism" in some black people even as we reject the color-coding of depression as a "white" emotional disorder. The problem here is how to distinguish between the illusion and the reality of hardiness. Take, for example, the 1992 report that African American caregivers of demented patients were only half as likely to show signs of depression than their white counterparts.[246] A question not addressed by this report is whether the apparent absence of depression in so many of the black workers was due to the absence of depression or, alternatively, to a disinclination to acknowledge or an inability to recognize depression. We have already seen that elements of emotional stoicism are built into the lives of many people whom life "teaches" to endure pain or frustration, because they see no relief in sight. One might want to categorize the ability to tolerate this kind of suffering as "emotional hardiness." We confront the same conundrum in the case of a report that "found that older African-American women reported fewer depressive symptoms than their white counterparts even though they had more predictors of depression, including physical illness, perceptions of unmet need and low sense of control."[247] Could it be that "black emotional hardiness" is an adaptive ability to suffer without complaint, rather than the genuine absence of emotional suffering? The tradition of "the strong black woman" in African American life would suggest this is the case.[248] But acknowledging this kind of suffering will be difficult when stoicism mandates that depression be seen as "just being too weak in the 'white man's world.'"[249] Or as two southern white psychiatrists phrased this, "the attitude of tolerant suffering is considered a virtue in itself. . . ."[250] Here we see how easily black stoicism can be converted into a rationale for inaction on the part of doctors who might otherwise be less tolerant of untreated black suffering.

Manic-depressive illness, known today as bipolar disorder, was coded "white" a century ago, because blacks were regarded as too primitive to be vulnerable to affective disorders involving sudden mood shifts. The "social logic" of this bias is grounded in the racist doctrine of a "Negro personality" that was assumed to be both simple and predictable, a doctrine that enjoyed the status of received wisdom in American psychiatry well into the twentieth century. Racist humor about black behavior often took the form of an amused response to the inevitable consequences of blacks' inextinguishable appetite for chicken, watermelon, or sex; indeed, responses of this kind occasionally appeared in the medical literature. Predictability was important because the racial discipline of the Jim Crow South was predicated on the attempt to create and maintain fixed black character traits that would ensure that the oppressed practiced self-control.

The "Negro personality" was, therefore, dissociated from affective illnesses that appeared to require a more complex emotional life. The affective illnesses include unipolar and bipolar depression, generalized anxiety disorder, agoraphobia, panic disorder, social phobia, and obsessive-compulsive disorder. These conditions often involve sudden mood swings that suggest an unstable and unpredictable character structure psychiatrists saw as more typical of whites than blacks. Before the Second World War, many physicians regarded blacks as too mentally simple to be vulnerable to such disorders. During the 1960s the rationale for dissociating blacks from affective disorders took a psychodynamic turn. A new doctrine held "that since most blacks were deprived of self-esteem, material possessions, status, etc., they did not have what was required to experience a 'loss' which was the precipitating factor to trigger depression."[251] The rationale here was that poverty and the simple way of life it imposed on black people literally deprived them of the capacity to feel certain kinds of losses they allegedly did not experience. "What is clearly characteristic of the southern Negro," two psychiatric authors argue in 1962, "is his limited expectation, and this stands him in good stead in times of loss. . . . This really amounts to stoicism based in experience"—as fine a definition of emotional hardiness as one could ask for.[252]

There is little research on obsessive-compulsive personality disorder (OCPD) and race. It is likely that OCPD has been coded "white" and underdiagnosed in African Americans due to traditional ideas about blacks, their intellectual functioning, and their presumed lack of ambition.[253] The patient with OCPD typically demonstrates perfectionism and an excessive devotion to work, which are contrary to standard racist stereotypes about blacks. A 1960 psychiatric report, for example, alleges that black Africans lack "the traits of the anal personality—meticulousness, orderliness, punctuality, frugality, stubbornness and organizational ability."[254] It would be difficult to find a more efficient way to stigmatize a population as being unfit for modern civilization. Indeed, this stereotype is so powerful that the prominent black psychiatrist Alvin Poussaint once accepted a version of this : "Blacks do not have obsessive-compulsive neuroses, which is more of a puritanical thing," he told *Time* in 1970. "But they have more anxiety. I have a theory that blacks feel more depleted or worn out psychically than whites, but I don't know how to measure that."[255] The sheer power of the idea that blacks are not meticulous, orderly, or punctual can also be seen in the history of the "type A" personality model. The original formulation of the "overt behavior pattern A" included traits such as "excessive competitive drive" and "a severe sense of time urgency" focused on deadlines.[256] As late as the 1980s, as we have seen, the African American epidemiologist Sherman A. James was arguing that poor blacks as well as the middle and upper-middle classes were capable of developing a coping style that included "type A" behaviors. James's argument was yet another attempt by black health professionals to convince a predominantly white society that blacks possessed the character traits necessary "to cope actively with behavioral stressors" in a modern society.[257]

The white medical conception of black emotional hardiness has sometimes included the idea that homosexuality is less common in blacks than in whites. This presumed immunity to what was once called "inversion" derives from the black's imagined role as a kind of physiological noble savage who, for evolutionary reasons, remains closer to what Nature originally intended perfectly dimorphic male and female sexes to be. This was the view of the American endocrinologist Louis Lurie, who wrote in 1944: "Among primitive peoples and savages, homosexuality appears to be almost non-existent."[258] During the Jim Crow period, the idea that blacks were endowed with especially robust heterosexual instincts had to compete with the more common belief that black sexual impulses were essentially out of control and open to any available gratification. In 1936 the *American Journal of Orthopsychiatry* reported that "perversions are not common among colored children, older or younger. At least they are not admitted. In interview they are rather convincing in their positive belief that anything other than hetero-sexual is 'crazy.'"[259] Three years later a psychiatrist directly challenged this view: "This is not entirely in agreement with our experiences. We have observed every type of childhood experience and reaction to it. . . . In some instances the sexual experience and knowledge of preadolescent negro children were indeed a revelation, as was their ability to absorb such experiences."[260] At this time "many American doctors spent much time warning against such inverts' predilection for white lovers. More broadly, there was a distinct tradition in the United States to regard homosexuality as a nonwhite vice that was spreading into white communities."[261]

African Americans as a group have characterized the threat of homosexuality in very different terms. The spreading AIDS epidemic of the 1980s had the effect of intensifying black homophobia and denial to the point where the "gay" disease "was presented as a disease of white men."[262] While some other "white" diseases had been associated with high social status, here was a plague that offered positive status to no one. Many blacks, *JAMA* reported in 1988, "believe that homosexuality is a white phenomenon. While men (and women) may practice homosexual behaviors, they see themselves as heterosexual in orientation, making it difficult for them to accept AIDS risk-reduction messages aimed at the gay community."[263] This self-deluding sexual lifestyle eventually became known as the Down Low, a pattern of male behavior that has infected many unsuspecting female partners and wives. Most black men who have sex with other men refuse to identify themselves as gay, preferring to see homosexuality "as a white man's perversion."[264] The Down Low thus functions as an alternative sexual identity that enables this group of men to appear to fulfill their obligation to uphold black standards of masculinity, even as they engage in sex acts they consider effeminate when practiced by whites.

The myth of hyperstable black heterosexuality, like the myth of black stoicism, has served white and black constituencies with very different agendas in mind. During the first half of the twentieth century, the "natural" heterosexual orientation sometimes ascribed to blacks was invoked to suggest their arrested evolutionary development. Much later in the twentieth century, it was still possible to speculate in the scientific literature about the super-robust nature of black sexuality. In this case researchers observed that black women appeared to be "'inoculated' against severe gender identity pathology. But why should this be? Perhaps the black female's unique role as mother and provider within their matrifocal society allows them to exhibit appropriate levels of aggressiveness and assertiveness without compromising their femininity."[265] Two decades after the Moynihan Report had associated the black matriarch with black family pathology, these investigators call "the black female's unique role as mother and provider" a guarantor of mental health. This "strong black woman" demonstrates both gender stability and the devotion to family that has made her a revered (and sometimes resented) stoic type endowed with a legendary emotional hardiness.

Conclusion: How Human Organ Systems Acquire Racial Identities

The long and influential careers of "white" diseases and folkloric ideas about black "hardiness" confirm that racial interpretations of health and disease have pervaded our medical culture, even in the absence of overt efforts to promote this kind of thinking. The racial interpretation of human organ systems is an integral part of a symbolic system that continues to shape ideas about alleged differences between the minds and bodies of "white" and "black" human beings. The overt assigning of racial characteristics to human organ systems was more common in American medicine during the first half of the twentieth century. The medical racism of that era was a specialized version of the societal racism that encountered little resistance among influential white people and institutions. At this time the stigmatizing of blacks by means of medical diagnoses or public health edicts had the status of common sense. Following the Second World War, the public mores of American medicine changed at the same pace as the racial mores of the larger society, and this was typical of other American institutions, as well. The Boy Scouts of America, for example, did not embark upon racial integration until the Supreme Court led the way by ruling in favor of school integration in 1954. It may come as a surprise to some that the medical establishment did not play anything resembling a leading role in opposing or dismantling Jim Crow segregation. This lack of interest in promoting integration existed alongside of, and did not discourage, the habit of thinking in terms of "black" and "white" fluids, tissues, and organs, a tradition that in its more recent forms remains a part of modern medicine.

RACIAL FOLKLORE IN MEDICAL SPECIALTIES

A Century of Racial Pharmacology: From Racial Folklore to Racial Genetics

In a society that is preoccupied with defining racial differences, administering drugs to blacks and whites inevitably creates a racial pharmacology that expresses, or even makes novel contributions to, prevailing racial dogmas and folkloric notions about traits that are widely believed to be of racial origin. The racial pharmacology that developed over the course of the twentieth century began as a logical development of the racio-medical anthropology of the nineteenth century that described inherent anatomical, physiological, and psychological differences between black and white human beings. This doctrine of racial essences, most notably formulated in the writings of the plantation physician Samuel Cartwright, virtually required a racially differential pharmacology that would provide yet another demonstration of racially distinct physiological mechanisms in whites and blacks. The following prototype of race-conscious pharmacological thinking shows once again how easy it can be to conflate what is taken for science with the racial folklore of the era in question.

Almost a century ago, a Texas doctor named Robert E. House performed a pioneering pharmacological experiment that employed the drug scopolamine as a "truth serum" to interrogate two suspected criminals. Acting under the supervision of Dr. W. M. Hale, the Dallas County Health Officer, Dr. House administered a combination of chloroform and scopolamine, a powerful and dangerous sedative, to a pair of suspected thieves. The first was "a very intelligent white man" who afterward wrote a detailed description of his experience in this twilight state of consciousness. The second subject was "a negro of average intelligence" who remembered nothing, went to sleep for five hours after receiving the second dose of the drug, and was such a compliant talker under sedation that he "made a better witness under the drug than he did when sober."[266]

The racial pharmacology of the scopolamine trial performed in 1922 displays three paradigmatic and interrelated ideas about psychophysiological racial differences between blacks and whites, and these are ideas that remain influential to this day. First, there are the familiar and linked themes of differential racial intelligence and mental complexity; the results of the "truth serum" experiment presented yet another example of the classic contrast between white intelligence and black dullness. The response of the white subject was complex and unreliable, while the response of his "average" black counterpart was to speak compliantly while under sedation. This pharmacological event thereby confirmed a fundamental racist dogma.

The second psychophysiological paradigm that is evident in this event may be called the narcoleptic predisposition that has frequently been ascribed to blacks both inside and outside the medical literature: Black people have been credited with a supernormal ability to fall asleep. This special capacity includes, as we have seen, four ways of losing consciousness: falling sleep, anesthesia, hypnosis, and hallucinations. Blacks' alleged responsiveness to pharmacologically induced unconsciousness conforms, therefore, to the traditional folkloric idea that blacks possess a racial affinity for the unconscious state. Black and white psychiatrists have proposed that blacks are more likely to have hallucinatory experiences than whites.[267] The purported evidence of a narcoleptic disposition in blacks is linked to a set of related racial folkloric ideas about deficient black intelligence, laziness, passivity, and mental disorder. Putting a drug into a black subject, such as Dr. House's "average negro," can thus be interpreted as revealing a racial essence that might be less conspicuous when the subject is not under its influence.

The third paradigmatic idea about blacks associated with the "truth serum" trial posits a subordinate racial personality that is characterized by suggestibility, receptiveness, and a responsiveness to external influences that may include drug therapies. Dr. House's black subject exemplifies this kind of subordination by succumbing to the drug. His zombie-like testimony under sedation is one version of the totally submissive black man who meets the requirements of Southern racism. The enduring power of this (and other) paradigmatic conceptions of black personality suggest that even peer-reviewed observations of black subjects' greater responsiveness to drug therapies should be carefully scrutinized for their possible vulnerability to folkloric ideas about the black personality.

Categorizing racial pharmacology as a set of practices can be done in two ways. The first approach is to classify procedures according to whether they administer or withhold drugs, or employ different drugs, in racially differential ways. The second approach would involve distinguishing between racist and nonracist procedures, assuming that medical racism can be defined in a satisfactory way. I have found it more useful to adopt the first approach, while attempting at the same time to identify racially motivated variations on nonracist procedures for administering drug therapies.

Racial pharmacology has taken several forms over the past century. Doctors may *administer, overprescribe, underprescribe, or withhold* drug therapy to or from one racial population on account of clinical observations (which may be of uncertain value) or based on their assessments of patients' racial traits, whether these are behavioral or physiological. At their worst, such assessments can amount to medical neglect and indifference. Racial folkloric influences on clinical reasoning prevent us from making a clear distinction between practices based on clinical observation versus those based on malfeasance or incompetence (neglect or indifference). The *motives* of those administering or withholding therapeutic drugs, as best we can ascertain them, will determine whether or not one chooses to judge these practices as racist in intent.

Racially motivated administration of therapeutic drugs to blacks can be prompted by an intention to control the behavior of people whose personalities are regarded as potentially violent or more prone to psychosis than those of whites. "African Americans are treated differently in the mental health system," one observer noted in 1996. "They are more likely to be hospitalized, to be involuntarily hospitalized, to sometimes receive seclusion and restraints, and to be discharged earlier. . . . Factors such as greater perceived dangerousness and social distance may play a part in the excessive use and dosing of antipsychotic medication."[268] African American parents have interpreted administering a stimulant such as Ritalin (methylphenidate) to black children as an attempt to control or take away their children's spontaneity and creativity. Here one may encounter different cultural definitions of what constitutes "normal" behavior for children. While Ritalin is commonly prescribed for attention deficit/hyperactivity disorder (ADHD), black parents may also fear more than their white counterparts that Ritalin will serve as a gateway drug to other forms of drug abuse.[269] This intense fear of "drug" use in general derives from the devastation wrought by crack cocaine in many black communities during and after the 1980s.

Racially motivated overprescribing of therapeutic drugs, as these scenarios suggest, is largely a matter of cultural perspective. Whether one regards mentally disturbed black adults or restless black children as medically different from their white counterparts has a great deal to do with one's social formation. Social attitudes may also play a role in less explicitly racial scenarios. It has been reported, for example, that blacks are prescribed "first-generation" antipsychotic drugs (neuroleptics) such as Thorazine and Haldol more often than whites, who are more likely to receive "second-generation" antipsychotics such as Abilify and Risperdal. In the absence of clear evidence that one of these drug classes is more effective for the treatment of schizophrenia than the other, the appearance of racially differential prescribing is striking. One study suggests that physicians prefer to prescribe first-generation neuroleptics to patients who have a substance abuse disorder, and doctors may determine or simply assume that black patients are more likely to be abusing drugs. Alternatively, physicians may not prescribe the second-generation drug clozapine for blacks "due to greater perceived risks of clozapine-induced diabetes and agranulocytosis among black patients."[270] The second rationale would appear to be less related to stereotypes of blacks than more socially charged assumptions about drug abuse by blacks.

There is an important distinction between over- and underprescribing drugs. African Americans are more likely to feel over- rather than undermedicated, because they are more likely than whites to feel under assault by drug therapies that remind them of the ravages of heroin and cocaine and that may seem (like birth control) to be a scheme formulated by whites to control black people's lives. At the same time, different drugs inspire different degrees of overt protest against perceived overmedication. Black parents' feelings about Ritalin involve many children whose treatment can be discussed in an accessible public forum like the schools. In fact, African American children are prescribed much less Ritalin than their white counterparts.[271] It may be that the number of black people with strong feelings about the excessive use of antipsychotic drugs on black patients in hospitals is limited, because this procedure is less socially conspicuous than the mass medication of school children with stimulants.

Racially motivated underprescribing of therapeutic drugs is entirely plausible, because it conforms to a larger pattern of undertreating black patients with a variety of beneficial procedures.[272] The practice of prescribing drugs less often to black patients includes psychotropic drugs in general and asthma drugs.[273] Black veterans with bipolar disorder are less likely to be treated with lithium and SSRIs (selective serotonin uptake inhibitors).[274] The failure of medical professionals to provide black patients with pain relief comparable even to the (often inadequate) analgesia offered to whites has been documented over and over again.[275]

Why underprescribing occurs is not always clear. For example, blacks are prescribed less antidepressant medication than whites. It is possible that this physician behavior has been influenced by the racial folkloric idea that blacks enjoy a degree of immunity to depression due to a "happy-go-lucky" disposition. There is no reason to assume that this conception of Negro character does not live on today in the minds of many psychiatrists who make choices about how (and whether) to medicate black patients who may be suffering from depression. It is also possible that "rates of depression among Blacks may be underestimated as Blacks may experience or express depressive symptoms in a manner not well measured by standard diagnostic instruments."[276] Unfamiliarity with how many black people express their feelings will make it more difficult for psychiatrists to recognize and treat their mood states.

Racially differential underprescribing may also be caused by factors that are not directly related to how white physicians think about their black patients. There is, for example, the question of how black patients feel about specific medications or the idea of being medicated at all. It has been reported that "African Americans find medical treatment of depression less acceptable than Caucasians."[277] This is one reason why black patients are less "compliant" than whites: less willing to acquire and take the medications that are prescribed for them.[278] The tricyclic antidepressants (TCA) that are prescribed more often to blacks are generally regarded to have more severe side effects than the SSRIs that are more frequently prescribed for whites, and this in itself might account for less compliance by black patients. Why physicians prescribe the older medications to blacks in a disproportionate manner may be a sign of the medical neglect of black patients that has been amply documented in a variety of medical specialties.

Perhaps the best-known examples of therapeutic drugs that may be underprescribed to blacks are the beta-blockers and ACE inhibitors that are given to heart patients to regulate heart arrhythmias, lower blood pressure, and prevent second heart attacks. Given that high blood pressure and heart failure affect a disproportionate number of black people, the availability of these highly regarded medications to the African American patient population is of real medical significance.

The idea that beta-blockers and ACE inhibitors have different effects in black and white patients has been debated over the past decade. "Those of us who went to medical school before a certain time were told that black patients did not respond well to ACE inhibitors," a physician observed in 2006.[279] The prevailing (but not unanimous) opinion among medical authors has been that some ACE inhibitors as well as certain beta-blockers are less effective in blacks than in whites.[280] Researchers have made conflicting claims, for example, about the value for black patients of the ACE inhibitor enalapril.[281] Among the beta-blockers, carvedilol appears to be equally effective in whites and blacks, whereas bucindolol has been described as ineffective in black patients.[282] A recent and dramatic discovery has shown that a gene variant that confers a beta-blocker–like physiological capacity on far more African Americans than whites may account for the apparent ineffectiveness of these drugs in clinical trials of African Americans. This group will presumably include a disproportionate number of people (estimated at 40 percent) who carry the altered gene that mimics the beta-blocker effect. These subjects will appear to derive no benefit from this class of drug. At the same time, the 60 percent of African American subjects who do *not* carry this gene variant may well benefit as much from beta-blockers as whites do.[283]

Claims that there are heart medications that work better in blacks than in whites rarely appear in the medical literature, the prominent exception being the antihypertensive drug combination BiDil that was approved in 2005. It is possible that this racial imbalance derives from the historical predominance of white participants in clinical drug trials. Skewed racial samples may have prompted investigators to eliminate candidate drugs that appeared to be ineffective or caused adverse reactions in white clinical trial subjects, but that might have proven to be more effective in other racial populations.[284]

Racially differential prescribing of heart drugs based on clinical trials can be problematic for several reasons. The response of obese individuals with reduced venous capacitance (who might be overrepresented among black subjects) could make the ACE inhibitor being tested appear more ineffective than it would be in non-obese patients.[285] Black subjects may be sicker than white subjects.[286] Black subjects may be underrepresented in clinical trials. Physicians may also have to consider different doses for white and black patients; one response to claims about the ineffectiveness of ACE inhibitors in blacks has been to recommend that they be given higher doses. The African American cardiologist Elijah Saunders has identified nebivilol as a particularly valuable beta-blocker for black patients and has encouraged its use.[287]

It is now widely accepted among medical researchers that racially differential drug responses originate, to a significant degree, in genetic polymorphisms that code for varying proportions of different versions of drug receptors or drug-metabolizing enzymes in racial populations. "Black Americans and Africans have a high frequency of a CYP2D6 allele that encodes an enzyme with impaired activity," one scientist wrote in 2001 in an oft-cited editorial. "This allele is virtually absent from white and Asian populations."[288] This is the promising scenario that makes it possible for us to imagine a pharmacogenomics that will "abolish" racial identity within the medical realm by prescribing drugs for individual genomes and thus render the entire race concept irrelevant to therapeutic treatment.

The ideal of postracial drug therapy is thus utopian in the sense that it dissolves the race factor in medicine and, therefore, the likelihood of biased diagnosis and treatment. In the absence of this sort of utopia, the current ideal posits a racially unbiased medicine that still must wrestle with conflicting data and—although medical authors rarely acknowledge it—racial folkloric ideas that can influence how physicians imagine the physiological and psychological traits of their black patients. In the absence of an overt critique of the (unconscious) motives that might cause physicians to undermedicate black patients, differences of opinion seldom violate the polite conventions that govern medical journal discourse.

An interesting deviation from the polite norm appeared in a letter to the *New England Journal of Medicine* in 2001, in which two cardiologists took strenuous exception to the practice of denying ACE inhibitors to black patients:

> Although we cannot be certain that this belief [that black race should constitute an accepted reason for not prescribing ACE inhibitors] is common, it is disturbing that it exists at all. This simple-minded

interpretation of the study by Exner et al. is not only distasteful, it is dangerous, potentially placing blacks at risk for inappropriate treatment. The data presented in the report are provocative but not definitive. They should inspire further research, not change accepted practice.[289]

Medical authors who are willing to criticize a clinical judgment as "disturbing," "simple-minded," and "distasteful" raise important questions about the thinking of physicians who make "dangerous" recommendations and what can be done to discourage racially differential drug therapy that is based on speculation rather than data. The conventions of this professional literature simply do not accommodate the kind of analysis that might offer plausible hypotheses about where a recommendation to undermedicate might come from. If the clinical data do not support the administration of lower doses to blacks, then what might account for these clinical decisions? How can one identify extra-medical factors that might lead to the "simple-minded" dosing of racially labeled patients?

Traditional racial interpretations of the black human organism deny it "normal" biological status in comparison to the white body, its physiology, and its organ systems. Traits identified as "black" are typically found to exceed or fall short of white norms that take on the status of benchmarks for normal human functioning. We have already seen how the prescribing of a wide variety of modern therapeutic drugs—antipsychotics, antidepressants, antihypertensives, and stimulants like Ritalin—has conformed to this model of racial pharmacology. The basic paradigm, then, is that of biological racial difference that permeates every aspect of human physiology.

This bipolar model of the black organism's differential sensitivity to drugs appeared long before our own era. A retrospective survey of the medical literature shows that earlier researchers categorized blacks' responses to drugs in a bipolar way, meaning that they were found to be either hyper- or hyporesponsive to the influence of some drugs. This racially distinctive sensitivity pertains to both psychoactive and other drugs. The standard responses conform to de facto white norms, and there is very little commentary favoring the assumption of a universal human physiology that would rule out racially differential drug effects.

A statement on behalf of a universal (pan-racial) drug response was actually published in *JAMA* in 1955. Given the impact of tuberculosis (TB) on African Americans, a report in 1949 that black patients benefited only temporarily from streptomycin, the first drug shown to be effective against TB, was cause for alarm.[290] Doubts about the value of streptomycin for blacks may have prompted the query from a New York physician who asked the editors of *JAMA* whether there were "any differences between the Negro race and the white race in their responses to antibiotic therapy." Their reply discounted purported racial differences: "There is no evidence that there are any appreciable differences in the responses of the various races of the world to antibiotic therapy. The results have been more or less uniform with respect to efficacy and reactions in all parts of the world."[291]

This medical proclamation, so reminiscent of the racially egalitarian UNESCO Statement on Race that had been issued five years earlier, was exceptional in its universalism. More typical of published commentaries is the racial dichotomizing pioneered by the crude empiricism of Dr. Niles back in 1913, which has reappeared intermittently ever since. In 1937, for example, invoking a familiar axiom of nineteenth-century racial anthropology, an anthropologist claimed that different nervous systems accounted for the purported fact that "the negro is less susceptible than the white man to the central action of atropine."[292] As late as 2000, a team of medical authors noted that the confirmation of atropine's effectiveness in black Africans "contradict[ed] earlier reports of its absence in the negroid race."[293] It is sobering to think that a racial folkloric fatalism about the therapeutic value of this drug to black patients may have affected their treatment for most of a century before this potentially deadly form of therapeutic nihilism was discredited.

Findings of low responsiveness to drugs have alternated with some claims that black patients demonstrate a supernormal pharmacological reactivity. As a believer in the narcoleptic predisposition of Negroes, Dr. Niles found them more sensitive to sedatives and "hypnotics." As this case shows, the interpretation of how black people react to drugs can be influenced by racial folkloric ideas about their personalities. Another experiment, reported in 1955, involved observing the effect of amphetamine on black and white prisoners. What the investigators observed was that "the Negro addicts seemed to have a greater incidence of pleasant reactions from amphetamine, the whites a higher number of unpleasant ones."[294] Given what we know about how often white psychiatrists have misread their black patients, it is worth asking how much these investigators knew about how to assess the reactions of black prisoners. In this case, we should take into account the racial folkloric theme of black hedonism, of the Negro's helpless surrender to the pleasures of fried chicken, watermelon, sexual pleasure, and a lazy disposition. Similarly, when black subjects are credited with a greater placebo response, a more rapid rate of clinical improvement in response to drug therapy, a greater sensitivity to antidepressant effects, or a more treatment-responsive form of ADHD, one must factor in the possible role of racial fantasies or wish fulfillment in making such clinical judgments.[295]

How racial stereotyping can affect clinical judgment is evident in the following assessment of antidepressant effects in black and white male in-patients. Speculating on why the black subjects had responded so poorly to chlorpromazine, the authors suggest that the personalities of these lower-class black men "were organized about the use of physical activity and self-assertiveness," while other personalities "were organized around intellectual activities and introspective concerns" that were unlikely to be of interest to black men of this social class.[296] The working assumption is that physical and assertive men do not tolerate the side effects of chlorpromazine as well as more cerebral types, hence their poor response to treatment with this drug.

This reasoning relies on a stereotype of black male physicality that owes much to popular culture imagery (black athletes and rappers) and little to data about the sedentary habits of the black population. This appearance of the physically assertive black male in the pharmacological literature recalls a similar appearance of the "muscular black male" as a medical type in the *American Heart Journal* in 1984. In this racial type, according to the author, a certain abnormally high physiological variable "may be normal."[297]

Pharmacology is fertile ground for the study of the race factor in medicine because drug therapy expresses the physician's thinking about diagnosis and treatment. The choice of a drug and its dosage follows the medical evaluation of the patient, a process that will sometimes incorporate thinking about racial differences of which the physician remains unaware. The racial dimension of psychopharmacology is especially important due to the traits and symptoms we routinely associate with both "drugs" and the medical (and moral) evaluation of black human beings: intoxication, hedonism, addiction, violent behavior, hallucinations, loss of self-control, and (impaired) intelligence. In this sense, as we have seen, therapeutic drugs have long served as instruments of both medical and social policy, sometimes helping and sometimes hurting the intended beneficiaries.

The Role of Racial Folklore in Obstetrics and Gynecology during the Twentieth Century

Twenty-five years before he was appointed surgeon general of the United States, Dr. David Satcher published a commentary on relations between white doctors and black patients in the 1973 volume of the *Journal of the American Medical Association* (*JAMA*). In the course of describing some of the effects of racial stereotypes on these relationships, he recalls in particular a series of gynecological examinations that had illustrated with graphic clarity the imbalance of power between white practitioners and the black women they were assigned to examine. "Black patients," he writes, "are almost invariably called by their first names and they are frequently exploited for teaching sessions. One black woman related to me that she had had nine pelvic examinations by physicians and students and had never been told whether her pelvis was normal or abnormal."[298]

How can we account for such behavior on the part of white physicians? On the one hand African Americans belonged to a medical underclass throughout the twentieth century. The social invisibility of black women subjected to unethical examinations or surgeries was consistent with their low status in a racial caste system. At the same time, the treatment (and mistreatment) of black patients has been influenced by racial folklore about black minds and bodies that Western medicine both absorbed and nurtured over the past two centuries. In this sense, the medical caste status of black patients combines inferior social status along with alleged psychological and biological traits that have often been granted the status of a racial essence. Black women who allegedly enjoy a racial immunity to pelvic endometriosis—a "constitutional racial factor," as *JAMA* surmised in 1951—will receive less monitoring and treatment of this disease than their white counterparts.[299] If black women enjoy a "lessened sensibility to pain," they will be less entitled to pain relief when giving birth.[300] These are only two of the ways in which biological rationales have influenced the medical treatment of women. The purpose of what follows is to describe how a system of such ideas about purported psychological and biological racial differences have influenced the diagnosis and treatment of black women by obstetricians and gynecologists.

The claims about obstetrical hardiness that have appeared in the medical and anthropological literatures almost always refer to black women. "The easy labors of primitive women are not entirely fictitious, as is shown by many authentic observations," as one medical author wrote in 1929. "Furthermore, our present civilization with its artificial refinements and customs has made women less able nervously and physically to stand the strain of a hard, prolonged labor."[301] The fundamental dichotomy that marks the presence or absence of obstetrical hardiness is a distinction between the primitive and the civilized, and this is not always a distinction between black and white. There is, the *British Medical Journal* noted in 1948, "a robust and primitive type" of woman who "will tolerate no inhaler" while giving birth, because she does not need that kind of pain relief.[302] When a U.S. Senate committee asked the popular science writer

Paul de Kruif to explain in 1942 the heroic Russian resistance to the Nazi invasion of their homeland, he replied as follows: "The Russians are hereditarily a healthy lot. The Russian women do not seem to have much trouble in bearing children, because of the rapidity of parturition. They bear children very quickly. The childbirth takes less time than it does in many other western countries, and consequently you cannot say that it was the medical care that did it, because they are such tough, good people, you see."[303] For de Kruif, obstetrical hardiness was just one aspect of an ethnic toughness that could be ascribed to "primitive" whites as well as blacks.

White obstetrical hardiness is, however, exceptional, because a principal function of medical folklore about sex and reproduction has been to reinforce the traditional division between "primitive" blacks and "civilized" whites in biological terms. Africans and African Americans are combined into a single racial type that is said to demonstrate a special stoicism during childbirth. "I believe, given the same type of care, that the colored woman is on the whole better fitted to endure the ordeal of pregnancy and parturition than is her white sister," an American physician comments in 1932. Why? Because "the colored woman, because of her lessened sensibility to pain, is willing to endure a prolonged labor when a white woman would hours before be demanding relief."[304] In a similar vein, a 1947 report from South Africa observes that "the European requires assistance at delivery more often than the Bantu," since "it has been proved that the Bantu in her own home is a more efficient parturient than the European woman."[305] "During labour no form of analgesia is asked for or given," reads a 1944 report from Nigeria. "It is rare to hear more than the grunts of bearing down. Tears are uncommon and never serious in extent."[306] All blacks are to be counted among the "'stoic' savage races" that are characterized by a "lessened sensibility of the general nervous system to pain and shock."[307] The anatomical explanation ascribed ease of birth to smaller infants that fit through the smaller pelvic openings of nonwhite mothers. A smaller pelvic aperture could accommodate "the small size and softness of the head of the Negro."[308] Ease of birth thus implied a second and apparently "racial" anatomical characteristic of the infant.

The idea that pelvic measurements were a racial variable was challenged by a sociohistorical perspective that linked pelvic size with nutrition and work habits. The increased incidence of contracted pelvises typically associated with black women could also be attributed to the urbanization that caused workingwomen to contract rickets.[309] Indeed, "the overwhelming majority of pelvic contractions are due to childhood rickets," a socioeconomic factor the racial theory of pelvic size had overlooked.[310] With the passage of time, the idea that pelvic size was a racial variable became less influential. In 1941, for example, two authors questioned the obstetrical significance of pelvic size, given that "no clinical pelvic racial variation occurs that is not well compensated for by other factors." They also refer to the role of hearsay evidence in the medical discussion of pelvic measurements: "While a contracted pelvis is generally accepted as more frequent in the colored race, nature apparently produces a termination of pregnancy that is as effective as in the white patient."[311]

Obstetrical hardiness included other alleged aspects of black women's pregnancies and birthing experiences that seemed to imply biological advantages of evolutionary origin. "We believe," one physician wrote in 1924, "that labor is more readily induced in the negro than in the white woman."[312] The fact that the author apparently saw no need to offer a rationale for this judgment suggests that he saw it as a natural consequence of a racial biology his colleagues would recognize and understand. Such comparisons of robust Africans and fragile Europeans belong to the authentic language of colonial medicine, which transforms the unspoiled Noble Savage of the eighteenth century into the physiologically noble savage of the twentieth. Obstetrical hardiness became an influential racial folklore within medical theory and practice because it harmonized so well with the racial ideology that had already shaped Western thinking about racial differences. The smooth transition from limited observation to confident generalization was typical of Western medical reasoning about hardiness.

The doctrine of obstetrical hardiness was frequently contested in the medical literature. The idea that African American women generally experienced problem-free childbirth was contradicted, for example, by a "rather unexpected finding" in 1932 that they underwent longer labors.[313] Colonial physicians, too, were often capable of not romanticizing African patients into specimens of hardiness. "In spite of the rapid growth of antenatal clinics and hospital obstetrics," wrote the British doctor in Nigeria, "the vast majority of African women still have no medical obstetric attention. It is surprising the rarity with which emergencies are admitted but there is no knowledge of how many women die in the 'bush' from native medicine."[314] "There is a current myth which states that primitive women have babies with greater ease and less pain than do modern women," two authors wrote in *JAMA* in 1950. "Examination of the anthropologic literature shows that there is absolutely no factual basis for this notion."[315]

The substantially higher maternal mortality rate among black women was reported without reference to their alleged hardiness or stoicism.[316]

Reports of pelvic inflammatory disease emphasized its disproportionate effect on black patients: "Not only are such diseases more common in the negress, but the rapidity and extent of their ravages are incredibly greater. Even when the disease is checked, the restoration of normal anatomy and function, common in white women, is seldom observed."[317]

Claims that black women benefit from a relative immunity to nonobstetrical disorders of the reproductive organs fall under the category of gynecological hardiness. Endometriosis, a frequently painful disorder that involves the growth of endometrial tissue outside the uterus, is a clinically important disease that shows again how ideas about race and class can shape physicians' thinking about disease. The labeling of endometriosis as "a twentieth century disease"[318] already identifies it with a modern civilization that has frequently been assumed to incubate "white" diseases from which blacks supposedly enjoy a kind of racial protection. As the *Textbook of Black-Related Diseases* pointed out in 1975: "As recently as thirty years ago students of gynecology were taught that endometriosis in Black women was practically unknown. This led one to believe that there might be an actual racial immunity to the condition; and indeed, one rarely saw endometriosis in the Black population. It was also observed concurrently that the incidence of endometriosis in the White indigent patient was much less than in the private White patient. This suggested that more than simple racial immunity played a part and that contributing influences such as malnutrition, pelvic inflammatory disease, and early and frequent childbearing might be important considerations."[319]

The gradual discovery that endometriosis was not "a white woman's disease" was also addressed by William F. Mengert in 1966. "[U]ntil about 15 years ago," he wrote, "I did not believe that endometriosis as recognized in the Caucasian ever appeared in the Negro." Subsequent experience had persuaded him that the protective factor was earlier pregnancies among black women.[320] While Mengert ascribes perceptual error to physicians in the case of softheaded black infants, he treats endometriosis differently. In this case, he suggests, physicians saw much less pathology in black women, not because they were biased, but because the pathology did not exist. It was left to a later commentator to offer a different, and less flattering, explanation of white physician behavior. Socially conditioned to regard all black women as promiscuous, "gynecologists would almost automatically diagnose a black woman with symptoms of endometriosis as having pelvic inflammatory disease" as a consequence of her sexual behavior.[321] Dorothy Roberts reiterated this interpretation as late as 1997; rather than think of black women as vulnerable to endometriosis, "gynecologists are more likely to diagnose Black women as having pelvic inflammatory disease, which they often treat with sterilization."[322]

The myth of black hyperfertility expresses a legendary reproductive hardiness that dates from the early encounters of Europeans and Africans during the Age of Exploration. Its longevity has been guaranteed by the Western fascination with African sexuality that has combined erotic and reproductive powers into a single biological force. Fantasies about super-fertile black women became deeply embedded in Western thinking about racial differences.

The medically and socially harmful consequences of the widespread pre-occupation with black fertility have been profound. These responses have included forced sterilizations, medically hazardous birth control schemes employing the insertion of subcutaneous Norplant capsules or Depo-Provera injections, unnecessary hysterectomies, and possibly the denial of pain relief to drug-abusing black women who are giving birth.[323] System-atic medical abuses of this kind have been possible because they have been regarded as antidotes to irresponsible black childbearing that threatens so-cial stability. In addition, the fertility stereotype operates in a synergetic relationship with medical stereotypes about racial pain thresholds and the black child. It would be surprising if racially inequitable pain relief does not extend into hospital birthing rooms.[324] Maternal drug abuse, generally as-sociated with black women, intensifies this response by creating powerful images of the morally deficient mother and the medically damaged child: "Public expectations of 'blighted' children fuel controversial punitive poli-cies directed toward addicted mothers."[325]

There is evidence of the continuing influence of the hardiness paradigm in obstetrical medicine. Stereotypes of racial immunity to pain may help to account for the lesser degree of pain relief (oligoanesthesia) adminis-tered to patients of color who are giving birth. As late as 1998, anesthe-sia was being denied to women during childbirth in California hospitals based on their ability to pay in advance, a stipulation that would affect many women of color.[326] Los Angeles County eventually paid $24 million to settle claims filed from 1992 to 1997 by poor women on Medi-Cal who were forced to have vaginal deliveries rather than more costly caesarian procedures, thereby crippling or killing dozens of women and children. In a similar vein, black and Hispanic women are much more likely than whites to undergo vaginal breech deliveries rather than the safer caesarian sec-tions.[327] Employing a medical euphemism, the researchers who conducted this study refer to "unmeasured factors or processes" in order to account for the endangered status of women of color. They make no attempt to associate their findings with ideas about racial biology that might contribute to an understanding of the doctor-patient interactions that produce racially differential results.

The decline of overtly racial biology in the obstetrical and gynecological literature does not signify the end of racial biology as a factor in medical thinking and practice. To assume otherwise would require us to imagine a medical culture that has been severed from its own history and from the society within which it operates. This is why it is not surprising that *JAMA* once suggested that pregnancy after menopause was subject to racial variation.[328] It could not be otherwise in a world in which *every* human biological phenomenon is subject to racial differentiation.

4. Medical Apartheid, Internal Colonialism, and the Task of American Psychiatry

INTRODUCTION

This section of the book presents two related topics: the African American medical condition as a form of "internal colonialism" and how American psychiatry has treated African Americans over the past century. This exploration of American "internal colonialism" and its consequences for white psychiatrists and black patients precedes the book's analysis of race and American psychiatry for three reasons. First, the comprehensive demoralization that inheres in the colonial experience makes colonial status a state of mind and an emotional complex as well as an economic and political condition. The most dramatic description of the emotional predicaments in which colonial subjects find themselves remains Frantz Fanon's *Black Skin, White Masks* (1952). While Fanon focuses on the black colonial subject, this book examines the predicaments of both black patients and the white psychiatrists who have often been unprepared to help them. Second, among physicians it is the psychiatrist one might expect to be most inclined to practice the kind of self-examination we associate with conscientious anthropologists who enter cultural worlds to which they do not belong. Whether inside or outside the medical realm, race relations that allow people to share tasks and experiences in civil and productive ways depend in part on introspection and the self-knowledge it makes possible. White psychiatrists constitute an overwhelming majority within this medical specialty, and offering competent treatment to black patients requires an understanding of the social and emotional barriers that separate American blacks and whites. Finally, there is the role of the black psychiatrist, who for many years has served as an advocate for black humanity in the broadest sense of that term. A primary social task of the black psychiatrist, as we shall see, has been to insist that the minds of black people are as deep and complex as those of whites, and that blacks should have access to the full range of psychotherapies that are available to serve white patients. Indeed, the idea that blacks are less complex human organisms than whites is as "colonial" a doctrine as one can imagine.

The idea that African Americans have been subjected to a form of colonial medicine will seem improbable to many readers. Colonialism, after all, has been associated with the domination and exploitation of people who are geographically and culturally remote from our society. Similarly, the use of the term *apartheid* to describe African American status in the United States today seems counterintuitive. We assume that *apartheid* was a form of South African racism, roughly comparable to the racist Jim Crow system in the American South, and that is now extinct. What is more, the application of these ostensibly extreme terms to the world of medicine in particular seems harsh and overly judgmental. Surely, one might argue, the racial integration one sees today in hospitals, medical schools, and physicians' waiting rooms is remote from the practices of colonial medicine. Today, we tend to assume that most African Americans enjoy legal protections and an economic security that provide them with access to doctors and medical technology on a par with other ethnic groups. To assign colonial medical status, or colonial status in its larger sense, to black Americans in this day and age might therefore seem an anachronistic and misleading portrait of the African American condition.

There are, however, good reasons to argue otherwise, as previous authors have noted. Andrew Hacker's *Two Nations: Black and White, Separate, Hostile, Unequal* (1992) made this sort of argument two decades ago, employing the term *apartheid* and describing a "pervasive and penetrating" separation of the races that has cast African Americans as "aliens" in their own country.[1] The legal scholar Dorothy Roberts has shown how the historically unprecedented mass incarceration of African American men has produced a state of "political subordination" while inflicting "devastating collateral damage on black communities." Other scholars have equated black distrust of the criminal justice system with "a kind of civic isolation, in which the workings of the state are seen as alien forces to be avoided rather than services to be employed."[2] The Harvard sociologist Orlando Patterson pointed out in 2009 that, outside the prison complex, "we still live in a racially fragmented society," and that "in the privacy of homes and neighborhoods we are more segregated that in the Jim Crow era."[3]

The "colonial" status of African Americans has been complicated by the separation of this population into dramatically unequal social classes. While it is hard to imagine black professionals and other members of the black middle class as colonized "natives," no such difficulty prevents us from thinking of the so-called black "underclass" as a "colonial" population. Black and white commentators alike have argued that the "internal colonialism" most evident in the racially segregated ghettos of American cities is in some ways no different in kind from the classic colonial scenarios we have come to associate with the exploitation and brutalization of black African and other dominated ethnic populations.

Opponents of the colonial thesis might thus argue that medical care is linked to social class. It is true that the black middle class, like the white middle class, has better access to medical services than the black or white poor. Nevertheless, what separates the African American relationship to the medical world from that of whites is that elevated social status does not eliminate racial stigma and estrangement that has persisted since emancipation. African American estrangement from the medical profession has differed in important ways from the similarly dysfunctional situation of marginalized whites who, like marginal blacks, have been neglected, left medically ignorant, and have received inferior care.

In fact, most African Americans do not inhabit the same medical universe as the majority of whites who are not poor or indigent. Black and white patients may attend many of the same medical facilities, yet they will frequently have different attitudes toward medical treatments, experience different levels of stress, and have different kinds of relationships with predominantly white (or international) medical personnel. We have already confirmed that racially differential diagnosis and treatment are widespread in American medicine. Indeed, the estrangement of African Americans from the health care system in the United States has been cited so often in the medical and public health literatures that its deleterious consequences are simply accepted as a fact of life in American medicine. To be sure, the "Negro medical ghetto" described in *Pediatrics* in 1949 is gone.[4] Yet "medical apartheid," according to the *Journal of the American Medical Association*, still existed in the United States in 1991. Having described the health hazards of the South African "townships" and "homelands" reserved for blacks, these authors ask: "Who can read this description and fail to recognize the haunting similarity to America's inner cities, the *colonias* of south Texas, or our Native American reservations?"[5] As late as 2002, the African American physician-authors of a monumental history of American medical racism were citing the 'health colonization' of inner-city and largely Black communities.[6] But the relevance of the medical colonial model is not limited to the black residents of the inner cities. Alienation from our medical system has become one aspect of the African American condition that extends across socioeconomic classes.

The colonial and apartheid analogies are useful because they convey the stigmatized status, the dependency, the vulnerability, and a degree of estrangement from the societal mainstream that remain a significant dimension of the African American experience in general and the basis of the African American medical condition in particular. A public health policy that conflates the medical status of blacks and whites as though they constituted a single patient population is, therefore, sociologically inaccurate, strategically counterproductive, and morally indefensible. An important factor in this regard is the fact that traditional racial images of African Americans continue to influence how laypersons and doctors think of them in relation to sickness and health.

Colonialism is the imposition of political and economic domination upon a subordinate and racially stigmatized population. This means that colonial status is more than a state of political and economic submission that is imposed upon a subject people. Colonial status means that one has been identified and classified as a racially inferior type of human being. Colonial subjects are "primitives" or "savages" who have failed to climb the evolutionary ladder in the manner of "civilized" peoples. This degraded status distorts all human relations between colonizers and the colonized. The dominant group legitimates various forms of surveillance and discipline by invoking the inferior capacities of the dominated, who may respond with various forms of resistance. "Colonial domination," said Franz Fanon, "gives rise to and continues to dictate a whole complex of resentful behavior and of refusal on the part of the colonized."[7] As we will see, the resentments that result from a colonial imbalance of power have an especially profound effect upon medical relationships between white doctors and black patients.

The idea that African Americans have experienced a form of colonial domination in the United States has been expressed repeatedly over the past century, and especially during the 1960s, at a time when open black self-assertion took on a dramatic new role in American public life. The "colonial" status of African Americans during the era of Jim Crow segregation is clear in retrospect and was evident to some contemporary observers. In his famous polemic *The Mis-Education of the Negro* (1933), the black historian Carter G. Woodson invoked the theme of white colonial dominion over blacks to shame his people out of what he saw as their lethargy during this period. American Negroes, he says, are "the most docile and tractable people on earth," and it is no wonder that "European nations of foresight are sending some of their brightest minds to the United States to observe the Negro in 'inaction' in order to learn how to deal likewise with Negroes in their colonies."[8] In a similar vein, the black sociologist E. Franklin Frazier described the segregated schools of this era as a form of internal colonialism: "The relation of the Negro heads of schools and of other segregated institutions depending upon white support to the Negro educated class amounted to what is known in the field of colonial administration as a system of 'indirect rule.'"[9] Both men regarded American Negroes as comparable to the colonized Negroes of Africa.

White interpretations of the "colonial" status of American blacks have come from both ends of the racial political spectrum over the past century. Identifying black people as the equivalent of colonial subjects required the "Africanization" of African Americans as both biological and cultural subjects. In 1928, to take one of many examples, Alex Hrdlicka, editor of the *American Journal of Physical Anthropology* and even today a revered figure in anthropological circles, noted in an article on "The Full-Blood American Negro" that the subjects he approached "were not eager to be measured. It is quite a different thing to measure among the pliant, trusting savage, and then among the semi-civilized, suspicious, scattered free laborers and servants of a big city."[10] The difference between black American and black African "savages" was that the cultural development of the latter remained arrested at the level of ignorance and innocence, while their counterparts in the New World remained embittered by the fetters of Jim Crow segregation and thus refused to divulge their thoughts and feelings to inquisitive whites. That this estrangement between colonizer and colonized applied to both of these black populations was noted in 1932 by a South African doctor: "There is in the States a persistent effort by the negro to conceal his thoughts and feelings—there appears to be a similar diminishing contact in South Africa also."[11] Colonial status was, therefore, a state of mutual estrangement between puzzled whites and resentful blacks, a dysfunctional relationship that persists to this day in the United States and other multiracial societies both inside and outside of the medical world.

This estrangement and other forms of "Africanization" of the American Negro became a standard feature of the American psychiatric literature during the first four decades of the twentieth century. Constant invocations of African "primitivism" in the media and popular culture, from *Tarzan of the Apes* (1912) to the images of political and medical catastrophes in Africa that often appear in newspapers and on television screens today, connect African Americans to the continent of their origin in ways that have haunted and embarrassed them over many years. "At the time that I was growing up," James Baldwin wrote in 1961, "Negroes in this country were taught to be ashamed of Africa." The Negro, the white sociologist Thomas F. Pettigrew commented in 1964, "has shared much of the naïve conception of Africa as the dark continent of wild and naked savages."[12] These pathological images of Africa have been conjoined with the theme of medical disaster since the nineteenth century, from the disease-infested jungles of that era to the ravages of AIDS and the army of orphans it has left behind. This association between Africa and disease is the biological dimension of "colonial" identity in the modern age.

Descriptions of the African American condition as one of colonial submission and confinement peaked during the 1960s in commentaries from both white and black activists and observers. In his influential book *Crisis in Black and White* (1964), which includes a chapter on "The Revolt against 'Welfare Colonialism,'" Charles Silberman offered a portrayal of the inhabitants of American inner cities that could have come right out of Franz Fanon's account of the oppressive colonial medicine practiced in Algeria during the French war of occupation.[13] "It is not surprising," Silberman writes, "that the 'child-adults' who inhabit the slums hate the colonial administrators who come to 'uplift' them through 'social discipline,' or that they try to sabotage the disciplinarians' program."[14] The message he delivered upended the prevailing assumptions of liberal paternalism in a shocking way:

> The result is that the do-gooders, to their amazement and consternation, find themselves attacked instead of welcomed. When, a few years ago, Mayor Robert F. Wagner of New York City proudly announced a bold new program of mental health for Harlem, he was greeted by an explosion of anger; Harlem leaders forgot their own bickering long enough to unite in an attack on "welfare colonialism" and a demand that any new programs be developed by the community itself. In city after city, in fact, supposedly supine Negroes have been turning on their benefactors with such slogans as "we refuse to be planned for as though we were children," "we're tired of being guinea pigs in sociological experiments," and the like.[15]

A similar "colonial" scenario played out two decades later in New York City, as public health officials undertook to rescue African Americans from the ravages of AIDS. The white authorities were unpleasantly surprised when they encountered massive resistance among black citizens to a proposed pilot needle-exchange program. Even the black police commissioner, Benjamin Ward, protested on the grounds that as a black man he felt "a particular sensitivity to doctors conducting experiments, and they too frequently seem to be conducted against blacks." "Why," asked the Reverend Reginald Williams of the Addicts Rehabilitation Center in East Harlem, "must we again be the guinea pigs in this genocidal mentality?"[16] The medical missionaries who came to save Harlem from its bad habits did not recognize the nature of the colonial drama, intensified by its medical theme and the catastrophe of black drug abuse, in which they were playing a starring role. In fact, the authority to protect the public health is an intrinsically "colonial" authority precisely because it includes the authority to classify (stigmatize) and quarantine (segregate). The updated medical colonialism that came to Harlem to deal with AIDS arrived long after the stigmatizing and segregating of Harlem's black population were already a fait accompli. The new element on this occasion—the modern face of medical colonialism—was the combination of good intentions and the naïve disappointment that resulted when the expected interracial collaboration was rejected by its intended beneficiaries. What the white public health officials had not included in their strategy was a way to engage and disarm a profound black distrust of medical authority of which they seem to have been unaware. During Jim Crow this estranged relationship had been obvious to many white physicians, who confessed their ignorance of what black people were thinking and feeling and called upon black personnel to bridge the racial divide. In the 1980s, however, this sort of candor—and, therefore, any official acknowledgement of medical colonialism—was out of the question.

Over the course of the past two centuries, medical colonialists have arrived with good intentions and the promise of expertise than can benefit the "native," "primitive," or "underdeveloped" people they have come to serve. In the modern era, expertise is the ideal form of authority because it can dispense with overtly coercive methods in favor of the persuasive techniques that are compatible with liberal democratic norms. But what if black people feel threatened and insulted by white experts? As the movement for black self-assertion gained momentum during the civil rights decade of the 1960s, black intellectuals and others bitterly criticized a white social policy intelligentsia that was now sounding the alarm about the problems of the urban black ghettoes. By the mid-1960s, previously "supine Negroes" were now revolting against what they regarded as a new type of colonial mastery that wielded the findings of sociological research studies rather than cruder coercive techniques. A resentful and sometimes bitter critique of social science and its alleged defamatory effects on the image of black people reached a crescendo following the publication in 1965 of Daniel Patrick Moynihan's government-sponsored report on *The Negro Family: A Case for National Action.*[17] Even politically moderate elder statesmen of the black intelligentsia protested what they described as the intrusions of white social scientists into the lives of black people who resented this sort of attention. Ralph Ellison denounced what he called "specialists in the 'Negro problem'" who operated "that feverish industry dedicated to telling Negroes who and what they are."[18] The writer Albert Murray riffed on the African theme, identifying the intrusive social scientist as a new version of the "white hunter" who "is regarded as an expert on U.S. jungle manners and mores, but his natives are no longer referred to as savages. They are 'culturally deprived [i.e., non-white!] minorities.'" The most rigidly segregated space in the United States, Murray said, was to be found in the "behavioral science surveys, studies, and statistics" that portrayed black people as afflicted and inferior. "There is little reason," he concluded, "why Negroes should not regard contemporary social science theory and technique with anything except the most unrelenting suspicion."[19]

The idea that African Americans are colonial subjects appears in the writings of both black and white commentators during this turbulent period. The most prominent black psychologist of his generation, Kenneth B. Clark, stated: "The dark ghettos are social, political, educational and—above all—economic colonies. Their inhabitants are subject peoples, victims of the greed, cruelty, insensitivity, guilt, and fear of their masters."[20] In *The Crisis of the Negro Intellectual* (1967), Harold Cruse describes one generation of black intellectuals as victims of "the most thorough brainwashing that Western civilization has ever perpetrated on the non-white colonized mentality." Black Americans, he says, have never fully accepted the fact that they have been subjected to "a special kind of North American domestic colonialism."[21] In his widely read manifesto *Black Power: The Politics of Liberation in America* (1967), the radical activist Stokely Carmichael titled one chapter "White Power: The Colonial Situation" and argued that "the social effects of colonialism are to degrade and to dehumanize the subjected black man" in the United States and elsewhere.[22]

White sympathizers also endorsed the idea that American blacks were living in colonial conditions. The radical journalist I.F. Stone called the

African American predicament "a unique case of colonialism, an instance of internal imperialism, an underdeveloped people in our very midst."[23] William Ryan, a Boston College sociologist who became the most vocal white critic of the Moynihan Report, played sardonically upon the theme of Darkest Africa by calling the sociologists' analysis of black social distress "the popular new sport of Savage Discovery," whereby "savages are being discovered in great profusion in the Northern ghetto."[24] Ryan's intention was to mock the Tarzan-era images he employed in jest and thereby separate Black America from the traditional racist caricatures of Black Africa. The same rhetorical technique of mockery-by-imitation of colonial intentions appears almost a half century later in Robin D. G. Kelley's *Yo Mama's Dysfunktional: Fighting the Culture Wars in Urban America* (1997). Criticizing the progressive social scientists of the late 1960s who attempted to rescue poor blacks from their status as mere victims, Kelley casts them in a colonial role in which they surely did not see themselves: "With the zeal of colonial missionaries, these liberal and often radical ethnographers (mostly white men) set out to explore the newly discovered concrete jungles."[25] Finding caricatured versions of Africa in the ghetto experience—both white and black—was as easy as stepping off the train at Harlem's 125th Street station and ogling the "natives" in front of the Apollo Theater. The more difficult problem, then as now, was distinguishing between the anthropological observer capable of contributing to knowledge and the anthropological voyeur whose insights did not transcend stereotypes.

"AFRICANIZING" THE BLACK IMAGE

The images of "savages" and "concrete jungles" that persist in American racial discourse show that African Americans have never been allowed to shed their involuntary role as imaginary African "natives." This image has established itself among even racially sophisticated black and white Americans. In 1966 the civil rights leader Bayard Rustin called America's ghettoes "man-made jungles." In a speech delivered on October 29, 1965, the Reverend Martin Luther King, Jr. employed the jungle analogy as follows: "The Negro family lived in Africa in nature's jungle and subdued the hostile environment. In the United States, it has lived in a man-made social and psychological jungle which it could not subdue."[26] For many years these images and locutions evoking a primeval "Africa" have led parallel yet different lives inside the heads of black and white Americans. While caricatures of blacks as "African" primitives have long served whites as a form of entertainment, they have had a traumatizing effect on the many African Americans who have been acutely aware of Africa's image as a continent of savages. The black historian C. Eric Lincoln described this disturbing experience in 1968:

> "The Picture" is a universal experience in the life of Negro Americans. It is the picture of a black savage with a bone through his nose, hoops in his ears and discs in his lips. There are feathers around his knees, and circulets around his ankles. His teeth are filed to points, and his face is horribly marked with tribal scars. His countenance sags under the weight of ignorance and stupidity.[27]

This racist caricature has been replaced by a variety of softer versions that continue to "Africanize" American blacks in sometimes subtle and unexpected ways. (President Barack Obama was caricatured in this manner on the Internet during 2009.) Indeed, we have already seen that blacks as well as whites have employed these stereotypes about themselves. For example, referring to young black males as "an endangered species," as one black psychologist did in his influential book, inadvertently naturalizes these men into an imaginary "African" universe of primordial life forms and pitiless evolutionary competition in which their human complexity dissolves.[28]

The "colonial" status of African Americans is due in large measure to these deeply rooted associations with an imaginary African world. Bringing the benefits of civilization to the "dark ghetto"—the pathological urban form of the "dark continent"—has been a colonial project in all but name since the 1960s. These attempts at social engineering—and the paternalism that has helped to limit their effectiveness—make sense to many whites precisely because they appear to target a social disorder of African origin. "Outsiders consider a place like this a kind of zoo or jungle," one black Chicago clergyman remarked in 1964; "they mean well, but they choke us. It seemed to us that any effort would be futile unless our own people could direct it. . . ."[29] We must also recognize that images of zoos and jungles connote more than social disorder. These are also biological images that convey doubts about the evolutionary capacity of "slum-dwellers" as a species. In retrospect, it can be surprising to read some of the language white liberal reformers have used to describe ghetto blacks. Theodore H. ("Teddy") White, one of the most popular journalists of his day, won a Pulitzer Prize for *The Making of the President, 1960*. In the successor to this best seller, which includes a chapter on the summer race riots of 1964, White addresses in a loaded biological idiom what he calls "the awful Negro tragedy" of the urban ghettos. The "collapsing"

Negro community represents "biological anarchy—a decomposition of family life and family discipline" that includes "a pattern of mating and breeding" that imposes an intolerable burden on American society. From "the zoological tenements" in the "concrete jungle" come the "junior savages" who prey upon "the decent Negro families" trapped in the ghetto.[30] The reckless fusing of biological essence and social status is summed up in the grotesque idea of "zoological tenements," whose denizens would seem to require the services of veterinarians rather than doctors. The extremism of this language reminds us that the "dark ghetto" is as exotic an environment in its own way as are the jungles of the "dark continent." Colonial status, in summary, combines a racially coded biological essence with a subordinate and degraded role in the social hierarchy. This is why the "colonial" status of African Americans is especially evident in the medical context.

Colonial status is a state of mind that can persist over generations even as upward social mobility occurs, as in the case of African Americans who have remained estranged from a "white" medical system even as their social status has risen. The colonial medical predicament this group has experienced over the past century has promoted estrangement by putting them on the defensive against the complaints of public health personnel, who have claimed that they were dirty, infectious, and irredeemably flawed in a biological sense. Mordant humor about the syphilis-ridden Negro was common in the medical literature prior to the Second World War, and it is unlikely that an awareness of this sort of commentary by white doctors was limited to black physicians. The mandatory sickle-cell testing laws passed in twelve states and the District of Columbia during the early 1970s had demoralizing and destructive effects on black people that the African American physician Charles F. Whitten described at the time in the *New England Journal of Medicine*. "Some of the statutes do not require concomitant education and counseling," he noted, "so that there is no real opportunity for those affected to understand the implications of having sickle-cell trait, or to be relieved of the anxiety and apprehension that this knowledge frequently engenders."[31] Many people (and some doctors) falsely believed that carrying the trait was equivalent to having the disease. By subjecting the entire black population to testing and implicitly limiting reproductive rights, white legislators and public health officials conveyed to blacks the message that the entire "race" was sick. By exaggerating the incidence and importance of sickle-cell anemia, ostensibly concerned whites "failed to dissociate themselves from the contagious disease model through which the black body had been understood since the nineteenth century."[32] The stigmatizing potential of this public discussion reached a nadir in 1968 when the great chemist and Nobel laureate Linus Pauling wrote in the *UCLA Law Review* that young sickle-cell carriers should be "tattooed on the forehead" to prevent them from "falling in love with one another" and having diseased children.[33]

African Americans experienced the public discussion of sickle-cell disease as a violation of their privacy. Many found the sudden white interest in a black health issue suspicious. There was something unseemly about the haste with which white lawmakers and doctors rushed to enact legislation and testing programs whose disadvantages for blacks had not been thought out in advance of their implementation. The revelations about the Tuskegee Syphilis Experiment announced in 1972 only exacerbated an already tense situation. White legislators' anxieties about bringing the black population under medical control was evident at the Senate Subcommittee on Health hearings on sickle cell that were held on November 11 and 12, 1971, where Senator Edward Kennedy addressed the following question to a black doctor from Los Angeles: "What is the willingness of the members of the community to take these tests? Do you find that there is an interest in it? Are they willing to take these tests if it is given at a decent time and under adequate kinds of circumstances and in clean facilities? . . . Do they want to know about sickle cell anemia?"[34] In these remarks the liberal senator from Massachusetts expressed the white doctor's traditional concern about the noncompliant black patient whose ignorance or carelessness will frustrate the doctor's best-laid plans.

The racial biology that underlies African American "colonial" status has included an evolutionary narrative that appeared in the medical literature as accepted doctrine during the first half of the twentieth century. The idea that there is an evolutionary link between black humans and animals appears repeatedly. An American physician argues, for example, that "the negro pelvis shows a reversion toward the type found in the lower animals."[35] The "comparative rarity of hemorrhoids in the negro" exemplifies "an immunity common to primitive races" and "the lower mammals."[36] Other publications conjoin blacks and animals through skin diseases or the shape of the teeth.[37] It is not hard to see how the idea that black and white human beings had evolved at different rates might affect a doctor's treatment of his black patients. A gynecologist in Dallas, while conceding that he was "not biologist enough to say" whether "the negro" was somehow "nearer to the childhood of the race," was nonetheless willing to offer his own clinical experience and that of some peers as impressionistic evidence that indicated retarded Negro evolution. He as well as other clinicians, he said, had found that the Negro's "nervous system exhibits a lessened sensibility to pain and shock, and that the pure black type is the safest surgical risk to be found in our hospitals. . . ."[38] The undertreatment of pain in black patients remains a problem to this day.[39] Medical publications reporting this racially differential oligoanesthesia never refer to the history of racist thinking about pain susceptibility in the earlier medical literature. It should be emphasized that the introduction of evolutionary racism into medical thinking came, not from racist eccentrics, but from people with medical and academic credentials.

AMERICAN PSYCHIATRY AS RACIAL MEDICINE

The colonial subject is a primitive whose political role is to illustrate the absolute difference between the "savage" and the "civilized." This primitive status is reinforced in the biological realm by the colonial racist idea that the primitive individual amounts to little more than the needs and limitations of his or her body. "To suffer from a phobia of Negroes," says Franz Fanon, "is to be afraid of the biological. For the Negro is only biological." "The Negro symbolizes the biological."[40] A South African doctor reports in 1932 a colleague's opinion that "the Native is hopelessly deficient in logical processes, and that his energy is wholly absorbed in merely bodily functions, that there is stunted mental development."[41] To this day the predicament of symbolic entrapment in the black body remains. Paul Gilroy describes "Blacks who live 'in the castle of their skin' and have struggled to escape the biologization of their socially and politically constructed subordination," to "escape from bestial status into a recognized humanity."[42] This is why "black dominance" in popular global sports is, in the last analysis, a form of colonial entrapment that equates black talent with the black body and its apparently supernormal capacities.[43] African American dominance of professional basketball and East African dominance of distance running offer enormous global audiences the most dramatic, quantitative, and (therefore) persuasive demonstrations of racial differences to which modern people are exposed.[44] Survey data suggest that many white Americans endorse a genetic explanation of racial athletic aptitude.[45] Indeed, given the traditional identification of black people with their bodies, it would be remarkable if this were not the case. A major premise of this book is that the tendency to interpret perceived racial differences in biological terms remains the dominant paradigm in medical thinking about race.

Twentieth-century medical authors have often interpreted black people, their disorders, and their temperaments in terms of their physicality, and this has reinforced their "colonial" status as medical subjects whose physical organism is their primary anthropological characteristic. A psychiatrist at the Georgia State Sanitarium thus wrote in 1914 that "the negro race" is "active, boisterous, restless, manifesting increased muscular activity,"[46] implying that black self-expression is muscular rather than mental. The black men chosen for a study of vital capacity reported in *JAMA* in 1926 "were picked for their strength and ability to do hard labor."[47] In 1929 the *Transactions of the American Gynecological Society* refers to "the active and outdoor occupations habitual with the negro" as a possible factor involved in the rarity of gallstones in Negroes.[48] These medical authors make it clear that the physicality and the labor status of the Negro, and what they imply about his life and limitations, have affected how doctors think about him as a medical subject. As late as 1984, a cardiologist writing in the *American Heart Journal* refers to a clinical population of "muscular black males" in a study of enzyme levels and the diagnosis of myocardial infarction in black subjects.[49]

The fact that references to "muscular white males" do not appear in the medical literature suggests that some doctors, and perhaps many doctors, respond to the physical endowments of their patients in racially differential ways. Physical qualities that situate black people within the worlds of manual labor or athletic competition can affect how their doctors perceive and treat them as medical subjects. We have already heard my former student describe what she heard about black athletes from a medical student in Texas. It is hard to imagine how a medical student could have found a scientifically valid genetic basis for racial athletic aptitude, given that no scientist on earth has managed to accomplish this feat. The fact that he believed in the racial biology he conveyed to his tutees is what really matters. With media images of black athletic superiority filling his head, this young man translated his layman's grasp of genetics into ostensibly scientific conclusions he confidently transmitted to his even younger charges.

In summary, the role of physicality and what it seems to imply about black people "colonizes" these patients in a way that does not apply to white patients. A white doctor from Arkansas writing in the early 1950s expressed the "colonial" response to black physicality as follows: "I believe in strekt [sic] segregation. The average negroe [sic] is incapable of competing, mentally, with the average white person. Neither is the average white person capable of competing, physically, with the average negroe [sic]."[50]

Here is the segregationist dichotomy between the superior and inferior racial types who occupy dominant and submissive roles in a colonial society. One aspect of the African American predicament is that more literate and authoritative white professionals have promoted this distinction using more sophisticated language. Among these medical men have been psychiatrists from whom one might have expected a more sophisticated grasp of their own behavior.

THE RACIAL PRIMITIVE IN AMERICAN PSYCHIATRY

The "colonized" status of African Americans was evident in American psychiatry for most of the twentieth century. The idea that the Negro American was a primitive pervaded medical and social science commentaries prior to the Second World War. Psychiatric presentations of black people sometimes amounted to little more than recycled versions of contemporary racist folklore. In the view of a contributor to the first volume of *The Psychoanalytic Review* (1914), "the student of psychology working in the United States has access to a people the average level of whose development is lower than the white race and which furnishes numerous individuals showing psychological aspects quite similar to those of the savage." Negro psychology represented "a primitive type."[51] "It appears," a Georgia psychiatrist wrote the same year, "that the negro mind does not dwell upon unpleasant subjects; he is irresponsible, unthinking, easily aroused to happiness, and his unhappiness is transitory, disappearing as a child's when other interests attract his attention. He is happy-go-lucky not philosophical." Logical reasoning, introspection, and depression were foreign to the Negro personality.[52] "Less than three hundred years ago," the *American Journal of Psychiatry* reported in 1921, "the alien ancestors of most of the families of this race were savages or cannibals in the jungles of Central Africa. From this very primitive level they were unwillingly brought to these shores and into an environment of higher civilization for which the biological development of the race had not made adequate preparation."[53]

The consequences for the Negro of this involuntary migration were a reputation for inferior intelligence, sexual promiscuity, a fear of darkness, superstition, and a devotion to music and motion that produced dance-floor performances "suggestive of dances and orgies of the original African tribes."[54] Black people's attempts to speak sophisticated English made them sound ridiculous.[55] In 1935, a contributor to the *American Journal of Psychiatry* wrote that the followers of the charismatic Harlem preacher Father Divine are "not far removed from their savage ancestors with their primitive, tribal interest in the . . . more bizarre portions of religion."[56] A psychiatrist refers in 1941 to "the lower level of civilization and culture of the negro race, particularly in the South, and the comparative simplicity of their adaptations."[57] Life in the average American Negro community, the chief of psychiatric research at the Veterans Administration in Washington, DC, writes in 1954, "tends to be at a relatively primitive level of little restraint."[58] These depictions of American Negroes are colonial renderings of people whose American identity is essentially invisible, since it is dissolved in the constant images of savages and primitive tribes the psychiatrists had absorbed from racist images in the contemporary media. As the African American psychiatrist Rutherford B. Stevens put it in 1947, "many psychiatrists have been affected by the motion picture and newspaper portrayal of the Negro."[59]

Colonial commentaries on "natives" and "primitives" are typically animated by the instinctive self-confidence of the white supremacist, and some of this self-assurance is evident in the psychiatric commentaries cited previously. At the same time, among the striking characteristics of the psychiatric literature on black people during the Jim Crow era are the frequent confessions by these doctors that they simply do not understand their black patients. The dominated native who seems to submit to white authority can also be a sullen and evasive colonial subject who keeps his thoughts and feelings to himself.

The problematic Negro patient was a familiar figure in the medical and psychiatric literatures during the first half of the twentieth century. "The Negro is a peculiar and complex compound in temperament," the *Southern Medical Journal* declared in 1919; "if any psychiatrist has ever been able to determine his mental classification, the South awaits the verdict."[60] Three decades later it appeared little progress had been made. As two psychiatrists put it in 1947: "Investigators have found the Negroid personality hard to evaluate, the distinction between psychologic and psychopathologic relationships to be frequently obscure and the differentiation of the various psychoses difficult of accurate clinical appraisal."[61] The sociologist Gunnar Myrdal had pointed to "a mask behind which (the Negroes) conceal their true selves," and the best efforts of many white psychiatrists were defeated by this defensive screen. As Dr. Stevens, the black psychiatrist, commented with muted irony: "It would be extremely helpful if a magic formula for gaining rapport with the Negro patient could be presented to the white psychiatrist."[62] Alas, no such formula existed at the time, and the racial history of American psychiatry since the Second World War has not produced a solution to this problem beyond a greater awareness that it exists.

The Second World War marked a turning point in race relations within American society that left its own mark on the psychiatric profession. The military service of a million black men, even in racially segregated units, raised the civic status of African Americans in a way that made it impossible for whites to dismiss their demands for greater civic and economic rights in the traditional fashion. The drafting of these black men into the army and navy brought them into contact with white psychiatrists who were responsible for promoting their adjustment to military life to aid the war effort. Postwar psychiatric publications such as "Mental Illness among Negro Troops Overseas" and "Adjustment Problems of Selected Negro Soldiers" are instructive accounts of the difficulties white psychiatrists encountered in these relationships with black men who had good reasons to doubt the competence and good will of their white therapists. Black men who had already served under racist officers were not inclined to trust white authority figures of any kind.

Psychiatric assessments of black soldiers by white psychiatrists were impaired by factors of which they were often unaware.[63] Making white medical personnel aware of how race relations go wrong is a task that occasionally falls to a black professional who is better qualified to offer instruction in this regard. In the case of how to devise measures to prevent AIDS among African Americans, the breakthrough analysis was "AIDS in Blackface," by the Yale law professor Harlon Dalton, who served as a member of the National Commission on AIDS. The indispensable analysis of the predicament of the white military psychiatrist of the 1940s is Rutherford Stevens's "Racial Aspects of Emotional Problems of Negro Soldiers," in which he notes that one white psychiatric colleague with "a rather dogmatic opinion concerning the Negro" had "admitted that his knowledge was the result of eight years of contact with his office maid, who was a disciple of the [charismatic preacher] Father Divine." While this may appear to be an extreme case, the sheer naïveté of many of Stevens's white colleagues concerning the lives and mind-sets of their black fellow citizens should not be underestimated. Many military psychiatrists "felt insecure when dealing with the emotional problems of Negro soldiers," because they did not know black people and had absorbed false ideas about racial differences.[64]

The sharp contrast between "white" and "black" diagnoses of black soldiers and their problems at this time is evident when one compares Stevens's analysis of black troops with that of Lieutenant Colonel Herbert S. Ripley and Major Stewart Wolf, authors of "Mental Illness among Negro Troops Overseas," which appeared in the *American Journal of Psychiatry* along with Stevens's article in 1947. Ripley and Wolf cared enough about race relations to publish their observations in a professional journal, and were among the more thoughtful white psychiatrists who examined black troops during the war. They take seriously the possibility that the observed mental deficiency among Negroes may reflect an environmental "deficiency" imposed upon them. They saw that many white officers "were not suited to lead Negro troops" on account of their "temperament" or inexperience. And they understood that many black troops "felt they had very little to fight for," since "thoughtful Negroes, in view of their experiences at home, were not impressed by our national propaganda which justified our fighting on the basis of protecting the rights of men, preserving democracy and promoting individual freedom and equality."[65] In a word, Ripley and Wolf situated the predicament of these black men in a social and historical context that offered a better-informed alternative to the conventional racist ideas about the inherent inferiority of blacks that still circulated widely at this time.[66]

Yet even as Ripley and Wolf managed to transcend the worldview of the racist officers they interviewed, they recited without comment and with implicit approval a series of racist ideas about the black personality. A ludicrous 1914 paper on the simplicity of Negro dreams is presented as credible research.[67] That blacks do not belong to the "more highly civilized races," and that they have fewer emotional needs than whites, is taken for granted. Their stronger sex drives may have resulted from natural selection. And there are questions regarding blacks' ability to distinguish between "dreams and facts": "It is a common but probably mistaken idea that it is usual for normal Negroes to hear voices or see visions," they write, even as they proceed to weigh seriously the idea that black people make "less distinction between hallucinations and objective existence," since they may still be under the sway of their African origins.[68]

The black psychiatrist Stevens presents this troubled world of racially segregated regiments and racially integrated psychotherapy from a sharply different perspective. In retrospect, the principal weakness of Ripley and Wolf is their lack of interest in examining their own roles and limitations in the larger scheme of things. The euphemizing habit that turns white officers' racism into a matter of "temperament" is one sign of the racist indoctrination that caused them to embrace the "Africanized" view of the American Negro that preserves much of the mind-set of nineteenth-century racial anthropology. Stevens, unlike Ripley and Wolf, has no reason to employ euphemisms that signal a discomfort with acknowledging racism in the officer corps. Black soldiers, he says, "were frequently commanded by white officers whose attitudes toward race were to some degree fascist."

Like other black physicians before him, Stevens reminded his overwhelmingly white audience that "Negroes, like other minority groups, are hypersensitive about some things"—such as calling soldiers by their first names or nicknames—"which appear to be of little importance to the majority." He presents the emotional suffering and frustrations of these black men from their perspective. He challenges claims in the medical literature that as many as half of all Negro military patients had been diagnosed as psychopaths. And he notes the importance of making available to black men the black physician "who did not have to overcome those defenses [in the black patient] which the white psychiatrist was compelled to evaluate more or less blindly in arriving at his conclusions."[69]

The Negro soldiers of the Second World War were essentially colonial troops who bore the stigma of a racial inferiority that determined their roles in the war. This degraded status condemned most of them to lowly positions as servants or laborers, thereby depriving them of the more dramatic military experiences that could have elevated their civic status more than the mere fact of having been drafted into service. The military route to full citizenship was barred to them, and many black soldiers bitterly resented this racist maneuver during and after the war. Military psychiatrists played their own role in demoting the Negro soldier by often failing to distinguish between alleged race traits and the social and military racism that created symptoms they ascribed to inherent (and thus racial) defects of character and sanity. Given the choice between adopting the viewpoints of white officers or those of their black subordinates, many doctors chose to identify with those more like themselves, though this is hardly surprising given their social distance from black people and their susceptibility to the racial folklore of that era.

It is important to recognize that the wartime conception of the psychologically limited and deficient Negro represented mainstream medical opinion rather than the racist cranks of the day. By the end of the Second World War, and in part because of what some white psychiatrists had learned about race relations during their military service, American psychiatry was beginning to become aware of its participation in the mainstream racism of the larger society. It is not surprising that those psychiatrists who chose to describe their experiences and express their views on race relations in professional journals came from the racially tolerant end of the spectrum of psychiatric opinion. The military psychiatrist Jerome D. Frank, for example, who went on to become a well-known political progressive in the profession, went out of his way to look at black soldiers in a positive light. "It is greatly to the credit of the Negroes," he wrote in 1947, "that, despite the presence of many good reasons for a cynical attitude, the majority were good soldiers. This must be attributed to ingrained attitudes of conscientiousness and self-respect, coupled with the recognition that despite all discriminations they were still Americans whose welfare was identified with a United States victory."[70] By the standards of this era, these words demonstrated a generosity of spirit of which few medical men of that era would have been capable. Indeed, the idea that a white psychiatrist would devote himself to the care of Negro patients was regarded as nothing less than astonishing. The psychiatric clinic set up by Dr. Fredric Wertham in the basement of a Harlem church in 1925 was such an anomaly that it was covered by *The New Republic* in 1940 and by *Time* in 1947. There was a widespread view that black people did not require psychiatric care, and there were few qualified blacks to serve those who did. According to these reports, there were eight black psychiatrists in the United States in 1940 and fewer than 25 in 1947. "A white psychiatrist almost never accepts Negro clientele for fear of losing his rich white patients," the 1940 article reported. This was also "colonial" medicine in the sense that Fredric Wertham's presence in Harlem was no less remarkable in its way than the medical mission to the dark-skinned inhabitants of the Belgian Congo that made Albert Schweitzer a global celebrity. Wertham was fully aware of his special status, and he addressed the apparent gulf between racial worlds by asserting that the only difference between his black and white patients was that "here in Harlem the trouble is much more naked and obvious."[71] Most of his colleagues, having had less contact with black patients, would have regarded this claim as an exaggerated egalitarianism that derived from liberal good intentions. Regardless of how the beneficiaries of their care regarded them, both men were prime examples of the "Great White Doctor" whose medical skills and virtues incarnated the "philanthropic colonialism" that is analyzed later in this chapter.

An acknowledgment of psychiatry's absorption of popular racial folklore appears in the *American Journal of Psychiatry* in 1951. The author notes that "emotionalism, a capacity for so-called laziness, special musical abilities, impulsiveness, dramatization, and other singular [Negro] qualities *have been both popular conceptions and mentioned in various publications*" [emphasis added]. His personal response to these stereotypes is both candid and ambivalent: "The writer's own clinical impressions seem to confirm some of these conceptions. Regardless of the clinical diagnosis there did seem to be much emotionalism, a greater affective demonstration, more alcoholic intake, more exhibitionism, more motor activity in general, more psychopathic-like reactions."[72] More than a half century later, this conflicted postwar response to the idea of "black" behaviors will be familiar to thoughtful observers of race relations in the United States. Today we are more aware of our immersion in racially coded images that can affect how we interpret the traits and behaviors of whites and blacks. Much of this book, in fact, is devoted to demonstrating how deeply these images are embedded in doctors' thinking about the minds and bodies of their racially coded patients. At the same time, our self-awareness of such "unconscious bias" must compete with what we know about racially differential crime rates, educational deficits, professional employment profiles, and cultural styles (such as hip-hop) that are racially, and negatively, coded in the public sphere. Distinguishing between the stereotypes we have absorbed and the observations that we make about stereotyped people was even more difficult in 1950 than it is today, and at least some psychiatrists of this period were wrestling with this conflict. Two important differences between then and now are that ideas about racial essences are less influential today, as a new emphasis on cultural differences has to some extent displaced the dogmatic belief in biological differences that characterized traditional racism.

An awareness of psychiatrists' vulnerability to racial folklore has prompted some white practitioners to think about the racial dynamics of their interactions with black patients. We have already seen that many white doctors, dating from the early decades of the twentieth century, had become aware of the social and psychological abyss that separated them from the black population they might be called upon to serve. Prior to the Second World War, the response to this mutual estrangement was usually resignation to the social facts of life and a call to enlist black doctors and nurses to serve their own kind. During and after the war it became possible to be more ambitious about establishing what was commonly referred to as "rapport" across the racial divide that separated white therapists and black patients. A journal article on "The Negro Patient in Psychiatric Treatment" that appeared in 1950 offered the following advice to white colleagues whose nervousness about dealing with black men was often anticipated in such commentaries: "To avoid semantic errors in dealing with any patient who is sensitive because of race, the therapist must learn to be careful in his choice of words and learn to avoid seemingly harmless phrases. For example, a therapist who refers to Negroes as 'you people' or 'your people' calls attention to his own differences and makes the Negro patient suspicious, wary and fearful of being patronized."[73] Indeed, the racial sophistication of any doctor was already evident in how well (or how poorly) he understood that the racial dynamics of interracial therapy presented a minefield that was only beginning to be explored in a systematic way.

The psychiatric profession's monitoring of its own handling of race re-lations during the civil rights era was minimal at best. Individual thera-pists who cared enough to publish on the problems of the black patient or the hapless conduct of white therapists offered sporadic coverage where systematic self-scrutiny should have been the norm. "It is rare now that one hears any psychiatrist describe a Negro with a term like 'primitive' or 'uninhibited,'" one practitioner wrote in 1960, "though stereotypes—especially those unconsciously held—die hard. But every therapist finds himself faced with his first case of some unusual kind or other; and no matter what sophistications are voiced in the literature, he is prone to the same outrageous mistakes as his predecessors."[74] "Naïve papers continued to find their way into print," two psychologists commented in 1968 on the familiar claim that blacks suffered from more mental illness than whites, "but they are less common. Most authors now recognize the pitfalls in attempting racial comparisons regarding the kinds of behavior labeled as mental illness."[75] Both of these observers describe an age of transition dur-ing which white therapists groped their way toward a race-conscious code of conduct that would allow them to navigate their way through the racial minefield while causing as little emotional damage as possible.

By the end of the 1960s the American psychiatric establishment had witnessed enough racial turmoil to realize that the crisis in American race relations would persist into the indefinite future, and that the psychiatric profession might play a role in addressing racial tensions. How this was to be accomplished remained an open question to a profession that was not much better prepared to deal with the subject of race than most other white Americans. (Of the 17,000 psychiatrists in the United States in 1965, only about 300 were black. In 1972, 1.9 percent of those in psychiatric residency training were black.[76]) "The Psychiatrist's Role in Dealing with Social Turmoil," which appeared in the *American Journal of Psychiatry* in 1970, offers a series of clichés about "the current state of flux in American society" and a prediction that "the times ahead will be tumultuous." The author refers to race by noting that the status quo was being challenged "by the young and other minorities."[77] One participant in a 1971 panel discussion on "The Psychiatrist, the APA, and Social Issues" confessed that "we need an operational definition of social issues." Apart from brief ref-erences to "urban blight and ghettos," "racism," "race relations," and the "problem behavior of minority groups," there is no engagement with the race issue, let alone any suggestion that white psychiatrists might need to embark upon the sort of self-examination they were supposed to stimulate in their patients.[78] A 1975 survey on what a psychiatric curriculum for medical students should look like does not mention race at all.[79] It was not until 1978 that the American Psychiatric Association created a Task Force on Cultural and Ethnic Issues in Psychiatry under the direction of a white psychiatrist named John Spiegel. The mandate for this group makes a vague reference to cultural competence, but there was still no sign that white psychiatrists felt any obligation to take a hard look at their own professional relationships with black clients with an eye toward improving them. Possible problems related to interracial therapeutic relationships did not appear to concern them at all.[80]

This lack of commitment to taking the race issue seriously was evident in the *American Journal of Psychiatry* throughout the 1970s. Overjoyed to see an article by a fellow black psychiatrist in a 1978 issue of the *Journal*, James H. Carter of Duke University wrote a letter to the editor in which he noted "a three-year drought of articles about black mental health issues written by black authors. Could it be," he asked delicately, "that the process of selecting this type of work for publication should be scrutinized?" And he added: "This decline in the publication of work related to black mental health is apparent not only in the *Journal* but also at most annual meetings of the American Psychiatric Association." Finally, and in conformity with the etiquette of "the black physician as gentleman," Dr. Carter generously offered the opinion that "the American Psychiatric Association has probably been the most sensitive and forceful medical specialty group in recognizing the health problems of minorities, including women and the elderly."[81]

Over the decade that began in 1970 the *Journal* published a potpourri of about a dozen articles touching on the African American experience, including "Drug Use in a Black Ghetto," "Combat Neurosis in Inner-City Schools" (focusing on vulnerable teachers), "When the Psychotherapist Is Black," and "Time Orientation and Psychotherapy in the Ghetto," on the ability of ghetto dwellers to keep their appointments with their therapists. In other words, something like every hundredth article and report that appeared in the *Journal* over this period of time dealt with "black" issues.[82] Only two *AJP* articles during the entire decade addressed the problematic racial feelings and professional conduct of white therapists and what might be done to change them.

The antiracist *cri de coeur* of white liberal psychiatry appeared in the *AJP* in 1970. "Dimensions of Institutional Racism in Psychiatry," by Melvin Sabshin and two colleagues, proclaimed that it was "necessary for white psychiatrists to change the racist practices of their organizations and institutions." This critique offered a largely accurate condemnation of "white" psychiatry as racially unenlightened and socially negligent toward the black population. Whereas societal racism portrayed black people as *"innately lazy, unhealthy, unintelligent,* and *criminal,"* the psychiatric profession had generated "its equivalent racist stereotypes about the black psychiatric patient: *hostile* and *not motivated for treatment, having primitive character structure, not psychologically minded,* and *impulse-ridden."* From this critical perspective, "white" psychiatry is a form of "philanthropic colonialism," hence the authors' satisfaction at the "rude awakening" experienced by the "white 'liberal' mental health workers" whose "proposals to *do something for* poor blacks were rejected by blacks who wished to take leadership in program planning and implementation." It was time for these white liberals to recognize their own "paternalism and its racist roots" and learn how to respect the dignity and autonomy of their ghetto clients.[83]

This white practitioner's critique of psychiatric arrogance, ignorance, and incompetence can be understood as a wholly intentional contribution to the backlash against the so-called Moynihan Report of 1965. "The Negro Family: The Case for National Action," a 55-page essay packed with charts and statistics, had been prepared for a small circle of domestic policy advisers serving President Lyndon B. Johnson and was not intended for public dissemination. Once it was leaked to the press, however, the report's gloomy portrait of the Negro family and the "tangle of pathology" it represented generated a firestorm of protest against what many blacks and liberal whites regarded as racial defamation. The fact that the infamous "tangle of pathology" phrase had been borrowed from the prominent black psychologist Kenneth Clark was either unknown or ignored. Nor did Moynihan's salute to "the creative vitality of the Negro people" earn him any quarter from the (primarily white) critics who were labeling him a racist. "Three centuries of injustice have brought about deep-seated distortions in the life of the Negro American," Moynihan wrote. "At this point, the present tangle of pathology is capable of perpetuating itself without assistance from the white world."[84] This portrait of autonomous degeneration provoked bitter resentment in many blacks and much disdain in white liberal defenders of black dignity. Moynihan was interpreted by some to be arguing that the desperate state in which poor blacks found themselves was somehow independent of the cruelties and limitations inflicted upon them by the racist practices of white hospitals, school systems, banks, police forces, and real estate agents. What is more, the idea of autonomous degeneration might have seemed like an oblique endorsement of the old racist biology that regarded blacks as inherently diseased and beyond salvation.

At a certain point, as the African American historian Daryl Michael Scott has pointed out, "the assault on the report became a reflex." A more nuanced understanding of Moynihan's motives and proposals for social action on behalf of the black family became possible only years after his name had become synonymous with ham-handed and insensitive white intrusiveness into black life.[85]

Melvin Sabshin and his antiracist coauthors may have been unaware of the fact that several black leaders had expressed their approval of the Moynihan Report. "I could not understand the great shock that people were expressing over the report," said Robert Carter of the National Association for the Advancement of Colored People (NAACP). "Moynihan, it seemed to me, was making a comment on the results of discrimination in our society. It's an old story and not a startling discovery and not new. These things that he points out—the pathologies of the ghetto—are a result of discrimination." "It's kind of a wolf pack operating in a very undignified way," said Kenneth Clark of Moynihan's fiercest critics. "If Pat is a racist, I am. He highlights the total pattern of segregation and discrimination. Is a doctor responsible for a disease simply because he diagnoses it?"[86] These comments showed that self-respecting black observers, as well as Moynihan's white defenders, perceived an element of hysteria in the response to the controversial report. If the antiracist psychiatrists were aware of this complication in the racial politics of the Moynihan affair, there is no sign of it in their analysis of institutional racism. What they could *not* have missed, however, was the unprecedented public flaying of a white authority figure on the grounds that he had shown insensitivity toward abused and disadvantaged black people who deserved more respect than the Moynihan Report appeared to give them.

In this political climate, the use of certain code words made it easy to dissociate oneself from Moynihan's position without even mentioning him. Accordingly, the authors of "Dimensions of Institutional Racism in Psychiatry" expressed their disapproval of the controversial policy expert by accusing white psychiatrists of disseminating "mythical definitions of black psychopathology" and by describing mental health missionaries to the ghettos as the inventors and facilitators of damaging stereotypes of the black personality. "Many white mental health professionals," they wrote, "regard black communities as seething cauldrons of psychopathology. They create stereotypes of absent fathers, primitive rage, psychopathy, self-depreciation, promiscuity, deficits in intellectual capacity, and lack of psychological sensitivity. Gross pathological caricaturization ignores the enormous variation of behavior in black communities."[87]

For politically aware members of that generation, the use of the word *pathology* remains even today a sure way to raise the ghosts of the Moynihan affair from out of the now remote world of the radical sixties and the utopian fantasies that included a black "revolution" that would liberate African Americans from American racism. The neophyte radicalism of these antiracist psychiatrists can be heard in phrases such as "the white power structure of psychiatry" and the epithetic use of the phrase "white liberal," as if for some reason this term did not apply to the authors themselves. While headlong flight from the ideological shame of whiteness was common enough at the time, participation in a form of self-rejection that sometimes took on masochistic overtones was not a sign of personal or political maturity in psychiatrists or, for that matter, in any other professionals involved in race relations. "White 'liberal' mental health workers," like their black clients, deserved to be understood in terms of their strengths as well as their weaknesses. Reducing them to caricatures that cast them as involuntary racists was an unnecessary concession to the hyperemotional white antiracism of this period.[88]

The really difficult challenge for mental health workers and social scientists alike was to produce a psychosocial analysis of the ghetto poor that described their problems accurately and sympathetically without reducing them to distorted images of their real selves. Sabshin and his coauthors, like many white commentators before and since, evaded this challenge by reporting the alleged beliefs of their offending colleagues in quotation marks that implied disapproval or ridicule: "seething cauldrons of psychopathology, absent fathers, primitive rage, psychopathy, self-depreciation, promiscuity, deficits in intellectual capacity, and lack of psychological sensitivity." The dishonesty of this rhetorical device lay in its implicit claim that none of this was true, and that the problems of ghetto blacks were no more severe than those of middle-class whites. The sheer implausibility of this position went unacknowledged by white authors determined to rehabilitate the black image in this fashion. After all, if the residents of Harlem were no worse off in terms of their mental health than most other Americans, then what was it that made racism the scourge it was claimed to be? Why had James Farmer called black life in America "a living Hell"?[89] How was it that "racist oppression" did not produce psychological "damage"? In fact, the claim that the "pathologies" of the black poor were simply an illusion being propagated by naïve or mean-spirited white professionals like Moynihan was an emotionally convenient pretense for whites who found it unbearable to think of blacks as damaged people and objects of their pity.

One positive result of the backlash against the Moynihan Report was the critical scrutiny of stereotypes about blacks in general and the black poor in particular. From the vantage point of our own era of rampant divorce, it is striking to see Moynihan expressing alarm about the fact that 23 percent of urban black women were "divorced, separated, or living apart from their husbands," although this concern becomes more understandable in light of a corresponding figure of only 8 percent for urban whites. More importantly, the report's emphasis on "the deterioration of the Negro family" was too categorical, the author's qualifying comments about successful black families notwithstanding. "There is no one Negro community. There is no one Negro problem," Moynihan wrote. But this sensible observation was drowned out by the emotional response to a carelessly written document that alternated between sweeping generalizations that were followed by second thoughts about the need for more nuanced perspectives about the diversity of black life.[90] Finally, there was the tone of the report. Despite its enlightened moments and the author's good intentions, Moynihan's document conveys a philanthropic colonial tone typical of his professional class that alienated even some of the black leaders who refused to impugn his motives. His claim, for example, that the destruction of the Negro family under slavery "broke the will of the Negro people" was an embarrassment. If this was the case, then how had black people managed to create a civil rights movement that changed American society in profound ways that served their interests?

The notoriety of the Moynihan Report opened the portals to a flood of criticisms that were intended both to put this white government official in his place and to invalidate the racist stereotypes he stood accused of promoting. In their 1970 essay, the antiracist psychiatrists were right to point to a kind of white voyeurism that feeds on perceptions of black life as primitive, uninhibited, or degraded—spectacles that gratify appetites that have no proper role in the understanding of culture and human behavior. They were right to accuse their white colleagues of being in denial about their own racial biases and "habitual ways of relating" to members of "the lower caste." They were right to suggest that blacks might possess some coping skills that were superior to those of whites. And they had good reason to caution their colleagues against equating black militancy with psychopathology (see the following).[91]

A traditional failing of militant white antiracism in the United States has been its tendency to homogenize black thinking and behavior for the purpose of assigning it an oppositional role vis-à-vis the white adversaries of the antiracists. Imagining that all thinking blacks think like white militants allows the latter to present themselves as ideological and political allies of oppressed blacks. The authors of "Dimensions of Institutional Racism in Psychiatry" create this imaginary unified front by disregarding what prominent black intellectuals were actually thinking and saying about the black experience at this time. Perhaps the white psychiatrists were unaware of Kenneth Clark's *Dark Ghetto* (1965), which provided Moynihan with the infamous "tangle of pathology" formula as well as an intensely pathological interpretation of the black ghetto experience. "The dark ghetto is institutionalized pathology," Clark writes; "it is chronic, self-perpetuating pathology. . . . The emotional ill health of the dark ghetto is a continuum ranging from the anxious but 'normal' individual to the criminally psychotic."[92] In retrospect it is clear that *Dark Ghetto* was a principal source of Moynihan's stern recommendations for rehabilitating the black family and the black condition. It is all here: the "pathology," "self-hatred," "damage," "psychological emasculation," the "self-perpetuating" degradation of the ghetto that Moynihan rephrased as "the present tangle of pathology [that] is capable of perpetuating itself without assistance from the outside world."[93] But the antiracist psychiatrists could not have reported Clark's account of the ghetto without exposing the myopia that prompted them to claim that it was "the white power structure of psychiatry" alone that was inflicting pathological images on ghetto blacks.

Whether or not they had read *Dark Ghetto*, these authors were aware of another important work in this genre that appears in their footnotes. By far the best-known commentary of this period about black mental health was *Black Rage*, published in 1968 by William H. Grier and Price M. Cobbs. Three years after the initial controversy over the Moynihan Report, these militant black psychiatrists managed to distance themselves from its white author while repeating several of the report's claims that had so inflamed its critics. "The Negro family is in deep trouble," they write. "It is coming apart and it is failing to provide the nurturing that black children need." Like Moynihan, Grier and Cobbs ascribed current black problems to the deforming impact of slavery, a theory some militants would come to reject as too "pathologizing": "The black man of today," they write, "is at one end of a psychological continuum which reaches back in time to his enslaved ancestors." Grier and Cobbs also argued that the black slave "had to be absolutely dependent and have a deep consciousness of personal inferiority"—an unmistakable echo of the theory of the "Sambo" slave personality that had landed the white historian Stanley Elkins in hot water years before. Moynihan found himself saddled with the same kind of notoriety. Both Moynihan and these black medical activists had decided to deploy the most disturbing forms of damage imagery to provoke action on behalf of an abused black population. Moynihan's mistake, they wrote, was to have spread the "simplistic half-truth" about the "emasculation" of black men and their domination by "matriarchal" women.[94] More striking, however, are the major ideas identified with Moynihan these black psychiatrists found indispensable for their analysis of the black predicament. The white antiracist psychiatrists dealt with the discomfiting similarities between the celebrated black psychiatrists and the much-resented white policy maker by pretending they did not exist.

The phobia that discourages white men's examinations of black people's sufferings has had lasting consequences. Shocked and awed by the rough justice that had been inflicted on the unfortunate Moynihan, white liberal professionals like Sabshin were not about to explore the sensitive topic of black disabilities and expose themselves to the prospect of being ostracized by their peers. It is also worth asking whether these practitioners knew very much about the black problems they did not want to confront. Sabshin criticizes white psychiatrists for creating "stereotypes of absent fathers, primitive rage, psychopathy, self-depreciation, promiscuity, deficits in intellectual capacity, and lack of psychological sensitivity." What this indictment overlooks is that the black psychiatrists of this period took the reality of these "stereotypes" for granted, because they were willing to acknowledge the seriousness of the "damage" that had been done. This is evident in the contemporary writings of three young black doctors who eventually became eminent psychiatrists. "Most psychiatrists and psychologists would agree," Alvin F. Poussaint wrote in 1966, "that the Negro American suffers from a marred self-image, of varying degree, which critically affects his entire psychological being. It is also a well-documented fact that this negative self-concept leads to self-destructive attitudes and behavior that hinder the negro's struggle toward full equality in American life."[95] "To a considerable degree," Charles A. Pinderhughes wrote the same year, "the intense self-devaluation experienced by Negroes in segregated circumstances stems from their identification of themselves with 'bad' suppressed thoughts, feeling, and body products. This identification occurs because they find themselves treated in the same manner in which 'bad' thoughts, 'bad' feelings, and 'bad' body products are treated."[96] "Our racist society," James H. Carter wrote in 1974, "has produced and perpetuated environmental circumstances for blacks that do not encourage the use of constructive patterns and that provoke fear and uncertainty and reinforce immature patterns of behavior."[97]

The accuracy of the "stereotypes" listed in "Dimensions of Institutional Racism" was taken seriously by black mental health professionals at this time, and they have lost none of their relevance today. *Absent fathers?* While Alvin Poussaint pointed to "illegitimacy" and "broken homes," Sidney B. Jenkins argued that "we must stop thinking of the black father as a nonentity, a breeder, a stud."[98] *Primitive rage?* Grier and Cobbs had produced a best seller by declaring that "all blacks are angry."[99] *Psychopathy?* In a speech given on October 29, 1966, the Reverend Martin Luther King, Jr. had declared that *the Negro family* was "often psychopathic."[100] *Self-depreciation?* According to Alvin Poussaint, the *self-hatred* engendered in the black child "molds and shapes his entire personality and interaction with his environment."[101] *Promiscuity?* "Whether Negroes are more active sexually than whites is of little importance," wrote William Grier. "The fact that *is* important is that Negroes conceive of themselves as more active, less inhibited, more capable lovers and that *white people* share this conception."[102] *Deficits in intellectual capacity?* The prominent black physician Paul B. Cornely wrote in 1968 about "inferior mental functioning" (mental retardation) as a fact of life among "the deprived."[103] *Lack of psychological sensitivity?* "Because blacks are so proficient in wearing the 'mask,'" James H. Carter noted, "psychiatric impairment can be extremely difficult to ascertain. Establishing the presence and severity of psychiatric disorders among blacks can be impossible for those who are unaware of black behavior patterns."[104] *Seething cauldrons of psychopathology?* Charles Pinderhughes and Kenneth Clark saw the black ghetto as a *pathogenic social structure* and as *institutionalized pathology*, respectively. In summary, Sabshin saw "stereotypes" as potential sources of racial defamation that could be inflicted on blacks by whites, whereas his black colleagues perceived them from a different angle that recognized their relevance to the black experience. Overcompensating for their whiteness, Sabshin's group embraced the sort of militancy that insisted on seeing "stereotypes" where black professionals saw public health problems that required solutions.

The assault on Moynihan and others accused of promoting ideas about "black pathology" persuaded most white doctors and social scientists that frank talk about damaged black psyches was better left to their black colleagues. It is instructive to compare the Moynihan affair with the publication in 1951 of *The Mark of Oppression*, a somber look at the emotional life of the urban Negro by two white psychoanalysts, Abram Kardiner and Lionel Ovesey. Writing a decade later in a new preface to the book, the authors recall the "great controversy" their book had caused when "many readers, especially among the laity, rejected the findings on largely emotional grounds because they found them too painful to accept. Most of these critics, we feel, eventually reversed themselves as they gradually realized that the end products of oppression could hardly be very pretty." The authors also confessed to having had "some concern about the impact of this work on the Negro, who may consider it an intrusion on his privacy on the grounds that much had better been left unsaid." They had rejected this option on the grounds that such "excessive precaution would mean to abandon a useful implement for social research because its conclusions hurt the sensibilities of those being investigated."[105]

The crucial difference between these two episodes is that the publication of *The Mark of Oppression* occurred before the advent of Black Power in its various forms during the 1960s, which included a revolt against white interpretations of black life. In 1968, Alyce C. Gullattee wrote that the Negro "most often learns who he is not through self-discovery but through an outside source whose perceptions may be distorted and/or naïve." Nor was Gullattee the only black psychiatrist to make this point.[106] It took the Moynihan affair to really bring this black perspective home to the many white experts whose viewpoints dominated the scholarly and medical literatures that diagnosed and interpreted black lives. Before the controversy over the report, white authors were often self-conscious but relatively uninhibited about touching on potentially sensitive points. As late as 1962, Kardiner and Ovesey could dismiss the strategy of "excessive precaution" to avoid offending black sensibilities with a calm self-assurance that would have been harder to muster only a few years later. Similarly, the rough edges that mark the tone of Charles Silberman's *Crisis in Black and White* would have provoked more comment had the book appeared after 1964. Following the Moynihan affair, the temptation for white experts to ride to the rescue of the black image proved to be overwhelming for a number of people whose emotional commitment to this task at times outweighed their ability to weigh the evidence in a balanced fashion.

THE TASK OF BLACK PSYCHIATRY

The canonical figure of black psychiatry during the 1960s was Frantz Fanon, whose mission was the rehabilitation of the black colonial personality. "What I want to do," Fanon wrote in 1952, "is help the black man to free himself from the arsenal of complexes that has been developed by the colonial environment." Even more than his Afro-American colleagues, the Afro-Caribbean Fanon was uninhibited in his descriptions of the black man's plight. "We must see whether it is possible for the black man to overcome his feeling of insignificance, to rid his life of the compulsive quality that makes it so like the behavior of the phobic. Affect is exacerbated in the Negro, he is full of rage because he feels small, he suffers from an inadequacy in all human communication, and all these factors chain him with an unbearable insularity."[107] Fanon's classic description of colonial medicine, based on his experience in Algeria during the French war of occupation, is an almost perfect description of the African American medical predicament as it has existed over the past century: the chronic mistrust of the doctor, the unwillingness to follow his instructions (noncompliance), the patient's refusal to communicate with the doctor, his ostensibly perverse refusal of certain medical services. Colonial domination, Fanon writes, "gives rise to and continues to dictate a whole complex of resentful behavior and of refusal on the part of the colonized."[108] Examples of such resentful attitudes and behaviors on the part of black patients have been described and deplored in the American medical literature for generations. The one important difference between North Africa and North America in this respect is the description of the native doctor as a turncoat who joins forces with the white oppressors. By contrast, African American doctors' aspirations to join the American medical establishment on equal terms have not signified a betrayal of their people. And there have always been black physician activists who have attempted to analyze and oppose medical racism in its various forms.

Any account of black psychiatric activism must acknowledge the tiny numbers of practitioners involved. In 1965 there may have been fewer than 300 black psychiatrists in the United States out of a total of 17,000. Of the 1,000 practicing psychoanalysts, there were *four* blacks who had completed formal psychoanalytic training and twelve more were undergoing psychoanalytic training. According to a black psychiatrist at the National Institute of Mental Health, "the present need [in 1965] is for 10,000 Negro psychiatrists to meet the needs of the Negro population."[109] (As of 1999, there were about 900 practicing black psychiatrists in the United States and almost no blacks involved in psychiatric research.[110]) This enormous disparity between those in need and those qualified to serve them has had its own impact on how psychiatrists have thought about how to treat mental disorders in black patients. These speculations have in turn raised some of the fundamental questions about purported racial differences between the psychological functioning of white and black human beings.

The hallmark of colonial status in general, and colonial medicine in particular, is a profound estrangement from the authoritative figures who exercise power in a society or, in this case, a medical subculture. African American estrangement from major social institutions like schools, hospitals, and police forces has produced many destructive consequences, including at times a refusal to accept medical treatments blacks have identified (and stigmatized) as "white." Black resistance to psychotherapy, for example, has been rooted in traumatic social and medical experiences. These choices express a deep cultural logic that is rooted in historical circumstances and the value systems they produce.

Therapeutic treatments in a racially divided society often have a racial logic. The law of bipolar stereotyping dictates that the black patient's relationship to medical therapy will assume one extreme form or another: The black patient will either be hypersusceptible or hyperresistant to treatment. Writing in 1913, a contributor to the *Southern Medical Journal* declares that, "Psychotherapy among the Afro-Americans is almost like planting good seed in virgin soil," thanks to "the emotions and the somewhat primitively developed mentalities of these people" that make them receptive to the doctor's suggestions.[111] This conception of the black person as a psychodynamic simpleton recurs many years later in a report by a British colonial physician in Africa. "The native mind is undeveloped," Dr. D.H. Sandell writes in 1945, "both by nature and lack of education, so that its approach to most problems is childlike. One therefore deals with the native as one would with a child. The complexes and inhibitions of civilization are absent so that psychotherapy often consists merely of a sympathetic unraveling of childlike troubles."[112] In the United States the infantilizing of the black patient was acceptable in 1913, before the advent of the New Negro movement of the 1920s, but less acceptable by the end of the Second World War. In colonial Africa, however, time had stood still, so that even as late as 1945 the passive Georgia Negro of 1913 was alive and well and reciting his "childlike troubles" to a white psychotherapist somewhere in colonial Africa.

By the 1920s, which saw the popularization of psychoanalytic thinking in the United States, a self-confident African American writer like George Schuyler could look at the "white" psychotherapeutic culture from a critical and acerbically "black" point of view and find it ridiculous:

> These so-called sophisticated whites leap from one fad to another, from mah jong to "Ask Me Another," with great facility, and are usually ready to embrace any cause that comes along thirsting for supporters. They are obsessed by sex and discuss it interminably, with long dissertations on their moods and reactions, complexes and sublimations. Life to them seems to be one perpetual psychoanalytical clinic.... It is difficult to imagine a group of intelligent Negroes sprawling around a drawing-room, consuming cigarettes and synthetic gin while discussing . their complexes and inhibitions.[113]

Schuyler's disdain for white shallowness and self-absorption must have provided him with a triumphal moment at a time when such gratifications were not available to most black men and women. But from the standpoint of improving the black image, the disadvantage of this critique was that it dissociated blacks from the "long dissertations on moods and reactions, complexes and sublimations" that signified mental complexity for a twentieth-century civilization in which the prestige of psychoanalysis was steadily climbing. Modern society was already broadcasting the message of black hypersimplicity through various cultural media, including racist films such as "Birth of a Nation." *The Psychoanalytic Review* had reported in 1914 that Negroes were "savage" and "primitive" and "a race whose psychological activities are certainly less complex than those of the Caucasian."[114] A widely cited psychiatric journal article that appeared the same year portrayed the black as *nonintrospective*, commenting that: "Self-study is a pastime which does not appeal to him."[115] And here too the early twentieth-century, mentally simple American Negro had his much later colonial African counterpart. The *British Journal of Psychiatry* reported in 1960 on "the Nigerian's apparent lack of need to engage in the elaborate introspections and soul searchings in the way the European does."[116] The stereotype of the anti-introspective black mind had survived into the decade of Black Power and has continued to exert its influence within the psychotherapeutic culture. Psychotherapy, after all, requires the capacity for introspection that makes new and potentially healing self-knowledge possible.

While whites had formulated the primitive and anti-introspective model of the African psyche to contrast with their own mental complexity, African Americans had developed a differential racial psychology of their own. One crucial difference between these white and black doctrines of racial character is that the folk psychology of the black masses has no way to reach an audience of psychiatrists or the other professionals who would be well served to know something about it. This black folk doctrine of contrasting racial characters can be studied in the anthology *Drylongso: A Self-Portrait of Black America*, where a group of working-class and self-respecting black people narrate life as they have known it in their northeastern urban areas to the black (and blind) cultural anthropologist John Langston Gwaltney. Perhaps the most striking finding that emerges from these conversations, which were conducted during the early 1970s, is that nearly all of these people mistrust or despise whites and are willing to say so with the sort of candor one does not associate with the public standards and expectations of a "racially integrated" society.[117] There is a permanent estrangement of incompatible sensibilities: "What excites the white man does not move most of us," says Ruth Shays. At other times these black informants display a superiority complex that is wildly at variance with the more familiar images of damage and deprivation and depression that prevail in the professional literatures. "As a race we are sturdier and made out of better material," says Ellen Turner Surry. "And if you think about it," says John Oliver, "you know that when it comes to most things, we are really better than they are." *Drylongso* was planned and executed as a dissent from what the white experts of the 1960s and 1970s were saying about blacks and their disabilities in the learned journals. As Gwaltney puts it: "I share the opinion commonly held by natives of my community that we have traditionally been misrepresented by standard social science." One informant tells the black anthropologist, "I've been telling you about wrong things about myself and my folks, but there is much more right about us than there is wrong."[118]

The *Drylongso* testimonies also address indirectly the problem of whether the standard psychotherapeutic methods are suitable for black patients who are treated by white therapists. According to the black anthropologist, there is "an endemic wariness that pervades core black culture," and this wariness is everywhere in the narratives he has presented in his book. How much blacks should or should not reveal to whites has been a constant and often perilous aspect of black life for centuries. The result has been a "wariness" whose depths few whites can grasp. "We are a very suspicious people," says Carolyn Chase. "We are a very private people," says Mabel Lincoln. "You simply cannot be honest with white people," says Grant Smith. "We know whitefolks, but they do not know us," says Porter Millington. These excluded whites have always included doctors. "These white doctors ain' nothin' but snakes, jus' like all the res' of they coluh," says Velma Cunningham.[119] Small wonder there are so many references in the medical literature to what a white psychiatrist called in 1951 "the difficulty in establishing rapport with Negro patients," who tended to be "either suspicious or submissive or both." "The suspiciousness would take many forms, such as uneasiness, a wary look, sullenness, a hesitancy and reserve, open and frank remarks questioning the doctor about his status, a tendency to avoid any mention of psychological material with a resultant emphasis upon physical complaints, silence, and the like."[120] This difficult situation contained two problems. First, white therapists faced the daunting challenge of winning the trust of their black patients; second, the therapists confronted the question of whether standard psychotherapeutic techniques were equally suitable for whites and blacks. At the same time, black people could talk to friends or family members who were therapists in all but name. "She sat me down and we talked about my feelings from all angles," Grant Smith said of his Aunt Pearl. "You see, nobody had ever made me do that before."[121] The relevant question in many, many cases was whether a white therapist with an advanced degree could do half as well.

In a 1966 article on the universality of the Oedipus complex, William Grier described an African American belief in separate and contrasting racial characters. Forty years after George Schuyler had heaped scorn on the faddish self-absorption of spoiled whites who were fixated on "their complexes and inhibitions," Grier found black people in the 1960s making a similar distinction between shallow and overprivileged whites and better-grounded African Americans who faced "real problems." "By far the overwhelming majority of Negroes," he wrote, "feel that there must be two psychologies, one for white people and one for Negroes. They say Negroes have real problems, like rent, food and discrimination while white people have some frothy, superficial senseless discontent with their favored place in society. They have so much leisure and comfort that they think up things to worry about. The Negro's worries are real."[122] Two psychologies and two sets of problems implied in turn a need for two psychotherapies. The problem was that psychological segregation of this kind would in all likelihood preserve the invidious distinction between simple (black) and complex (white) minds and emotions.

One rationale for different types of therapies is class differences that make long-term "introspective" therapy both unaffordable and inappropriate on account of different levels of social vulnerability. In the following passage, the black psychiatrist Chester M. Pierce describes a dichotomy between therapy for the middle class and therapy for the poor:

> White middle-class psychotherapy is based on an expensive, one-to-one model in which "defensive mechanisms" are negotiated, with much emphasis on the unconscious roots of anxiety. The poor black may need care based on other models such as the negotiation of "offensive mechanisms" (offenses done to him), with much emphasis on the conscious roots of self-image. The white middle-class mode is based on long-range, introspective analyses. The poor black mode might have to be based on short-term, confrontation techniques and more decided use of environmental manipulation. Diagnostic interpretation and nosology (classification of diseases) might be markedly different.[123]

One problematic aspect of this dichotomy is that higher and lower socioeconomic classes correlate with deeper and shallower mental strata. While the middle-class white patient has the time to pursue "the unconscious roots of anxiety," the poor and more vulnerable black patient must spend his time working on "the conscious roots of [his] self-image" to deal with what black psychologists and psychiatrists would eventually call the race-related "micro-aggressions" that black people may endure on a daily basis. White therapy takes time and money and the personal attention of the practitioner, while black therapy requires less time and ostensibly less subtle techniques such as "confrontation" and "manipulation." These distinctions raise the uncomfortable question of whether the psychiatric establishment has regarded black people as being worth the time, effort, and expense of psychoanalysis. As of 1969, according to one report, there was an "almost complete lack of Negroes in private treatment"[124] that derived in part from their lack of financial resources. Four years later, the black psychiatrist James H. Carter observed that: "Seemingly, most psychiatrists have found little satisfaction in treating black patients." Until the early 1960s, "the only sustained 'treatment' available to blacks was primarily through state mental hospitals."[125]

Whatever its causes, the widespread exclusion of black Americans from the psychotherapeutic culture amounts to a form of cultural apartheid. It would appear that Sigmund Freud's enormous influence on American attitudes toward therapy has largely passed blacks by. It is as if the popular culture of therapy, including therapist jokes and countless *New Yorker* cartoons featuring bearded psychoanalysts and their hapless patients emoting on couches, has not even existed for African Americans. (This cultural gulf recalls Spike Lee's puzzlement over Manhattan moviegoers "rolling in the aisles" during Woody Allen films, whose humor eluded him.) But lack of access to psychotherapy is not a joking matter. In 1965 a black physician noted the existence of a faction within the profession that thought of blacks' therapeutic potential as follows: "These people cannot respond to psychotherapy. They are dull and they are inarticulate."[126]

A year later Chester M. Pierce pointed out that racially differential psychotherapies was not an idea that whites had simply imposed on blacks. On the contrary, blacks too could endorse the idea of racially distinct psychologies and therapeutic approaches:

> It is a strange thing that many thoughtful Negroes and their white colleagues, even in our profession, express the opinion that the solidly validated psychoanalytic theory of human behavior does not hold completely true for Negroes. Many of our most respected practicing analysts and theoreticians feel that the historical and contemporary trauma that Negroes have been subjected to, makes them unanalyzable, exceptions to the technique and theory which holds for whites. They feel that the social castration of Negroness in America is the issue with which the therapist is presented, and they feel that *this* cannot be talked away.[127]

According to this interpretation of the black experience, the traumas of African American history had inflicted so much trauma on black people that psychoanalysis could not help to repair it. Speculation about the possible irrelevance of psychoanalytic thinking to blacks could also tap into the highly controversial issue of the "broken" or "pathological" black family and, in this case, the consequences of the absent father. "In the case of Negroes," a white sociologist wrote in 1967, "it seems likely that a great deal of standard psychiatric nomenclature would hardly even come into play, viz, where an orthodox Freudian is confronted with members of a group of which a large percentage have never even seen their fathers, how often would the concept 'Oedipus complex' come to mind?"[128] Once again, the crucial question was whether defining difference also meant assigning blacks a simpler mental apparatus that required less sophisticated treatments.

By now it should be clear that a primary task of the black psychiatrist over the past 50 years or so has been to defend black people's right to the full range of therapeutic treatments against the doubts of white and even some black practitioners. As the black psychiatrist Walter H. Bradshaw, Jr. pointed out in 1978:

> some black mental health professionals ... argue that dynamic psychotherapy is not suitable for black patients because it is too cold and intellectualized, that the average black person's needs are more immediate, and that it is not relevant to the patient's struggles in the world. This strikes me as being partially tinged by the unconscious adoption of some of the racist myths about black people that are prevalent in our society. These remarks have certain implications, e.g., that black patients do not have the ego strength to tolerate some forms of therapy, that they do not have the ego capacity to form a therapeutic alliance even when they receive an appropriate preparatory education by therapists about the way some forms of therapy are conducted, that they do not have the capacity to use insight in relation to their own personal dynamics, that they must be invariably and strenuously infantilized, and that they do not have the capacity to use therapeutic methods that are specifically designed to offer the maximum opportunity for ego autonomy and freedom from neurotic conflicts.[129]

The task of the black psychiatrist is thus to insist upon the full complexity of the black psyche as well as its capacity to undergo the healing processes offered by psychotherapy. At the same time, he or she must also negotiate the ideological struggle over black identity and the racially differential psychologies that reflect the two competing interpretations of what a "black" personality is. If "white" psychotherapy is "too cold and intellectualized," then "black" psychotherapy must be somehow warmer and "more immediate." Or "black" psychotherapy may be understood as a kind of sociopolitical procedure for the purpose of indoctrination. One black psychologist proposed in 1976 that therapy from "the black perspective" could be understood as "a process which is based on black culture and which gives instruction in black ideology and cultural identity." The relationship between therapist and client can thus be presented as "an appreciation of black culture or the African concept of the 'care syndrome.'"[130] Bradshaw regards the idea of a "black" psychology as a trap that reproduces some of "the racist myths about black people that are prevalent in our society." From his perspective, the self-consciously "black" approach to the African American personality underestimates what black people can bring to the therapeutic process, thereby depriving them of "the maximum opportunity for ego autonomy and freedom from neurotic conflicts." As has so often been the case, being "black" in this sense means skepticism toward, or outright rejection of, what is "white." For this reason the black psychiatrist occupies a delicate position between confirming his solidarity with his racial cohort and identifying with his profession's more universal conception of human nature.

The black psychiatrists' defense of black patients' right to treatment has also included insisting that lower-class patients in particular do not have a disordered relationship to time that makes them incapable of keeping their appointments or benefiting from long-term psychotherapy. Doubts about black people's ability to keep track of time have long been a part of Western racial folklore bearing on both African Americans and colonized African blacks, and it is important to understand the fateful consequences of this anthropological claim about the black man's relationship to clocks and schedules that constitute the framework of "civilized" life. In 1944 a contributor to Otto Klineberg's *Characteristics of the American Negro* noted that a catalogue of "What Every White Man Thinks He Knows about Negroes" would include the dictum: "He has no sense of time, never gets anywhere on time."[131] Yet the idea of "Colored People's Time" is also an element of black American folklore. In his classic *Blues People* (1963), LeRoi Jones wrote that, given the black man's "constant position at the bottom of the American social hierarchy, there was not one reason for any Negro, ever, to hurry."[132] The black critic Stanley Crouch has identified "being on time" as one of the behaviors many black youth reject as a form of "acting white."[133] We have already seen how the black psychiatrist James H. Carter acknowledged the reality of different time orientations while pointing to the difficult circumstances that necessarily change poor people's relationship to keeping time and keeping on schedule.

The time orientation issue has also figured in discussions of black patients' suitability for psychotherapy. "The ghetto patient," two white psychiatrists write in 1980, "is not likely to be considered a good candidate for long-term therapy for many reasons," including a high dropout rate that results in part from a relationship to time that differs from that of better organized middle-class patients. "Many of these people do not expect that tomorrow or next year will be substantially better than today. To them the world is a risky, treacherous arena, and one would be foolish to postpone gratification. . . . Appointments are never more than approximate schedules; they are kept according to 'black people's time' or 'Puerto Rican time.'" These authors also connect time orientation to some of the classic themes regarding the black personality associated with "damaged" and "pathological" personality traits. "The ghetto patient is less likely to observe himself or herself developmentally along a time axis marked by stages of individuation," thereby demonstrating a deficient capacity for introspection and for charting out the road to maturity and adulthood. Second, frequent emotional rejection by parents and the compensatory need for special relationships with parent figures means that these patients are "not raised for a future that include[s] a long-term, mutually respecting heterosexual relationship. Rather, they [are] raised to stay close to the parent figure," a claim that raises once again the specter of the dysfunctional black family and the bitter debate around this topic unleashed by the Moynihan Report. Third, the authors associate present-time orientation with "harsh punishments" and demands for "immediate obedience" that exclude a developmental approach to child rearing. In summary, the absence of the middle-class values that "foster an internalization of rather clearly defined developmental milestones" is a burden that some ghetto residents will manage better than others. The good news is that these therapists "have found many [ghetto] patients who respond to long-term therapy,"[134] thereby contradicting the deeply rooted stereotype about the futility of offering sophisticated therapies to black patients. Or as James H. Carter put it in 1979: "The implication that somehow the method of treating blacks must be relatively simple is appalling."[135]

This interpretation of time orientation in the ghetto provoked a forceful and disapproving response from the prominent black psychiatrist Carl C. Bell, who reported being "extremely disturbed" by an interpretation of black behavior that "left a bad taste in my mouth." The overt disagreement with his white colleagues was that, after ten years treating ghetto patients, he had "a hard time believing that their original lateness stemmed from an orientation toward time that was deeply rooted in their fundamental value system," a phrasing that evokes one of the classic objections to the Moynihan Report's critique of black "culture." Lateness to appointments, he said, signaled an emotional vulnerability requiring an appropriate therapeutic response that should convey, among other things, an insistence on punctual behavior:

> It has been my impression that the ghetto patient who casually floats in late to his session is being "cool." It is extremely important that ghetto patients maintain some sense of power and control; to maintain this "overcompensatory grandiosity" they may initially attempt to downplay the importance of the therapeutic relationship by casually floating in late to their sessions. This behavior will continue unless the therapist makes it clear that it will not be accepted. Allowing this behavior to go unchecked only develops and reinforces a defense that undermines the necessity of being on time for work.[136]

White therapists may be too intimidated to insist on punctuality from black clients, or they may "simply excuse the patient's behavior as being culturally appropriate"—a naïve form of unwitting condescension toward the black patient and the "culture of poverty" that has deformed his relationship to time. White therapists can also mishandle the situation by misinterpreting sexual and aggressive behaviors "as being signs of impulsive behavior and therefore superego deficits. I would hardly expect," Bell comments, "such therapists to simply state that if the patient is late, he will not be seen."[137] On the contrary, having exaggerated the significance of the sexual and aggressive behaviors in his black clients, the therapist would be inclined to favor the continuation of therapy for the purpose of treating these disorders.

It is important to recognize that black psychiatrists' response to the perceptions and therapeutic strategies of their white colleagues operates on two levels. In the foreground is an apparently straightforward disagreement about whether most "ghetto" patients are willing to respect the rules of punctuality and show up on time for their appointments. While Bell claims that compliance with this requirement is "fairly high," the white authors reply that their experience had been that "patients who are told firmly that they need to be on time before they have established a relationship tend to drop out in great numbers." On a less obvious level, it is clear from his commentary that black practitioners regard this interchange as more than a disagreement about facts. The "bad taste" in Dr. Bell's mouth is related in part to his judgment that references to "black people's time," and the manner of thinking this implies, amount to an "unacceptable" breach of professional conduct. (The fact that such expressions, e.g.,

"Colored People's Time," belong to the black vernacular is not mentioned.) His critiques of hypothetical misbehaviors by white therapists are clearly aimed, however obliquely, at his white interlocutors, whom he can easily imagine falling into the traps that await therapists who know little about black life and are, therefore, unprepared to serve the needs of black patients who expect empathy and understanding. Bell does not suggest, for example, that white therapists might have caused, however inadvertently, the large numbers of dropouts they had observed. In this sense, Bell's critique of his white colleagues' approach to black time management belongs to a tradition of commentaries by black physicians that have appeared in this book, including Rutherford B. Stevens's account of the white military psychiatrists he encountered in America's segregated army during the Second World War.

The psychiatric literature has also presented claims that blacks experience hallucinations more frequently than whites do.[138] Here, too, black and white psychiatrists have participated in the discussion, although in this case sparring between "black" and "white" points of view has not occurred. Yet even in the absence of such conflicting interpretations of an observed "black" trait, the implications of this finding offer their own potential threat to the idea that blacks are as psychologically competent as whites, given that psychiatrists designate hallucinations as a form of "disorientation."

Hallucinations, like time orientation, can be perceived as a sign or symptom of "black culture." "It is often considered," three white psychiatrists from North Carolina write in 1963, "that the Negro places particular emphasis on impressions and experiences. At times the Negro group emotionally reacts out of proportion to the stimulus and shows a lowered emotional threshold and heightened tension. . . . Southern Negro music and religion give some evidence of this reliance on emotionality."[139] Whereas these white psychiatrists do not take this folklore at face value, their professional doubts are of less importance than the folkloric power of the idea that Negroes are, in church and in song, literally out of their minds. In this vein, a contributor to the 1916 volume of the *Psychoanalytic Review*, whose fundamental premise is that "the colored race" remained close to "its stage of barbarism," had argued that "hoodooism" (voodoo) persisted among the Negro population and that "this primitive method of thought is an integral part of the race."[140]

Three decades later this theory was still being taken seriously in the *American Journal of Psychiatry*, where two psychiatrists noted "the apparent ease with which the mentally ill of the Negro race develop hallucinatory experiences and [that] ideas of reference may be related to the fact that they are but a few generations removed from a culture in which such mental 'abnormalities' are incorporated in the actual beliefs and practices of their every day lives."[141] Writing at the beginning of the postwar era of American race relations, at a time when doing something about the racial imbalance of power had become imaginable in a way it had not been before, these authors demonstrate an ambivalence toward racial folklore that is typical of the medical profession and of educated white attitudes in general. "It is a common but probably mistaken idea," they write, "that it is usual for normal Negroes to hear voices or to hear visions. However, certain psychological differences between the Negro and white man that bear on this question have been described." For these psychiatrists, the idea that blacks have trouble distinguishing between "illusion and knowledge," and hallucinations and reality, was worth taking seriously.[142]

It is a short step from images of uncontrolled Negro emotions and waking dream states to the idea that black culture is itself hallucinogenic. The Nigerian American psychiatrist Dr. Victor Adebimpe, for example, wrote in 1981 that religious delusions and hallucinations among blacks point to "a baseline of 'non-schizophrenic' hallucinations among blacks [that] probably underlies the higher frequency of this symptom in black schizophrenics."[143] Here the black psychiatrist appears to endorse the view that a nonschizophrenic (nonpsychotic) predisposition to hallucinatory experiences is part of being black, at least in the context of religious experience.

But what might a predisposition to hallucinations imply about "black" emotional life in a more global sense? "Some American psychiatrists," a sociologist wrote in 1981, "have asserted that Negroes are less able to distinguish between 'objective existence' and hallucinations, that is, objective or everyday existence for the Negro can be closer to what the hallucinatory state is for a member of another group. Those who have interviewed Negro patients or have read their personal histories cannot but be impressed with the role of the Negro's disastrous social milieu in influencing the patient's own norms." The "disastrous" conditions in which blacks live have impaired their ability to distinguish between what is real and what is unreal, and thus between what is sane and what is insane: "The Negro's unwillingness or inability to recognize mental illness in other Negroes has been indicated in research, while others have pointed out that Negro tolerance of illness in general is greater."[144] "Deviant and bizarre behavior may be better tolerated in the Negro culture," according to the white psychiatrists from North Carolina.[145] In *Dark Ghetto* (1965), the black psychologist Kenneth Clark had posed the same question: "Is the pathology of the dark ghetto so pervasive that mental disturbance does not stand out as clearly as it does elsewhere? . . . Is less illness reported—or even recognized *as* illness—by ghetto families and friends?"[146]

But what does tolerance of mental illness actually mean in this context? In 1968 two psychologists reported that, "Negroes were found to have a lower level of understanding of current theories of mental illness, a greater sympathetic understanding of children and of the aged, and a greater tendency to feel that the mentally ill person is responsible for his difficulties."[147] In other words, tolerance can express ignorance, or compassion, or indifference toward people who are seen as having caused their own problems. Tolerance of psychological distress may also be a kind of realism about black life itself, so that blacks may be less inclined than whites to interpret an experience like depression in medical terms. "It is possible that blacks may more frequently feel they have a reason to be depressed and consider their symptoms to be normal outcomes of everyday problems, stress, and strain."[148] Whether one calls this ignorance of medical norms or stoic realism, the result is yet another version of racially distinct experiential worlds whose definitions of "normality" will differ. It is also "colonial" in the sense that trauma is now established as the basic psychic condition of a subordinated group.

A frequently cited problem associated with defining which mental states are "normal" for blacks and whites is the challenge of distinguishing between "paranoia" and the endemic caution among African Americans that has been described previously. In 1970, at a time when politically conscious "black psychiatry" was still in its infancy, the following commentary appeared in *Time* magazine:

> As necessary, the black therapist also redefines mental illness. "There are some behavior patterns that one could call pathological," says Charles Wilkinson, a black psychiatrist and executive director of the Kansas Mental Health Foundation. "But it's a question whether they are really pathological or simply adaptive. If judged by the majority of the prevailing culture, they could be called pathological. But from the black person's standpoint, they have been patterns he has had to use to make it. It is scarcely paranoid, for instance, for the black to distrust and fear the white society." Says Dr. William Malamud Jr., a white psychiatrist in Boston: "What's labeled as pathology is very often psychic health in blacks. You can say: 'How else would you expect them to act?'"[149]

This cultural relativism within the field of mental health had been evident to observant white physicians for many years. "The Negro would seem to mistrust the white physician," one psychiatrist wrote in 1951. "This feature of suspiciousness might appear to give a paranoid coloring in some individual patients, but it was found to be so frequent and to be so separate from real paranoid material that it would certainly suggest that it is attributable to the fact of Negroes mistrusting and resenting white men, the therapist being white."[150] Three decades later the black psychiatrist James H. Carter was making the same point in an article on how to recognize symptoms in black patients. White clinicians' ignorance of black culture, he argued, "has resulted in the abuse of the diagnosis 'paranoia,' which is much too strong a name for what I believe is generally a healthy cultural suspiciousness, an adaptive response to the experience of racism."[151] Yet even if the white practitioner is able to see this "healthy suspiciousness" for what it is, the fact remains that the profession's recognition of this emotional estrangement, like the idea of a hallucinogenic black culture, is one more indication of the estranged status of an entire group of people.

By now it should be apparent that the psychiatric literature has accommodated, in some cases without controversy or debate, a series of diagnoses of black mental functioning that present images of psychological incompetence, disorientation, and arrested development that have been applied much too broadly to the black population. The fact that the black-edited *Journal of the National Medical Association* is rarely if ever cited in mainstream medical journals or newspapers has facilitated distorted diagnoses of black mental health. Black-white medical dialogue that might correct for bias has never been promoted by the major medical journals. In the last analysis, these assessments of black mental life effectively deny the capacity of many black people to function as citizens and workers and parents on a level comparable to that of their white fellow citizens.

This meta-diagnosis of the black condition portrays a population requiring special handling and supervision in a "colonial" manner, and it is important to understand how American psychiatry went about translating this socially sanctioned diagnosis into coercive or paternalistic forms of therapy that have been applied disproportionately to black patients. Disciplinarian therapy of this kind should thus be understood as an extension of societal attitudes toward black men in particular that combine apprehension about their allegedly disordered minds with therapeutic ambitions to make their behavior conform to socially acceptable norms.[152]

The belief that black males require close supervision by whites was evident for hundreds of years in the institution of chattel slavery and the prison chain gangs of the American South. The grossly disproportionate representation of black men in the criminal justice system today continues this legacy. "Although African American men make up approximately 6 to

7 percent of the total U.S. population," a black social scientist noted in 2001, "they represent more than 60 percent of the two million persons under correctional supervision. African Americans are imprisoned at seven times the rate of whites."[153] It is not surprising, therefore, that psychiatric thinking about, and the psychotherapeutic management of, black males has been influenced by what Jerome G. Miller has called "the criminalization of the majority of young African-American males."[154] The fundamental question here is to what extent such thinking and therapeutic practices are based on science or racial folklore.

The urban ghetto riots of the 1960s prompted at least a few psychiatrists to associate violent behavior with psychopathology and to speculate about medical treatments for rebelliousness. Vernon Mark, a psychiatrist who performed 13 "psychosurgeries" on violent epileptics during the period between 1963 and 1973, and the author of *Violence and the Brain* (1970), coauthored a much-noted letter on the "Role of Brain Disease in Riots and Urban Violence" that appeared in the September 11, 1967, issue of the *Journal of the American Medical Association*. "Is there something peculiar about the violent slum dweller that differentiates him from his peaceful neighbor?" these authors asked. Their answer was that "electroencephalographic abnormalities in the temporal region" of the brain were strongly correlated with "poor impulse control" and physical assaults on others.[155] A rebuttal from another psychiatrist, Seymour L. Pollack, called Mark's letter "very disturbing." "Unfortunately," he wrote, "the old superstition of associating mental illness and electroencephalographic abnormalities with violence still exists. . . . The incidence of violent behavior with certain types of electroencephalographic disorders has been exaggerated."[156] During the 1970s, Orlando J. Andy, the founding chairman of neurosurgery at the University of Mississippi School of Medicine, performed brain surgeries on black children who had demonstrated "behavior problems." According to this neurologist, "the kind of brain damage that could necessitate such radical surgery might be manifested by participation in the Watts Uprising." "Such people," he proposed, "could have abnormal pathological brains."[157] This was the sort of thinking that prompted Melvin Sabshin in 1970 to warn that blacks would reject mental health clinics run by anyone who implied "that militancy indicates psychopathology."[158]

In 1998, it was revealed that the New York State Psychiatric Institute had administered intravenous doses of fenfluramine—a diet drug that was later banned—to 34 black and Hispanic boys between the ages of six and ten who were the younger brothers of delinquents and whose mothers were suspected of "adverse rearing practices." The theory was that serotonin levels in the brain might predict violent behavior. "Is there or is there not a correlation between certain biological markers and conduct disorders or antisocial behavior?" asked Dr. John Oldham, the director of the Institute. In 1999 the Mount Sinai School of Medicine and the Research Foundation of the City University of New York were criticized for injecting fenfluramine into sixty-six boys with a diagnosis of attention deficit/hyperactivity disorder. While those in charge defended these studies as ethical and socially responsible research, the specter of racial biology and its potential dangers hung in the air.[159] How far was American society prepared to go in the direction of preemptive "treatments" for potentially violent black and brown children? As the African American political scientist Ronald Walters put it: "If there is a reason for this kind of research, the aim is to find a drug. And if you begin using drugs to pacify young black males, as is often done with Ritalin for hyperactivity, you're creating a regime of social control."[160]

The discovery that medical researchers had been injecting a drug into 100 disproportionately minority children as a possible prophylactic against violent behavior caused a scandal. Yet the fact is that disproportionate use of psychotropic drugs in adult black patients has been the norm for many years. A 1967 report comparing the psychiatric treatment of black and white patients noted that blacks were 50 percent more likely to be given *drugs only* (without accompanying psychotherapy), corresponding to the treatment of lower-class patients in general.[161] "Black psychiatric patients," James H. Carter commented in 1984, "have historically received larger amounts of powerful psychotropic drugs without ancillary forms of intervention, and this also applies to the black elderly."[162] This racial imbalance has also been observed outside of the United States. The *British Journal of Psychiatry* reported in 1990 that "black patients are more likely than whites to receive psychotropic medications." During the 1980s in Britain, there was "concern over the apparent increase in the rates of compulsory treatment, police involvement, and prescription of long-acting neuroleptics among Afro-Caribbean immigrants and their descendants with psychotic illness."[163] A 2004 report in the *British Medical Journal* found that "Africans and Afro-Caribbeans were over-represented in the mental health services, received a more coercive spectrum of care, were more likely to be regarded as dangerous, and were more likely to be over-medicated.[164] A year later, the African American medical journal quoted a black mother concerned about "an inexperienced white teacher who wants to drug children into compliance."[165] The social impact of medication policies is thus magnified by black distrust of the whites who administer them.

It is important to note here that the black patients who were given more psychotropic drugs also received less psychotherapeutic treatment than whites.[166] One explanation for these racially differential treatments can be found in the theory of medico-racial folklore presented in this book. The black human organism has long been regarded as less evolved and thus less complex than its white counterpart. Doubts about offering psychotherapy to blacks, and a greater willingness to use drugs to sedate and control them, presume a less complicated psyche that is less inclined to therapeutic dialogue and more suited to a chemical intervention intended to turn the mind off and inhibit unpredictable behavior. Psychiatric treatments of this kind extend social or police authority into psychotherapeutic space and reproduce the surveillance and control procedures long associated with the administration of colonial subjects.

COLONIAL MEDICAL STATUS

The "colonial" status of African Americans within the American medical system has now been documented in a variety of ways. According to the classic definition of Frantz Fanon, colonial medicine is based on the estrangement of the dominated population from the medical personnel of the dominant authorities, who regard colonial subjects as less entitled to humane treatment; that is why their pain is discounted as unimportant. These "natives" are a source of various kinds of trouble—a theme that has appeared often in the American medical literature. The "Negro patient" of yesteryear was a misunderstood and frequently caricatured subject of the Jim Crow period. Today, African American children are seen as "normally more active than their peers from other ethnic backgrounds," show higher levels of "conduct disorder," and yet (according to a 1998 study) are less than half as likely as white children to be prescribed psychotropic medication. This example of racially differential diagnosis and treatment—more disordered behavior treated with less medication—defies therapeutic logic but exemplifies the political logic that governs the status of the colonial subject.[167] Neglecting the medical needs of the disordered racial other confirms that he is alien to the community that excludes him. Similarly, the denial of equitable pain relief to African American patients today subjects them to another version of "colonial" status.

The colonial medical subject, whether African or African American, feels the "endemic wariness that pervades core black culture," in the words of the black anthropologist Gwaltney.[168] As neglected medical subjects, African Americans resemble in their own way "the inarticulate peoples of the Colonies," as a British doctor described Africans in 1948[169], and this vulnerability has created a degree of suspiciousness about white motives and behaviors that can take the form of extreme views most whites would regard as irrational or even paranoid. Conspiracy theories of this kind include both highly eccentric claims by outspoken individuals as well as beliefs about the victimization of blacks that millions of African Americans hold, as many surveys confirm.[170]

The notorious murders of 29 black children, adolescents and adults in the Atlanta area between 1979 and 1981 inspired the activist and comedian Dick Gregory to suggest "that the Atlanta Centers for Disease Control were kidnapping and murdering black boys to harvest the anticancer drug found in the tips of their penises."[171] The most eccentric category also includes the 1988 claim by a black activist in Chicago that Jewish doctors were injecting the AIDS virus into black children.[172] A decade later a self-styled Afrocentric health expert told a rally in Harlem that AIDS was a creation of the white man and that black parents should "be very careful when you take your kids for the polio vaccine . . . because [the white medical establishment] are seeding the vaccines with germs to reduce our population."[173]

Many African Americans have believed and continue to believe that medical strategies such as contraception and anti-HIV/AIDS initiatives are actually intended to reduce or eliminate the black population. Long-standing conspiracy beliefs about birth control services offered to black women still persist into the twenty-first century.[174] A national telephone survey conducted in the early 1990s found that 20 percent of the black respondents agreed with the statement: "The government is using AIDS as a way of killing off minority groups." Two-thirds of blacks (as compared with one-third of whites) believed that "the government is not telling the whole story about AIDS." A 1993 report found that between 17 percent and 38 percent of black respondents "believed that there is some truth in reports that the AIDS virus was produced in a germ-warfare laboratory." More that 25 percent of black church parishioners in Louisiana agreed in 1996 that AIDS was "intended to wipe blacks off the face of the earth."[175] An even greater proportion of the African American population either believe or are willing to take seriously such claims of medical genocide. Black celebrities such as the rapper Kool Moe Dee, the actor Will Smith, and the filmmaker Spike Lee have endorsed similar ideas.[176]

Here, too, there is an important commonality between African and African American resistance to white medical authority. The devastating medical effects of conspiracy beliefs about AIDS have been most graphically evident in South Africa as a consequence of the disastrous AIDS policies the former president Thabo Mbeki pursued. These policies dismayed Western scientists, activists, and politicians. Over a decade, Mbeki refused to distribute the anti-AIDS drug AZT to pregnant women, welcomed American academics who denied that HIV causes AIDS, and employed a health minister who endorsed a cheap "miracle" cure for AIDS.[177]

Mbeki's intransigence can be understood as a bitter rejection of Western thinking in favor of an African approach that refuses to accept the authority of Western science—hence his fraternizing with the handful of AIDS scientists considered hopeless eccentrics by the great majority of their peers. This provocative behavior toward the Western medical establishment can also be seen as a postcolonial response to colonial-era medical racism and its legacy in postapartheid South Africa. The tragedy is that, in acting out his anticolonial resentments, Mbeki condemned thousands of South Africans, most of them women and children, to premature and painful deaths.

At its deepest level, colonial medical status is a diagnosis of the racial alien—a medical status report that describes his limitations and pathologies and prescribes therapeutic measures to remedy these deficiencies. From this perspective, African Americans have been colonized "natives" in all but name since Emancipation, and many blacks have been well aware of this colonized status and their related role as objects of study. When the American Association of Physical Anthropology and the National Research Council established a "Committee on the Negro" in 1926, there was nothing blacks could do to respond to this loss of autonomy. The racial imbalance of power could be protested only when black professionals attained positions from which they could promulgate their own views. Two decades later, when a group of American rabbis held a round table discussion on "The Negro in the United States," the black psychologist Kenneth Clark commented that "the question arises as to what Jews and others would think if a conference of Negro leaders were to devote a round table to the problem of 'The Jew in the United States.'"[178] Some professional white observers of black life of this era took note of the racial imbalance of power and expressed concern about the effects of their own studies of black lives. The authors of *The Mark of Oppression*, an influential and controversial study of the effects of racism on the Negro personality, acknowledged that the Negro might "consider it an intrusion on his privacy on the grounds that much had better been left unsaid."[179] But what were conscientious white sociologists or psychoanalysts like these authors to do? On the one hand, they wanted to put their knowledge to work on behalf of oppressed blacks. The problem was that being black and being studied—or, put more bluntly, being treated like a specimen—might well come at a cost to the dignity of people who had already absorbed far more than their share of emotional abuse.

By the 1960s, black protests against being treated like research subjects had become vocal. In particular, black intellectuals expressed impatience with what they regarded as intrusive and voyeuristic attitudes that expressed an unwholesome interest in black life. The civil rights leader James Farmer declared in 1965, for example, that "the cocktail hour on the 'Negro Question' is over," and "we are sick unto death of being analyzed, mesmerized, bought, sold and slobbered over while the same evils that are the ingredients of our oppression go unattended."[180] Black psychiatrists joined in this chorus, noting the loss of black autonomy that resulted when whites arrogated to themselves the role of defining black identity. "Too long," Chester M. Pierce declared, "has America relied on interpretations and forecasts by white scientists on the meaning of being a Negro. As is nearly always the case, most of what is written about Negroes has been written by whites and published through white channels."[181] "The 'experts' on the Negro are almost exclusively non-Negro," Alyce C. Gullatee noted in 1969. "The Negro, therefore, most often learns who he is not through self-discovery but through an outside source whose perceptions may be distorted and/or naïve."[182] A cautionary note about black resentment directed against "the overstudy of ghetto residents by government and university researchers" appeared in the *American Journal of Psychiatry* in 1971.[183] "Small wonder that the black community is fed up with being 'researched' by investigators who can see only the deforming marks of oppression," Alexander Thomas and Samuel Sillen noted acerbically in their *Racism and Psychiatry* in 1972.[184]

Colonial medical status has always meant being subjected to an intrusive scrutiny that describes the disorders of black minds and bodies. In this sense the Moynihan controversy of the late 1960s greatly expanded the diagnostic approach to black life and extended this public diagnosis to the black family and psychological problems in children and adults alike. The aftershocks of this controversy over decades prevented much serious research into the African American experience from being done, thereby leaving the field open to conservative interpreters of black life such as Charles Murray and his influential volume *Losing Ground* (1984), which argued that welfare programs for black families were useless.

Colonial medical status for African Americans now meant either being stigmatized by an overemphasis on "pathology" or neglected on account of researchers' fears of being called racists if they studied black problems. "It was as if, somehow, to discuss the Negro family in public were a breach of good manners," Irving Howe wrote in 1968. "What these whites were saying in effect, without realizing how deeply condescending they were, was that while blacks in the U.S. were oppressed, anyone pointing to the visible damage resulting from that oppression was an enemy of the Negroes."[185] Even the term *damage*, as a description of the consequences of racism, would eventually become a target of opprobrium, as if accepting such damage as real amounted to stigmatizing or "blaming the victims."[186] Two decades later, the prominent black sociologist William Julius Wilson was reiterating Howe's point, noting that there is "a potential danger for serious scholarly research from the fallout over the underclass debate. We need only to be reminded of what transpired following the controversy over the Moynihan Report on the black family in the late 1960s. The vitriolic attacks and acrimonious debate that characterized that controversy proved to be too intimidating to scholars, especially to liberal scholars."[187] At the end of the day, the argument over how and whether to discuss "damage" and "pathology" only reinforced a widespread conviction that the emotional damage was real.

5. A Medical School Syllabus on Race

INTRODUCTION

"It is an open secret that physicians dislike certain patients," a team of medical authors wrote in *JAMA* in 1979.[1] This oblique reference to the emotional vulnerabilities of physicians, and to the medical consequences of misjudgments and misconduct that can result from the dysfunctional personality traits or beliefs of doctors, opened a door through which not many medical authors have chosen to step. What is more, those who have stepped over the threshold into this territory have demonstrated a reluctance to penetrate too far into a *terra incognita* that presents a clear threat to the self-image of the medical profession. "Physicians have long been members of a special moral community," wrote former president of the American Medical Association, the late Ronald M. Davis, in 2008. It is noteworthy that this reference to moral community introduced Dr. Davis's *JAMA* commentary on the official apology of the American Medical Association (AMA) to African Americans and African American physicians for the profession's "dishonorable acts of omission and commission" that constitute the history of medical racism in the United States. That this official apology did not arrive until after the turning of the twenty-first century speaks to what Dr. Davis called "the group's current moral orientation," which continues to get far less attention than it deserves.[2] Dr. Arnold Epstein, then chairman of the department of health policy at the Harvard School of Public Health, had commented on the silence around medical racism a decade earlier in 1998. By this time the medical literature had clearly demonstrated that black patients were getting inferior medical care. "What is striking," Dr. Epstein said, "is that the findings are not subtle and that we as a country have done nothing about it."[3] More than a decade and hundreds of additional publications later, the medical profession has still not confronted medical racism in a committed and systematic way. The well-intentioned but piecemeal and inadequate attempts to change the racial thinking and behavior of medical students via curricular reform are described and analyzed in this final chapter.

It is the contention of this book that the current orientation of the medical profession regarding racial issues continues to preserve some dysfunctional habits. Transforming these habits for the purpose of improving medical treatment is the responsibility of the medical educators who supervise the training of medical students.

First and foremost among these old habits is that of paying little attention to black people, including black physicians and their interests. Indeed, one of the striking features of the medical literature on race and medicine that has appeared over the past several decades is the lack of interest in soliciting and presenting the views of African American physicians whose knowledge of race relations is likely to differ from, and in certain ways exceed, that of most of their white colleagues. Dr. James L. Potts, an internist at the Meharry Medical College School clinic, made this point in 1998: "It was necessary for me to learn about white Americans to survive. For white doctors, I'm not so sure the reverse is always true."[4] While this knowledge gap is of great practical significance to the practice of multiracial medicine, readers of the mainstream medical literature will find few African American perspectives to guide them through the intricacies of black-white relationships in the medical context. Contributing to the invisibility of the black physician is the invisibility of the *Journal of the National Medical Association (JNMA)*, the nation's primary African American medical journal. As of 2008, the *JNMA* had an Impact Factor rating of 0.9, equivalent to that of the *National Medical Journal of India* (0.9) and below that of the *South African Medical Journal* (1.0) and the *Croatian Medical Journal* (1.1). The *New England Journal of Medicine* (50) and the *Journal of the American Medical Association* (31.7) were orders of magnitude more influential than their African American counterpart. This gap represents a medically costly disparity in a society where African Americans bear a disproportionate burden of disease and have demonstrated limited trust in the medical establishment. The lowly status of the *JNMA*, citations of which are seldom encountered in either the medical literature or mainstream media, is one symptom of the lack of interest in black life that the medical profession should finally address and correct. In his commentary, Dr. Davis asserted that "the AMA's apology builds on an increasingly strong NMA-AMA collaboration in recent years."[5] It would be instructive to know the forms this collaboration has taken and what black physicians and patients can expect in the way of benefits. The long-standing disregard of black interests is typified by a survey of "American Medical Education 100 Years after the Flexner Report" that appeared in 2006 in the *New England Journal of Medicine,* the world's most prestigious medical journal. The racial dimension of American medicine, including the teaching of "cultural competence" to medical students, is simply absent from this report. The authors' closest approach to the race issue is their observation that, although "it can be hard to teach messy real-world issues" in medical school, it is still necessary to do so. The "messy real-world" issues remain unidentified. A passing reference to "the hidden curriculum of the practice environment" shows that the authors are aware of the oral transmission among medical personnel of potentially harmful stereotypes outside the formal medical curriculum, but this theme remains as intangible as race itself.[6]

The AMA's long-standing lack of interest in African American problems is directly related to physicians' feelings and beliefs about race and how medically dysfunctional these traits and syndromes can be. This is demonstrated by the documented consequences of racially differential diagnosis and treatment that can compromise black health and cost lives.[7] The racial folklore that has infiltrated medical thinking along with the rest of our society fills the heads of doctors just as it permeates the general population; the difference is that stigmatizing racial folklore can do special harm in the medical context. At the same time, the profession has never inventoried this racial folklore or attempted to calculate its effects on doctor-patient relationships. Medical education has shown little interest in promoting the acquisition of emotional self-knowledge by medical students and doctors, even though the idea that medical personnel can benefit from psychotherapy has occasionally appeared in the medical literature since the 1970s. The "multiple mini interview" procedure for vetting potential medical students demonstrates a new interest in interpersonal skills but does not address race relations.[8]

THE DOCTOR-PATIENT RELATIONSHIP

Concern in the medical literature about the doctor-patient relationship is usually dated from L. J. Henderson's "Physician and Patient as a Social System," which appeared in the *New England Journal of Medicine* in 1935. It would have required a white physician of rare courage and moral imagination to take up the race issue during the Jim Crow era, and this was not the author's purpose. On the one hand, Henderson saw "the personal relations" between doctor and patient being undermined by "the new and powerful technology of medical practice." But his primary purpose in this essay was to dispense some practical advice to doctors about the management of their own emotions. Doctors must not allow themselves to be manipulated by the "sentiments" of their patients, he advised. In addition, the doctor should weigh his own words carefully, since "the patient will eagerly scrutinize and rationalize what you say" and try to extract "shades of meaning that you never thought of." It probably did not occur to this Harvard professor that the virtue of doing "as little harm as possible . . . with the expression of your sentiments and emotions" would have special significance while treating black or female or homosexual patients.[9]

Henderson's advice to doctors about the value of self-scrutiny opens the door to a series of questions about the education of physicians. When did medical authors begin to see the need for *a self-analytical procedure* that might enable doctors to better understand themselves and their relationships with their patients? When did medical authors begin to write openly and frankly about the *"difficult" patients* they encounter, and which kinds of patients have been assigned to this category? When have medical authors pointed to *a lack of research* on the doctor-patient relationship? Have medical authors acknowledged the *sociological naïveté* of many physicians and its medical costs? And how many medical schools have tried to develop *pedagogical approaches* for initiating their students into the racial dimension of medicine?

A survey of the medical literature suggests that sustained interest in understanding the doctor-patient relationship did not appear until the 1970s and 1980s. This new emphasis on the interpersonal dynamics of medical relationships signified a retreat from the traditional model that featured two well-established roles: that of the authoritative physician, whose clinical conduct was assumed to be of high quality and thus went unexamined, and the patient who was assumed to be the source of any dysfunctional aspects of the doctor-patient relationship.

Several factors may have contributed to this "shift to more of a medical egalitarian model in the late 1970s and early 1980s." For example, a diminishing educational gap between doctors and patients would be expected to promote more collegial and less paternalistic relationships between clinician and client.[10] But this change in the nature of the doctor-patient relationship involved more than doctors encountering better-informed patients. In 1984, Barbara Gerbert noted "two general trends in the literature of physicians' decision-making. The first has been a shift from viewing decision-making purely as a response to patients' signs and symptoms to acknowledging that the process is influenced by patient characteristics that are unrelated to disease. The second trend has been to recognize, and begin to document, that physicians' feelings about their patients have a distinct effect on their treatment decisions."[11]

THE PROBLEM PATIENT

This overdue scrutiny of the doctor-patient relationship was driven in part by medical authors' newly found interest in finding ways to handle particularly troublesome patients for whom there already existed a collection of standard epithets (as follows). Doctors estimate that about 15 percent of the patients they see belong in the category of especially troublesome patients who were now described by various terms: "the obnoxious patient," "the undesirable patient," "the hateful patient," "the problem patient," "the heartsink patient" [British], "the frustrating patient," and "black holes." Looking back on James E. Groves's classic paper, "Taking Care of the Hateful Patient" (1978), a group of medical authors in 1991 asserted that this essay "provided sanction for physicians to discuss the previously taboo subject of their feelings of dislike and frustration toward certain patients."[12] As we will see, Groves presented four types of "hateful" patients whom doctors had to confront. "Admitted or not," he wrote, "the fact remains that a few patients kindle fear, despair or even downright malice in their doctors. Emotional reactions to patients cannot simply be wished away, nor is it good medicine to pretend that they do not exist."[13]

The discussion catalyzed by "Taking Care of the Hateful Patient" did more than simply allow physicians to vent about patients they resented or even hated. Groves's essential point was that physicians had an obligation to do something about their own hostile emotions to better serve their patients. "Sometimes the physician may feel uncomfortable about discussing emotional issues," Douglas A. Drossman wrote in 1978. "He then overtly or covertly conspires with the patient not to consider it further."[14] "All doctors," Richard Gorlin and Howard D. Zucker wrote in 1983, "however humane, will at times have negative or positive feelings and impulses that can interfere with optimal professional action or judgment. . . . Each of us, after all, has special vulnerabilities, usually with unconscious roots. By acknowledging his or her own emotional position, the doctor is able to consider the relationship with the patient more objectively."[15] A decade later medical authors argued that the problem patient was no longer to be regarded as the flawed protagonist of a difficult doctor-patient relationship. More useful was "an approach which explores the difficulties of the clinical transaction itself, rather than the supposed failings of the problem patient."[16] What mattered was the clinical relationship "rather than the more traditional expectation that the patient's 'pathology' is the target of intervention."[17]

A striking aspect of some of these commentaries is the confident assumption that doctors were capable of recognizing and dealing with these troubling emotions by themselves. According to Gorlin and Zucker, it is "the physician [who] identifies feelings in himself or herself that are likely to interfere with effective professional judgment and behavior."[18] Solomon Papper comments in 1987 that "perhaps it is helpful to acknowledge to ourselves that there are times when we, as individual physicians, participate in patient care in a manner that we really think and feel is not optimal. Honest recognition should stimulate and enhance a sense of self-discipline that minimizes the numbers of patients who become Undesirable."[19]

Other medical commentators were more skeptical about whether doctors were capable of recognizing and processing these negative feelings by themselves. In "Doctors Have Feelings Too" (1988), William M. Zinn pointed out that the existing studies of doctor-patient interactions were inadequate, because they had been "written by social scientists or psychiatrists who did not have access to the day-to-day medical encounters between patients and physicians"[20]—a research deficit that persists to the present day in the case of interracial encounters. A decade later Dennis H. Novack warned: "Unrecognized feelings and attitudes can adversely affect physician-patient communication. . . ."[21] For these observers, "honest recognition" of the emotional problems provoked in doctors by patients was not a self-analytic procedure of which every physician was capable. What was more, patients were being put at risk when doctors assumed unmanageable emotional burdens and refused to ask for help.

The obvious alternative to this sort of isolation was psychotherapy. Interestingly, the idea of doctors seeking counsel appears nowhere in "Taking Care of the Hateful Patient." Advising doctors who have been driven to the point of rage or despair by their intolerable patients, Groves never mentions the therapeutic option. His recommended coping strategy is that doctors should respond to provocation by changing their thinking through an act of will. Two decades later, Novack proposed that doctors recognize their similarity to mental health professionals who must constantly monitor their own emotional states for the purpose of facilitating the therapeutic process: "Because medical practitioners routinely work with patients in emotional pain, frequently discuss sensitive issues, and counsel people experiencing minor and major stressors, it would seem essential that they have similar training."[22] In fact, one finds very little talk about doctors in therapy in the medical literature, just as one finds no specific information about how doctors think about race. These two deficits are linked in that both preserve the personal and professional privacy of the physician. What, then, might justify psychotherapeutic intervention in the life of a doctor? One answer to this question was proposed in David R. Levy's pioneering 1985 article on "White Doctors and Black Patients": "For psychiatrists who lack the empathy needed for work with all groups of people, psychoanalysis has been recommended to erase distorted perspectives concerning race or at least to enable them to become more aware of when their irrational attitudes might impede the treatment process."[23] In the last analysis, trying to remove whatever hostility toward or contempt for blacks the psychiatrist might bring to the psychotherapeutic process was only an option, not an obligation. Monitoring the racial beliefs of physicians was not on the agenda.

MEDICAL AUTHORS' AVERSION TO RACE

Why does the "problem patient" literature never include black patients, given that the "Negro patient" had often been presented as a "problem patient" since the era of emancipation? He is absent from this roster of undesirable patients in part because the new racial etiquette of the post–civil rights era ended the causal stigmatizing of black patients by physicians; the new protocol prescribed nonjudgmental observations about emotional "barriers" between black patients and their white doctors. But the absence of blacks from the "problem patient" literature is more than a matter of etiquette. It also points to a race-aversive attitude on the part of medical authors that has done much to retard the improvement of race relations in medicine. Whereas the "problem patient" conundrum prompted the more introspective doctors to examine their own psychodynamics, it did not require them to confront their feelings about race. For this reason, while the "problem patient" discussion in the medical journals liberalized medical education by making the physician's personality a legitimate topic for examination, it simultaneously perpetuated the disinterest in blacks by promoting the idea that white doctors could examine themselves and their professional conduct without having to deal with the potential complications involved in treating black patients.

Black patients were thus written out of the liberal program to humanize physicians' attitudes toward "difficult" patients. Common terms employed by doctors and medical students for their most resented patients have included "self-pitiers," "crocks," "hits," "gomers," "geeks," "dirtballs," and "the enemy."[24] The omission of racial tags from many doctors' descriptions of "problem patients" was in all likelihood the result of three factors. First, physicians' deep resentment of such aggressive and obnoxious behaviors may simply overwhelm any special feelings the doctor might have about the alleged characteristics of minority patients, so that the "race" of the offender becomes irrelevant. Second, today's racial mores forbid the denigration of black people as a group. The third factor involves the fundamentally different relationships to the medical profession that whites and blacks have experienced over the past several generations. These differences have been so profound as to have largely excluded blacks from the standard "problem patient" category.

The four types of "hateful" patients Groves described in 1978 are "dependent clingers," "entitled demanders," "manipulative help-rejecters," and "self-destructive deniers." The "dependent clingers," caught up in their "self-perception of bottomless need," demand "all forms of attention imaginable." The "entitled demanders" may attempt to intimidate the doctor and "exude a repulsive sense of innate deservedness," a "sense of innate and magical entitlement to everything that is wanted." The "manipulative help-rejecters" are pessimists who project a depthless emotional need and seek "an undivorcible marriage with an inexhaustible caregiver." The "self-destructive deniers" seem "to glory in their own destruction. They appear to find their main pleasure in furiously defeating the physician's attempts to preserve their lives."[25]

There can be no doubt that physicians encounter some black patients who exhibit these behaviors. At the same time, it is probable that African American patients are underrepresented in this group for the following reason. All of the difficult, eccentric, and egocentric patients Groves described share a warped sense of entitlement to the time and attention from physicians that African Americans have long been denied. Over many years, African Americans have had to adapt to the chronic absence of doctors and medical services, as demonstrated by their persisting distrust of the medical profession and the resulting doctor-avoiding behaviors. If anything, the African American "problem patient" may be an uncommunicative person who represents the inverse of the "hateful" white patient who feels entitled to unlimited time and attention from medical personnel.

Medical educators should, therefore, be aware that black patients can present a different kind of "problem" for the many white physicians who know little about the black experience or have not experienced significant relationships with black people.

The lack of attention to race relations and black patients recurs over and over again in the medical literature that addresses the emotional predicaments of physicians. The finding reported in 1979 that a "physician tended to like best the patients that he thought he knew best" prompted no mention of racial barriers.[26] In "Doctors Have Feelings Too," William M. Zinn describes physicians' emotional discomforts as follows: "These problems are often, but not always, idiosyncratic and represent the individual physician's psychological, cultural, and educational history. Common areas of difficulty are those subjects that are problematic culturally for everyone but that are compounded in the medical encounter because of their repetition and intensity. They include issues of death, separation, sexuality, control, integrity of self, and dependency." For whatever reason, race was not included on the list of "those subjects that are problematic culturally for everyone." While Zinn is among the most thoughtful of these medical authors, and a keen promoter of self-analysis by physicians, race does not make it onto his agenda. "Sometimes self-analysis is enough," he writes, "but an important, though underused, tool is the sharing of experience through peer consultation. The world of medicine," he notes, "is not a culture in which it is easy to share personal emotional experiences."[27] One wonders whether this therapeutic "sharing of experience through peer consultation" might ever have involved consulting a black medical colleague.

Race is entirely absent from a *JAMA* article on "Personal Awareness and Effective Patient Care" that appeared in 1997. These authors avoid the race topic on repeated occasions in an otherwise thoughtful essay. "Unrecognized feelings and attitudes," they write, ". . . may preclude or distort meaningful discussions with patients about dying, sexuality, *and other difficult topics . . .*" [emphasis added]. None of four "common dysfunctional beliefs of physicians" has anything to do with racial thinking or beliefs. The authors' proposed exercise in self-examination for doctors is limited to feelings about gender roles: "Useful questions include, 'What messages did I receive from my family and society about sex roles? How have my attitudes contributed to instances of miscommunication with others of the opposite sex? Are there any differences in the way I respond to male and female patients? In the way male and female patients respond to me? Do I respond differently to feedback from male or female colleagues?'"[28] One wonders why these authors chose not to include analogous introspective exercises such as: "What messages did I receive from my family and society about racial differences?" Or "Are there any differences in the way I respond to black and white patients?" The only attention paid to nonwhites is devoted to Indian and Pakistani medical residents. The chronic aversion to confronting American racial problems is a way to keep private physicians' beliefs and feelings about race; and this strategy has been abetted by the medical profession's refusal to conduct the kinds of studies that would produce information about physicians' racial attitudes that might catalyze research that could really reform medical curricula.

Professional interest in the racial feelings of doctors requires a more general interest in the physician's psyche, its vulnerabilities, and what might be done to promote emotional health in the professional who is responsible for promoting the health of others. Some medical authors of the past decade have acknowledged the deficiencies of the medical literature in this respect, and medical students should be made aware of how medical journals' evasion of racial issues has affected medical curricula. As one team of authors reported in 2002: "While a small editorial literature addresses the concept of race as it is used in medicine and medical education, few data have been published to examine the actual patterns of use of racial and ethnic identifiers and their impact on student learning. Our literature search yielded only two studies of the use of racial and ethnic labels in case presentations."[29] A year later other authors pointed to the need to "bring a critical perspective that has largely been ignored by most research to date or that has circumscribed cultural inquiry into the differences between patients and physicians' 'beliefs.'"[30] A 2004 report, for example, concludes that "the literature lacks comprehensive studies that simultaneously examine patients' and physicians' beliefs and attitudes" in relation to invasive cardiac procedures."[31] In the meantime, amid all of this ignorance and uncertainty, there persists a hope that reforming medical curricula can somehow bestow "cultural competence" on the doctors of the future.

RACE AND MEDICAL EDUCATION: THE SEARCH FOR "CULTURAL COMPETENCE"

The reports from medical authors who have written about bringing racial enlightenment and "cultural competence" to medical education will not reassure those who, like this author, believe that such initiatives are essential for improving the quality of medical care in the United States. Part of the problem is that the topic of race relations in medicine should be part of a medical ethics curriculum that has never become a standard part of medical education. As Frederic W. Hafferty and Ronald Franks reported in 1994, "most medical schools (and faculty) appear satisfied to locate the content and teaching of medical ethics as a second-order priority relegated to odd hours in the formal curriculum."[32] Ten years later a survey of medical ethics education at U.S. and Canadian medical schools found that little had changed over the previous decade, that "practicing physicians and medical students alike have voiced their concerns that ethics curricula often fail to address the stage-specific needs of students." At a time when revocations of physicians' licenses were increasing, medical administrators had still not made ethics education a first-order priority.[33] Similarly, a 2003 report notes: "Training physicians to work with culturally diverse populations has often been seen as a commendable goal, but not as pressing as other issues. Offering cultural issues as electives in medical school demonstrates the often weak support the study of these topics has in the medical establishment."[34]

Medical authors have observed that resistance to changing the culture of medical education is a deeply rooted phenomenon. "Medical schools," write Hafferty and Franks, "have long been known for their resistance to curricular change."[35] "Why are medical schools what they are today?" Samuel L. Bloom asked in 1988. "Why is change in these schools all but impossible?" In part, he says, because the medical school "is above all a variant of modern corporate bureaucracy," and its "mission statements," like those of other bureaucracies, are a kind of "window dressing" that conceals the influence of deeper forces that have nothing to do with reform.[36] As for medical schools and racial issues, a group of black psychiatrists pointed forty years ago to "the white institution's concept of itself as liberal, unbiased, and nondiscriminatory."[37] This self-image remains intact, despite the contrary evidence that has been accumulating in medical journals since the 1980s. Even the medical liberals who are "troubled" by evidence of bias have consistently given medical institutions the benefit of the doubt on the issue of systemic racial bias.

Medical students are the primary audience for "cultural competence" training, and they can benefit from a competently presented introduction to the racial realities white professionals find it easy to avoid. How much do we know about the racial attitudes and behaviors of medical students? According to several Harvard-affiliated authors writing in the 2003 Institute of Medicine report, "political correctness appears to be the normative order in public discussion. Medical students with whom we spoke note they never hear overtly negative racist comments in the hospital or among classmates."[38] It is easy to believe that most medical students have either the scruples or the practical sense not to make openly racist remarks in a medical environment. The problem is that this reassuring, and perhaps overcredulous, assessment does not come to grips with the actual racial attitudes of the medical population. H. Jack Geiger, for example, points out in the same 2003 report that "openly pejorative racial comments on ward rounds have been described by many observers."[39]

Medical students can acquire such attitudes from their supervising faculty. In 1988, medical students at the University of Pennsylvania "stated their concerns over perceived insensitivities—inappropriate behavior or comments—expressed by faculty toward women and minority students within the classroom setting."[40] According to a 1990 study, half of the nonwhite and Hispanic medical students "reported experiencing racial or ethnic slurs" from classmates, clinical faculty, residents, and interns.[41] A 2003 report in *Academic Medicine*, which appears to serve as the social conscience of the medical profession, points to "a derogatory term [unspecified] widely used by students and faculty members to refer to patients from the skid row area of the city."[42] More generally, the 2003 assessment does not address the oral medical culture that includes expressions of contempt directed toward a variety of "undesirable" patients as well as medical students themselves. It is thus unlikely that any medical students are insulated against the effects of denigrating remarks about patients and medical students that have been described in the medical literature over the past thirty years as being virtually ubiquitous.[43]

Medical students need to know what can go wrong with doctor-patient relationships and interracial relationships in particular. Their need for instruction is clear from what is known about racial attitudes in the general population from which medical personnel come. "White America has an appalling lack of knowledge concerning the reality of black life," the Reverend Martin Luther King, Jr. told the American Psychological Association in September 1967.[44] Four years earlier a *Newsweek* survey of white Americans' beliefs about Negroes had found large majorities endorsing claims that black people "laugh a lot," "tend to have less ambition," "have looser morals," "keep untidy homes," and "smell different."[45] Whites who had at least some "social contact" with blacks were somewhat less likely to share these views.

There is no reason to assume that whites' knowledge of black lives has substantially improved since the 1960s, and black medical personnel are among those who have made this point over and over again. In 1982, for example, a black psychiatrist pointed out that "a white psychiatrist may not be sufficiently knowledgeable about black culture to identify the existence or severity of depression."[46] Whites, including doctors, who inhabit a media universe that features large numbers of black entertainers, athletes, and criminals, are likely to believe that they know more than they actually do about the personal lives and qualities of their black fellow citizens. The fact that changing racial mores have discouraged the collection and publication of graphic and intimate data about white racial beliefs does not mean that these beliefs have undergone substantial change since the *Newsweek* data were collected. In fact, the apparent liberalization of the attitudes toward blacks that whites are willing to acknowledge has made it more difficult for whites to admit to racial beliefs they find embarrassing.[47] It is, therefore, not surprising to read in a 1992 study that "White male students at all levels of racial awareness held racist beliefs and attitudes, whereas White female students tended to be most racist when their level of racial awareness was so low that they ignored or denied existing race differences."[48] This is, of course, the university student population that fills medical school classrooms.

That future doctors bring societal attitudes about socially marginalized people to medical school was already evident in the 1970s, at a time when medical schools were admitting few female students. As Mary C. Howell, MD, PhD, and an associate dean at Harvard Medical School wrote in 1974, it was not surprising that misogyny was an "approved" attitude in the medical profession at this time. "How could it be otherwise? In the first place, such attitudes about women are pervasive in society, and, secondly, the medical profession has been virtually a male province." "Assumptions about 'women's nature' and 'women's place,'" she noted, "are part of the fabric of society; we often fail to note that many of these assumptions are unfounded, and that they appear to convey malice."[49] Every aspect of this medical misogyny has its racial counterpart in the medical world: the sheer scope of the prejudice; the oral tradition of biased and inaccurate gossip; denial of pain relief; denial of surgery; distrust of the patient's judgment ("unreliable historians"); and speculative reasoning by the physician based on presumed biological differences, such as an alleged resistance to cardiovascular disease.[50] The painful irony for blacks is that, despite these shared stigmas, the influx of women into the medical profession has dwarfed the much smaller increase in the numbers of African American medical students and physicians since the 1970s. Despite their lowly status in the eyes of the medical power elite, white professional women gradually acquired a sociopolitical leverage over access to the professions that African Americans have never been able to match despite the monumental achievements of the civil rights era of the 1960s.

By the end of the 1960s, medical educators began to realize that the racial education of the nation's overwhelmingly white medical personnel was overdue.[51] In 1970, a group of African American psychiatrists who had recently finished their medical training presented this argument in the *American Journal of Psychiatry*. White psychiatrists, they wrote, were unable to relate effectively to black patients or their black colleagues. Black psychiatrists were required to adapt to the beliefs and behaviors of these uncomprehending white colleagues, even as their black identity was ignored or highlighted in awkward ways. They proposed training programs that would enable white physicians to reflect upon the clinical significance of their white middle-class origins and the limitations of the psychoanalytic orientation that was excluding black patients from psychotherapeutic treatment. They also suggested that "lectures, seminars, and small group discussions" would introduce doctors to sociological and anthropological perspectives along with opportunities to hear black patients talk about their own lives.[52]

We have already seen that, while most of this program remains unaccomplished, various medical authors would eventually endorse the idea that physicians should examine their own values and personalities. The crucial difference was that, while the black psychiatrists proposed that white psychiatrists engage directly with the race issue, the commentators of the late 1970s and 1980s consistently evaded the race question, preferring to invoke generic challenges such as "those subjects that are problematic culturally for everyone." Still, the new focus on doctors examining themselves produced a number of pedagogical projects that were, at least theoretically, relevant to race relations within medicine. Richard Gorlin and Howard D. Zucker reported in 1983 that they were engaged in "humanistic medical teaching," during which "one of us confronts the students by asking how the presenter or the others feel about the particular patient, illness, or situation under discussion. When the students hesitate to discuss their feelings, one of us may volunteer his own reaction and thus legitimize the discussion."[53] A 1984 publication on doctors' feelings about their patients reports that one (unspecified) medical school was now offering "a program designed to teach trainees to recognize their feelings toward patients and then to modify their behavior accordingly."[54] In 1988, William M. Zinn refers to "the proliferation in medical schools of programs to teach humanities and humanistic behavior." Although questions had been raised about their "focus and efficacy," these initiatives were "vitally important because it is not clear that even the most perceptive students would have the insight and ability to objectively monitor and analyze the significance of their emotional reactions."[55] Over the next decade the teaching of ethics would become "medicine's 'magic bullet' for the 1990s."[56] How the teaching of medical ethics has actually affected the practice of medicine remains uncertain.

Over the past two decades some medical educators have attempted to promote the teaching of ethics by means of "cross-cultural" initiatives that are commonly referred to as "cultural competence" programs. Determining how much ethical and cross-cultural instruction has been offered in U.S. medical schools over this period of time is a daunting exercise. Assessing the quality of these programs is even more difficult, since the many publications on this topic share a standard list of laudable goals along with a reluctance to identify and examine the racially motivated physician behaviors and misjudgments that are treated very gingerly in the medical literature. As for quantitative assessments, a 1994 survey found that "only 13 of 78 responding institutions offered cultural sensitivity courses designed to improve understanding of diverse ethnic groups, and all but one of those courses were elective."[57] A survey by the Association of American Medical Colleges published in 1998 found that "86% of U.S. medical schools provide at least one opportunity in multicultural education."[58] In 2002 the Office of Minority Health of the U.S. Department of Health and Human Services published a long report on "Teaching Cultural Competence in Health Care" that contains almost no quantitative information and examines not a single racial scenario involving white doctors and black patients (see the following section). A 2004 "Survey of Medical Ethics Education at U.S. and Canadian Medical School" published in *Academic Medicine* found that "only 55%" of the medical schools surveyed "had a mandatory introductory ethics course. Furthermore, although the majority of deans agreed that being a physician was not sufficient background to be an effective teacher of ethics, many deans also reported a lack of funding for ethics teaching at their institutions."[59] This article never mentions race as a topic for medical ethics instruction. A 2006 article reported that cultural competence programs had "proliferated in U.S. medical schools in response to increasing national diversity, as well as mandates from accrediting bodies." At the same time, the authors' assessment of these programs is generally negative; they find, for example, that "little consistency exists among training programs, and it is difficult to conclude what method and duration of training is most effective."[60]

TWO OFFICIAL VERSIONS OF "CULTURAL COMPETENCE"

"Teaching Cultural Competence in Health Care: A Review of Current Concepts, Policies and Practices" was released by the Office of Minority Health in March 2002. A striking aspect of this American document is the absence of a black presence. The words *race* and *racial* seldom appear and always within a familiar formula such as "racial and ethnic disparities." The word *black* never appears. The document's most forceful language addressing racial problems within medical practice appears in references to "lack of cultural sensitivity and cultural competence on the part of physicians and other health care workers" (p. 14) and "barriers of mistrust toward physicians and hospitals" felt by "minority groups" (p. 15)—in a word, the standard jargon. This is a stylistically sanitized document of a type we have encountered before. Here is a medical world from which open bigotry, clinical bias, and abusive treatment of patients and medical students are somehow absent. Apart from an oblique reference to "the power dynamics" of the physician-patient relationship, the familiar euphemistic formulas that gentrify racial or homophobic unpleasantness are the only evidence of their existence. Nine out of ten gay, lesbian, and bisexual physicians have heard medical colleagues disparage such patients, and more than half of them have "observed colleagues provide diminished care or deny care to patients because of sexual orientation."[61] Perhaps this is why the professional treatment of homosexual patients is not addressed in the document under discussion or in many others that offer curricula to encourage "cultural competence."

The exclusion of race from this document is evident in three specific instances. The first example is found in the "1999–2000 Liaison Committee on Medical Education Annual Medical School Questionnaire." Its categories include language training, use of traditional healers, use of alternative therapies, cultural beliefs related to death and dying, and cultural practices related to intercultural communication (44). No topic pertaining to race was included. The second example is found in the pages of coverage devoted to the task of providing of translators who mediate between doctors and patients who do not speak enough English to be safely treated by monolingual physicians. To facilitate these relationships, the document offers a list of "guidelines for working through an interpreter." These helpful instructions include how to address the patient, the importance of paying complete attention to what the patient says, being aware of conceptual differences based on culture, being alert to the possibility of "cultural misunderstandings" comments that might be "culturally inappropriate," and the virtue of patience (33). An analogous set of instructions, based on what is known about black-white clinical interactions from the medical literature, could have been included in this document but was not. The third example illustrates once again the common preference for studying "racial" scenarios that do not involve African American patients. "For example," a visiting medical ethicist led a discussion following the viewing

of a documentary that presented the dilemma of a Canadian-Indian family whose newborn infant developed life-threatening liver failure, but did
not choose to comply with the recommended liver transplant because of
cultural and spiritual beliefs. The medical students were challenged to find
a culturally sensitive solution" (51). African American patients and their
families have faced equally interesting and heartrending scenarios that
involve organ transplantation, but these dilemmas will not be found in
"Teaching Cultural Competence in Health Care." Instead, this cross-racial
medical drama was displaced into the Canadian wilderness.

In 2005 the Association of American Medical Colleges (AAMC) published a report, titled "Cultural Competence Education," that presents a
comprehensive list of goals for medical students to meet over the course of
their medical education.[62] The projected "cultural competence curriculum,"
created by "experts in cultural competence and medical education," lists no
fewer than sixty-seven objectives, including the development of interpersonal skills and the acquisition of relevant kinds of knowledge about a broad
range of topics within the area of race, ethnicity, and the practice of medicine. Having developed the Tool for Assessing Cultural Competence Training (TACCT), the AAMC's purpose was now to "assist medical schools in
their efforts to integrate cultural competence content into their curricula."
Absent from this report, along with other kinds of important information,
is an account of what kinds of efforts have been made in this direction.

As an official document, "Cultural Competence Education," like "Teaching Cultural Competence in Health Care," presents its own version of the
optimistic liberal model offered by the Institute of Medicine report (*Unequal Treatment*) that appeared in 2003. The 2005 report presents many
admirable goals in the absence of any specific procedures for achieving
them; equally important is the absence of any sense of how the history of
medical racism, the social phenomenon that has made this report necessary
in the first place, is to be taught to medical students or, for that matter, to
faculty who are likely to know as little of these matters as medical students
do. A single reference to the "history of stereotyping" points to one racial
topic among others that have not found a place in the medical curriculum.
How this major pedagogical objective will now be achieved is not addressed
in this report. Where, for example, are the academically qualified instructors who know enough about the racial dimension of medicine to teach
such courses?[63] And without such instruction, how are medical students
going to "learn to recognize and appropriately address gender and cultural
biases in themselves or others"? Over the past several decades at least, a
few medical authors have pointed out that the self-assessment of racial

biases is not enough to achieve independence from racially motivated ideas and feelings. But this perspective is not mentioned in a document that is otherwise filled with all sorts of details about administering the program and somehow verifying its expected benefits.

In short, this report offers a curricular framework but no curricular content, such as examples of the racial folklore that has infiltrated and influenced the practice of medicine over many years. Specific scenarios of this kind are necessary to bring such a curriculum to life and make it of practical value to medical students and physicians who want to avoid making racially motivated mistakes in diagnosis and treatment. This report, in contrast, offers empty categories that lack examples of how racial folkloric beliefs have distorted medical judgments to the detriment of black patients. The production of "cultural competence" thus remains a hypothetical exercise, aimed at inculcating appropriate standards of conduct to be applied to generic and ethnically anonymous patients. An alternative procedure would include an inventory of the unpleasant and emotionally threatening racial folklore these students bring to medical school with them. Combining this information with what is known about the medical consequences of certain racial folkloric beliefs would enable instructors to offer medical students practical advice about how not to commit certain errors of judgment under the influence of folkloric stereotypes.

Like the 2003 Institute of Medicine report, "Cultural Competence Education" employs the familiar euphemistic jargon that has long served as a defensive rhetorical strategy in the medical literature. The purpose of these verbal formulas is to insulate medical authors from the discomfiting aspects of American race relations that doctors may experience in their encounters with black patients. "Institutional cultural issues" may refer to institutional racism practiced in hospitals or to the so-called "hidden curriculum" of medical training this report should but does not mention; "cultural discord" may refer to racial hostility between blacks and whites (or between Afro-Caribbeans and African Americans); "barriers to eliminating health disparities" may include sheer resistance to change on the part of white physicians, who may not take kindly to the prescribed engagement in "reflection" that is intended to address their "personal susceptibility to bias and stereotyping." Medical students, however, are expected to embrace the process of self-examination: "Medical students must learn to recognize and appropriately address gender and cultural biases in themselves or others."[64]

Finally, published assessments of cultural competence programs in the medical literature tend to focus primarily on their limitations. For example, in 2000, two authors found that "the literature on cultural competency has, by and large, not linked cultural competency activities with the outcomes that could be expected to follow from them."[65] A year later an assessment in *Academic Medicine* concluded that the impact of "the establishment of medical ethics and humanities teaching in the majority of medical schools" had proven to be "generally minimal" and that such curricula are "irrelevant unless they can produce a substantive and continuing impact on hospital culture."[66] In 2006 another team of researchers agreed that cultural competence programs had "proliferated in U.S. medical schools in response to increasing national diversity, as well as mandates from accrediting bodies." The problem was that not all programs appeared to be effective, they were being accorded little curricular time, they were not being integrated into students' clinical rotations, and there was no consensus on how to teach them. Cultural competence programs could have beneficial effects, but "there is limited evidence demonstrating that the current models of education lend themselves to positive outcomes and implementation in clinical practice."[67] In 2009 the psychiatrist Jonathan M. Metzl pointed out that the overdiagnosis of schizophrenia in African American men and the use of higher dosages of antipsychotic medications in these black patients were racial disparities that had proven to be "remarkably resistant to interventions such as 'cultural competency training' or 'standardized' diagnostic encounters."[68]

This evidence suggests how little is known about the racial "competence" of American physicians. A striking aspect of the 2006 study referred to previously is the authors' anxious concern over their finding that "20% to 25% of recent medical school graduates feel unprepared to provide specific components of cross-cultural care." Seen from another angle, another reason for concern is that 75 percent to 80 percent of these medical school graduates actually felt that they *were* prepared to deal competently with the racial dynamics of medical practice. Given what we know about racial attitudes among the general population to which doctors belong, there is little reason for this sort of optimism.

PHYSICIANS' BELIEFS ABOUT RACIAL DIFFERENCES: A (BELATED) STUDY

Nor does the clinical medical literature offer much reason for optimism about physicians' preparedness to transcend the racial barriers that are so often referred to in the medical literature. American medical authors' general lack of interest in race relations, and the tacit censorship enforced by the norms of professional courtesy, have ruled out serious scrutiny of physicians' thinking about racial health disparities in the pages of these journals; in a word, assessing the racial sophistication of physicians has never been a priority for American medical authors. The traditional avoidance of this topic becomes even more evident when we encounter a medical publication that documents, with a few pointed allusions to accountability to black patients, physician biases that can cost black patients their lives. Despite its use of the standard euphemisms and the standard abstention from pronouncing judgment on how doctors behave, "Physicians' Beliefs about Racial Differences in Referral for Renal Transplantation" (2004) takes a cautious step beyond the less penetrating studies that preceded it.

"Physicians' Beliefs" takes a hard look at how nephrologists decide whether or not to recommend black patients for kidney transplantation. Comparing the views of nephrologists with those of their patients, the authors found that doctors frequently misconstrued black patients' attitudes toward renal transplantation and underestimated the availability of living kidney donors for them. Only 38 percent of the nephrologists believed that "problems with communication and trust" between the (mostly white) doctors and black patients had anything to do with how black patients were evaluated as candidates for a transplanted organ. They were "much more likely to believe racial differences in referral for renal transplantation arise from differences in patients' preferences than from problems with communication, trust, or racial bias. . . ." But that is not what their patients thought. In fact, the more confidence physicians had in their interracial communications skills, the less likely their black patients were to report having been given substantial information about transplantation. Only one physician in eight (12 percent)—but one black physician in four—thought that racial bias played a role in access to transplantation. Like other medical liberals before them, the authors conclude that their findings "merit further study" and refrain from passing judgment on the beliefs and behaviors of their colleagues.[69] Their special innovation was to give black patients a role in assessing, however indirectly, the conduct of their white physicians.

A MEDICAL CURRICULUM ON RACE

There is an untested alternative to the standard "cultural competence" program that combines ethical idealism with sensible advice about understanding and communication across racial barriers. That alternative is the contents of this book. For example, two principal weaknesses of the standard program are its lack of historical perspective and its reliance on sanitizing and euphemizing language to describe racial attitudes and race relations in medicine. These basic aspects of the standard program are linked, in that an unawareness of the history of medical racism makes it much easier to believe that the great majority of doctors are racial liberals who do not share the problematic racial attitudes of their fellow citizens. The standard program relies on this operative fiction so as not to alienate medical personnel who may not welcome cultural competence instruction in the first place.

A historically informed curriculum offers its medical audience two kinds of information. First, medical students entering the profession can and should understand the value system and the social dynamics of the medical world they have entered; they should eventually understand the rules and mores of this medical world, including the dynamics of its race relations, better than most of the faculty who will be teaching them. This part of the curriculum should address the nature of power in medical settings, the complex of collaborative as well as unequal relationships that constitute the social reality of medical practice. Imbalances of power and their consequences are a primary aspect of medical relationships and are often relevant to relationships between black patients and white doctors.

The second kind of information consists of practical advice regarding how physicians can avoid certain kinds of predictable, and thus avoidable, errors that many doctors have made over many years to the detriment of many black patients. Most of this curriculum is embedded in the sections of this book and describes the racial differentiation of human organ systems and diseases as well as the misjudgments such racial interpretations of human biology have led to. The major examples of racially motivated diagnoses and treatments are reviewed below.

The first type of information, concerning what we may call the microsociology of the medical world, includes informing students about the traditional resistance to examining racial folklore and race relations within the world of medicine. The medical ethics establishment has shown little interest in medical racism, leaving it to medical schools to create and implement "cultural competence" courses to the best of their ability. This arrangement is inadequate, because these curricula do not address the racist history of American medicine or present the hard facts about race relations in the United States. The resulting ignorance of the racial past has had consequences. While the destructive effects of racially biased medical care have been demonstrated beyond any reasonable doubt, most white physicians "believe that the health care system does not discriminate against racial and ethnic minorities," while more than half (56 percent) of the African

American public believes otherwise.[70] In 2005 one in three cardiologists "believed that people received different care according to their racial/ethnic status," one in eight thought that racially biased care occurred at their own hospitals, and one in twenty believed that their own patients might get biased care.[71] A 2006 report showed that one cardiovascular surgeon in eight (12.5 percent) "believed racial/ethnic disparities in cardiac care in general occur often or somewhat often," while one in thirty (3 percent) thought that racially differential care occurred in their own practices.[72] A 2010 study reports that, while 75 percent of white doctors "believe people are never or rarely treated unfairly based on race and ethnicity," only one in five (20 percent of) black doctors agree with them. What is more, almost three-quarters of the physicians surveyed "explained unequal medical treatment in terms of Black patients' perceived shortcomings."[73] In summary, most white physicians hold views of racial bias in medicine that do not correspond to research findings about how physicians actually behave, and most of their black colleagues do not share their upbeat assessment of racial dynamics in medicine.

Medical students should understand the implications of these data, and this understanding requires knowledge of past forms of medical racism. As we have just seen, most medical personnel today find it difficult to believe that they or their colleagues are capable of racist feelings and behaviors, even those that result from unconscious motivation. Many prefer not to believe the published data or find it uncomfortable to talk about race at all.[74] This is not surprising, given that white medical personnel have been conditioned to see their profession as being free of racism. This conditioning has been made possible by their general ignorance of the profession's long-standing participation in the societal racism that doctors have absorbed along with their fellow citizens. Even many years later, it is disturbing to learn that in the 1940s "professors at a leading medical school regularly 'warmed up' their classes with anecdotes that included racial epithets and stereotyping."[75] Our instinctive assumption that practitioners of medicine are immune to seeking this sort of gratification has played an important role in insulating the profession from scrutiny of doctors' racial beliefs and behaviors. Researchers have noted the effects of this isolation from racial realities: "The general lack of awareness [among cardiologists] is a bit surprising given the extent of government agencies' and professional associations' efforts to make physicians more aware of this issue." The failure of this educational campaign suggests that cardiologists (among other physicians) are either not interested in or are resistant to absorbing information that points to medical bias. "If experience is any guide," these authors note, "educational strategies are likely to have only limited effectiveness."[76] In addition, medical education itself plays a role in fortifying doctors against accepting data that indicate racial bias. More than one observer has noted "a trend toward more conservative sociopolitical attitudes as students progress through medical training." This conservatism usually includes a refusal to take medical racism seriously as a professional issue.[77] Physicians who have acquired this outlook are likely to show little interest in "cultural competence" instruction that is supposed to make them more sensitive about interracial relationships.[78]

This lack of interest in racial matters suggests that the perspectives of black medical personnel should play a significant role in medical education. Judging from the coverage of "cultural competence" instruction that has appeared in various medical journals, there appears to be little demand for black physicians' perspectives on race-related behaviors in the medical world. Medical educators have not shown an interest in assigning a significant pedagogical role in medical schools to African American physicians or to the black psychiatrists who have offered published advice to their white colleagues over many years. White physicians' lack of familiarity with the published views of this group is consistent with the lowly status of the nation's primary African American medical journal. Both forms of neglect point to the "invisible" status that many African Americans have cited as a source of their alienation from whites. The small numbers and marginal status of black doctors will be evident to medical students, and they will draw their own conclusions about whether they need to acquire more racial expertise than they already possess. A 2004 study reported that three out of five medical students "believed that their schools have adequate curricula in place to teach them about disparities, but only a minority (36%) of African American students believed this. An even greater percentage of students, however, still desired more exposure to these issues (72%)."[79]

But what do these data really tell us about race and medical education? One wonders, for example, whether medical students are sufficiently informed to judge what constitutes an adequate curriculum in this area, given that the racial knowledge and stereotypes most of them bring to medical school would suggest they are not. One also wonders whether medical educators will take the opportunity to look into why more black students than white want more instruction in matters having to do with race. This difference between the viewpoints of black and white medical students recalls the difference already noted that separates the views of black from those of white physicians. Yet the study of racial differences in medical opinion has long been neglected. As late as 2004 the report on nephrologists and referrals for kidney transplantation could only draw the obvious conclusion that "these differences in physicians' beliefs . . . merit further study."[80] In fact, it is a scandal that medical authors and editors had not bothered to conduct and publish such research by the early twenty-first century. But this perspective never appears in medical journals, because the entire topic makes most white doctors uncomfortable, and because black doctors and their views remain marginalized within the medical profession. Attentive medical students will notice that even the research that does address physicians' views of race seems to have had little impact on medical behavior and instruction. In fact, the research just presented shows that most physicians discount the relevance of racial factors in medical relationships. The relatively few white medical liberals who are "troubled" by evidence of medical racism have been unable or unwilling to engage in the sort of activism that might produce more than cosmetic reforms in medical education.

PRACTICAL ADVICE FOR PHYSICIANS

Difficult relationships between white professionals and black patients are an important aspect of American race relations. Doctors, police officers, social workers, professors, and other trained personnel have interracial relationships that require a familiarity with the lives of their clients. Professionals should also know how interracial relationships can go wrong in unanticipated ways. David R. Levy observes that these relationships can be distorted by *ignorance* and *unconscious prejudice* on the part of the physician. Ignorance may prompt physicians to regard culturally appropriate or adaptive attitudes and behaviors as deviant, or it may lead doctors to assume that one person's psychopathology represents a racial trait. This type of error will be common in a society that has conditioned people to see certain "black" traits as expressions of a presumed racial essence. Unconscious prejudice can distort doctors' emotions in various ways. It can cause white physicians to overcompensate for the abnormal degree of social distance by becoming "overindulgent, paternalistic, and condescending." It can tempt physicians to discount the effects of racism and be "color blind" in such a way that "the black patient becomes a white patient with a black skin." Most perversely, physicians' unconscious prejudice can create "a conspiracy of silence" when doctor and patient tacitly agree that racial differences signify black inferiority, "and to discuss them would be tantamount to discussing a missing limb with an amputee."[81] In all three cases, doctors' overadaptation to racial difference prevents them from thinking of patients as "normal" human beings. The dysfunctional results are, respectively, an anxious overfamiliarity with the racial alien, an evasive denial of the social reality of racial differences, and a tacit position of white supremacy.

SOCIAL CLASS, MISDIAGNOSES, AND THERAPEUTIC FATALISM

Physicians are professionals who do not have the time (or, in most cases, the inclination) to become race experts or part-time sociologists who study the troubled lives of the poor. Over time many doctors do of course learn a great deal about the lives of their poor and troubled patients and how best to take care of them. There are clear advantages to preparing medical students for these relationships at the beginning of their careers, since an awareness of how white professionals can misperceive black people through the lens of social class as well as race can prevent some errors of medical judgment. For example, many whites are predisposed to see blacks as disordered or violent. This category includes the tragic example of a black radio and television journalist who "died of a virus after a hospital emergency room—seeing only a disoriented, disheveled black man—misdiagnosed him and sent him home to get 'more sleep.'"[82] ER personnel may assume black middle-class sickle-cell patients are drug addicts and deny them pain relief. Physicians assessing injuries to black children may be more inclined to suspect parental abuse than if the child were white.[83] We have seen that the image of the "physical" and "self-assertive" black man can affect antidepressant treatment.[84] In summary, we may assume that doctors make racially motivated and fallible or uncertain judgments, and that relatively few of these judgments are brought to the attention of the profession in medical journals.

Physicians should also be prepared to face the medical consequences of what racial segregation and poverty have done to some black patients. In the words of the former president of Meharry Medical College, "you have to reverse a whole way of being" to improve their health.[85] "Many patients," Levy notes, "may appear depressed, not because of personal psychopathology, but because of the effects of poverty. If they live in a world that is fraught with frustration, unrealizable goals, and hopelessness, the sadness is appropriate."[86] Medical students, most of whom have led privileged lives, should be prepared to deal with the feelings, whether of rejection, sympathy, or guilt, that these patients are likely to inspire in them.

Over the past century white physicians have often encountered passive resistance from such patients who were expressing their refusal to receive care from what they saw as a racist medical system. Some of these behaviors have continued after the period of Jim Crow segregation. As Levy wrote in 1985: "Patients may 'give up' and passively resist treatment by not keeping appointments, not taking medications, or not fully sharing their concerns, worries, and fears."[87] Both doctors and patients can act out their own versions of what we may call "therapeutic fatalism." Doctors do not want to offer therapies they expect will be wasted on noncompliant patients. Patients may not trust therapies, may simply resign themselves to illness and death, or may place their medical fate in God's hands.

Therapeutic fatalism is not limited to the poor and uneducated, because it can also be caused by the stress and fatigue that can be an integral part of the black experience. A study of folk medical beliefs among blacks reported in 1974 that "interviews with several hundred Harlem adolescents showed that three fourths of them believe an individual can expect a lot of sickness during his lifetime, and more than half think there is not much that can be done about it." At this time two-thirds of urban blacks said they usually "feel sick."[88] A 1992 report demonstrated that 36 percent of a nonrandom sample of African American men "considered themselves to be helpless with regard to controlling their health."[89] We may assume that this disproportionate sense of chronic illness, which is *not* hypochondria, still exists today.

Therapeutic fatalism is particularly dangerous when it delays the diagnosis and treatment of a potentially fatal disease. Cancer fatalism among African Americans makes people less likely to participate in cancer screening. "There is an urgent need to modify fatalistic perceptions among African-Americans," and medical students should be aware that even reducing the cost of screening by means of "educational interventions" does not modify behavior enough to resolve this problem.[90] For example, belief in fate or destiny among black women has been linked to the avoidance of potentially life-saving medical examinations. "Women who reported never having had a breast exam were more likely to believe in fate or destiny than women who did not have a belief in fate or destiny."[91] Such passive and, perhaps, self-destructive patients impose an unfair burden on the physician. In these circumstances medical students should understand the possible origins of what may appear to be bizarre and irrational behavior. They should understand the role of *demoralization* in the lives of many African American patients. What may seem to be a refusal of medical services may actually be an inability to ask for medical help on account of discouragement or depression.

Another form of resistance to medical treatment is the proliferation among blacks of pseudomedical conspiracy theories of which medical students should be aware. Urban myths about U.S. government plots to infect African Americans with the HIV/AIDS virus have run rampant through this population since the 1980s. Black activists animated by mistrust of white doctors have campaigned against standard childhood vaccinations and the "genocidal" administration of Ritalin, a stimulant widely prescribed for attention deficit disorder, to black children. "Antipsychiatry groups flood the African-American communities with slick, glossy, antipsychiatry propaganda," the black psychiatrist Carl Bell stated in 2001. Health education undertaken by white medical personnel is sometimes regarded as a form of "cultural imperialism."[92] In summary, anti-medical conspiratorial thinking among many black people is one aspect of a more general hostility toward the medical system that became an integral part of African American life during the twentieth century. Medical students must find a way to acknowledge this therapeutic predicament while devising ways to establish working relationships with black patients whose individual attitudes toward medical relationships will naturally differ while sharing this heritage of estrangement.

"CULTURAL COMPETENCE" AS KNOWLEDGE OF STEREOTYPE SYSTEMS

The essential point here for medical students and physicians is that the misdiagnoses described previously are not random or arbitrary events; they are rather the predictable results of a "coherent belief system" that has been created and sustained by American racial folklore since the era of plantation medicine. A major task of this book has been to describe the operating concepts of this belief system and its medical consequences. These concepts include *racialization*, the process that creates biological rationales for defining racial differences; the category consisting of *"white" diseases"* that are compatible with a folkloric "white" racial essence; the concept of *black "hardiness"* that presumes the special toughness and primitive status of the black organism; and, most fundamental of all, the *complexity principle* that presumes that black human beings are less complicated organisms than whites.

The racial folklore that continues to shape modern thinking about race has demonstrated a remarkable stability over the past two centuries, and this is why it continues to produce predictable effects inside and outside of the medical world. At the same time, the historical analysis of medico-racial folklore presented here does acknowledge changes in racial folklore over time; for example, many ideas about physical and mental racial differences that flourished in American medicine during the first half of the twentieth century have been discredited or have simply disappeared, while others have survived because modern researchers have either confirmed racial differences of medical significance, updated the relevant medical terminology, or eliminated offensive associations with the medical-racist past.

Explaining this model is important, because a principal objection to "cultural competence" instruction has been a well-founded disapproval of "the 'trait list approach' that understands culture as a set of already-known factors." From the perspective of this kind of cross-cultural instruction, "patients of a certain ethnicity . . . are assumed to have a set of core beliefs about illness owing to fixed ethnic traits. Cultural competency becomes a series of 'do's and don'ts' that define how to treat a patient of a given ethnic background."[93] Homogenizing patients in this way oversimplifies both them and the "culture" to which they belong and can hinder accurate medical diagnosis.

The explanatory model that is built on analyzing the racial interpretation of disease, the "hardiness" doctrine, and the "complexity principle" is cautious about identifying shared ethnic traits. What this model does assume is that African Americans share a common *predicament* as a result of slavery, racial segregation, and the history of stressors associated with being black in the United States. A disproportionate distrust of doctors is one aspect of this predicament. "Cultural competence" educators should bear in mind that cultural "traits" result from the collective consequences of group experiences that have accumulated over many years. Respect for the individuality of minority patients is entirely compatible with acknowledging shared responses to racial trauma and exclusion.

A second point is that, unlike the ethnic "trait lists" approach to "cultural competence," the model proposed in this book emphasizes the behaviors of doctors rather than patients. Both physicians and patients exhibit predictable attitudes and behaviors that can result in medical errors. While patients' attitudes have been studied for years, it is the "core beliefs" of doctors that require detailed attention they have not received. Indeed, a key limitation of the "cultural competence" approach is its exclusive focus on the observable traits and behaviors of patients; physicians participate in this dyadic relationship as ("competent" or "incompetent") observers who are exempted from being observed, apart from their ability or inability to interpret or misinterpret patients' problems. In the meantime, medical educators and "cultural competence" instructors continue to ignore medico-racial folklore that contributes to making today's diagnostic misinterpretations possible.

RACELESS HUMANISM: "MEDICAL HUMANITIES" AND THE EVASION OF DIFFERENCE

"The most common criticism made at present by older practitioners is that young graduates have been taught a great deal about the mechanism of disease, but very little about the practice of medicine—or, to put it more bluntly, they are too 'scientific' and do not know how to take care of patients." So wrote the legendary Francis W. Peabody, MD, the doyen of Harvard Medical School, in 1927.[94] The "common criticism" of emotionally inadequate doctors that Peabody endorsed in that bygone era has had a long career. The idea that physicians' attitudes toward their patients need to be more empathetic and "humanized" has circulated in medical circles for at least a century. This view has coexisted with a sense that physicians should also be culturally literate people. Almost a century ago, a character in Somerset Maugham's *Of Human Bondage* (1915) "complained that the young medical men were uneducated; their reading consisted of *The Sporting Times* and the *British Medical Journal*."[95] In this vein, the belief that "the humanities" have a more than semantic relationship to the humane behavior expected of doctors has persisted and has been incorporated in one form or another into most North American medical school curricula since the 1960s.[96]

Like the advocates of "cultural competence" programs, the scholars who have promoted the "medical humanities" have argued that their curricula can improve the quality of medical care by producing more thoughtful and sensitive doctors. But whether the study of literature ("narrative medicine") can actually fulfill its stated purpose remains unclear. As one commentary put it in 2008: "The medical humanities have been presented as a panacea for medical reductionism; a means for 'humanizing' medicine. However, there is a lack of consensus about the appropriate contributing disciplines and how curricula should be taught and assessed."[97] As a scholarly genre, the medical humanities have much to offer; the hundreds, or perhaps thousands, of published studies range widely throughout (Western) history and literature and make interesting forays into the realm of science fiction and the history of medicine, among other topics. In this sense, the medical humanities would seem to present an opportunity to explore the racial dimension of medicine in ways that would benefit the training of medical students.

In the course of almost a half century the medical humanities have produced very little on race and medicine. In fact, this copious literature has almost entirely ignored the African American experience and the relationship between black people and the world of medicine. The lack of interest in black life that prevails in the medical humanities is easy to document. An examination of fifteen years (1995 to 2009) of the journal *Literature and Medicine*, the official journal of the Institute for the Medical Humanities, demonstrates both the rarity of black-themed publications and the indirect methodological approaches authors almost always employ when they are writing about Africans or African Americans. Over these fifteen years, *Literature and Medicine* published only one article that bears directly on the modern African American experience, an important essay on the health-related consequences of the stereotype of "the strong black woman."[98] Another article examines the possibility that a fictional black character might be dying of rabies.[99] Two more articles deal with race and disease in late nineteenth-century colonial Africa.[100] Apart from "Genetics and 'Race' in *The Merchant of Venice*" (1999), these four articles constitute the sum total of the race-related publications that appeared in *Literature and Medicine* over fifteen years.[101]

The *Journal of the Medical Humanities* presents an almost identical picture. Over a thirty-year period (1980 to 2009) that saw the publication of more than 500 articles, only two essays relevant to contemporary African American life were published: one on the presentation of breast cancer in African American women's popular magazines, and the other a manifesto propounding an Afrocentric psychology to which many black psychologists and psychiatrists would not subscribe.[102] Two other essays examine medical racism in the American South during the age of Jim Crow.[103] One essay analyzes the image of Africa as a pathological environment that produces deadly viruses, whereas another presents a history of ideas about blood and racial identity that includes past episodes of medical racism in the United States.[104] Another article examines nursing in Africa during the colonial period.[105] A final article looks at grief in a novel by Toni Morrison.[106] In summary, just over one percent of these publications concern the lives of black people in any direct or indirect way. The authors' lack of interest in racial issues and African Americans is, as we have seen, typical of highly educated Americans who are physicians or who take a professional interest in the culture of medicine. What is more, even the few studies that do address the lives of African Americans tend to avoid the actual experiences of contemporary black people in favor of examining black lives that are either imagined or historically remote. Medical humanities scholarship is more interested in diagnosing fictional characters than real ones. Similarly, its studies of medical abuse of blacks are invariably reported from an era when medical racism was overt in ways it is not today. Diagnosing a case of syphilis in a character invented by Nathaniel Hawthorne is less discomfiting than discussing venereal disease in a racially stigmatized population such as African Americans today; and revisiting the infamous Tuskegee Syphilis Experiment that began in 1932 is less emotionally challenging than confronting evidence of racial bias among physicians today. Like most people, humanistic scholars are creatures of habit who operate according to an agenda that prioritizes certain kinds of research over others. While the study of literature and history has been a prestigious activity for centuries, the study of medical racism has only been underway for a few decades and has no ties to the realm of high culture.

The value of the medical humanities to medical practice is thus limited by the fact that the task of the humanities is traditionally seen as the study of cultural products rather than the lives of people with medical (or other) problems. Medical humanists have argued that "positive identification with the fictional other" can prompt medical students to think about the social origins of human suffering, and that reading literature "may lead students toward empathy not merely with the fictional other but subsequently with 'real' humans who share similar life circumstances or attributes."[107] It is, indeed, possible that some medical students identify more easily with fictional characters than with real people, and that emotional engagements with imagined people might improve their relationships with their future patients. But the use of "narrative medicine" as preemptive psychotherapy for future doctors seems like an uncertain and unnecessarily indirect response to the emotional deficits of people who will be practicing medicine.

The relevance of the humanities to the practice of medicine would be enhanced by a greater emphasis on other branches of the humanities, such as anthropological, sociological, and psychological approaches to the medical world and its inhabitants. The application of these disciplines would open up lines of inquiry into the racial dimension of medicine in various ways that would benefit medical training. That this deeper humanistic strategy has not been introduced at this late date represents a missed opportunity for medical education.[108]

This pedagogical deficit derives from the fact that neither the medical humanities nor bioethics ("medical ethics") have ever embraced sociological thinking about medicine and its social context. As the medical anthropologist Arthur Kleinman commented in 1983: "Biomedical practitioners believe that their domain is distinct from morality and aesthetics, and from

religion, politics, and social organization. . . . Social scientists discern inter-
connections between these domains, however, which practitioners usually
deny or ignore."[109] We have already noted Jerome Groopman's portrait of
physicians in *How Doctors Think* as sociological naïfs who tend to ignore
social context. A major argument of this book is that physicians must be
able to apply sociological and historical perspectives to their relationships
with black patients when this can improve care.

MEDICAL CURRICULUM CHANGE IS POSSIBLE: THE CASE OF ABORTION TRAINING

Skepticism about the prospects for reforming the medical curriculum is
deeply rooted in the medical culture. Medical humanists and other outsiders have sometimes felt, and with good reason, that they were visiting
the world of medicine on sufferance, and that they would encounter an
ingrained resistance to their efforts to broaden the minds and soften the
hearts of medical personnel. "I select my materials and tone to challenge,
but not goad, an already sensitive audience," as one feminist historian
put it in 1988.[110] "Yet for all our trying, we are usually marginalized in
the broad portrait of medicine," another medical humanist commented in
1992.[111] It was around this time the famous physician and medical essayist
Lewis Thomas offered a pointed comment on such attempts to humanize
medical education: "There is still some talk in medical deans' offices about
the need for general culture, but nobody really means it. . . ."[112]

The difficulties inherent in reforming a medical curriculum make it
clear that those who set about to expand the scope of medical training will
have to organize to achieve their goals. A successful example of such a
campaign to address a perceived curricular deficit concerns the training of
future abortion providers. This curricular innovation originated, not with
the senior medical educators who run medical schools, but due to the initiative of a medical student named Jody Steinauer, the founding member of
Medical Students for Choice, an organization whose membership of 10,000
includes more than 10 percent of the medical student population in the
United States. The result of this medical-political activism is that today
about half of the obstetrics and gynecology residency programs in the
United States offer instruction in abortion techniques in residents' regular
rotations.[113]

This remarkable achievement raises two questions for readers of this
book. First, which factors made it possible for medical students, the least
powerful cohort in the medical hierarchy, to bring about such fundamental

change? Second, why has nothing comparable happened to bring about effective "cultural competence" training for the treatment of black patients that would serve a large and historically neglected black patient population? Providing answers to these questions requires us to think about social phenomena such as popular demand for medical services, generating the political will to provide them, and the lack of professional status black medical students and faculty have had to deal with since African American doctors organized themselves into the National Medical Association in 1895.

The institutionalizing of abortion training in many medical schools, including some of the most prestigious, is particularly noteworthy in that this training has faced the opposition of powerful social forces that favor an outright ban on abortion. Several important factors account for what may appear to be the implausible success of this initiative. It required an extraordinarily dedicated organizer. It had the public support of one ally outside the medical profession, the National Abortion Federation, and the less conspicuous (but essential) financial support of the wealthy investor Warren Buffett. It won the crucial support of the Accreditation Council for Graduate Medical Education, which represents the medical profession, and a core group of high-status institutions—Harvard, Columbia, Johns Hopkins, Stanford, and University of California, Los Angeles—that provided the kind of respectability that most insurgent groups must do without.[114] This was, in short, an insurgency that shared a value system with a large and liberal segment of the medical establishment that was willing to accommodate an expansion of the medical curriculum that was compatible with its own norms. What is more, more than 50 percent of current medical students are women, a large constituency that included many who endorsed the abortion-training initiative.

The racial integration of American medical schools during the 1970s and 1980s coincided with a new interest in the dynamics of the doctor-patient relationship that helped to open the door to "cultural competence" training in its various forms. The problem for African American medical students and faculty has been that the ideal of introspective and "culturally competent" physicians never came to include a genuine interest in white physicians' racial attitudes and behaviors or the predicaments of their black colleagues. One factor that has enabled the development of race-aversive cultural competence programs has been the historical vacuum within which medical training takes place. Medical students learn nothing, for example, about the racist practices that have limited and deformed the medical education of blacks throughout most of the twentieth century. *The Flexner*

Report on Medical Education in the United States and Canada (1910) is the most influential document in the history of medical education; it was also an overtly racist blueprint for turning black doctors into a lower caste of medical servants who would specialize in "hygiene rather than surgery" for the purpose of containing the "infection and contagion" represented by Negroes, while whites would monopolize the more advanced medical specialties. One consequence of this segregated medical training was that black patients eventually "noticed a difference in skill level between black and white physicians. Because of inadequate clinical and surgical experiences, black practitioners were aware of their deficits and suffered from low professional self-esteem. In turn, black patients became skeptical of black practitioners and often resisted their treatment."[115] In their monumental history of American medical racism during the twentieth century, W. Michael Byrd and Linda A. Clayton have fully documented the professional damage that was inflicted on African American medical students and doctors over many decades.[116]

Most of a century after the publication of the Flexner Report, the effects of its recommendations were still in evidence, even as the medical establishment succeeded in preserving "the white institution's concept of itself as liberal, unbiased, and nondiscriminatory." Surveys of black medical students taken during the 1980s found that most were experiencing problems related to race: "Certain repetitive themes emerged. Blacks were treated as though they were intellectually less able than white students. Blacks felt they were 'invisible.'" Some black medical students "described themselves as shocked and disappointed at what they found, with one student stating that she thought medicine was 'above the petty stuff.'"[117] The problem was that medical schools had done little to protect black medical students from demoralizing encounters with some of their white fellow students and teachers.

This historical denigration of black medical personnel helps to account for why they have been unable or unwilling to demand medical curriculum reform comparable to that brought about by the white medical students who catalyzed a dramatic expansion of abortion training. Here we encounter the enduring power of nineteenth-century ideas about black human potential and their impact on professional careers. Whereas the stigmatizing of white women as intellectually and emotionally unfit to practice medicine did not survive the feminism movement of the 1970s, the status of black medical personnel has not risen in a comparable fashion, and part of the difference has to do with sheer numbers. Over the past three decades, white women have flooded into medical schools at a rate that far exceeds that of black males or females. Consequently, their status and influence over policy making has grown accordingly. In contrast, the status of black medical personnel has stagnated.

Medical Students for Choice succeeded in part because its members were overwhelmingly white. At the same time, other critical factors were required to graft a controversial medical procedure onto the standard curriculum. A national organization dedicated to the same goal served as an extramural ally. An enormously wealthy philanthropist funded the residency programs that made curricular reform credible to leading medical schools and made possible the advanced research programs that bring prestige to the institutions that sponsor them. The tipping point came when these assets acquired the critical mass that prompted the Accreditation Council for Graduate Medical Education to make abortion training a requirement for its approval.

Any African American initiative to put racial issues on the medical school agenda would require a similar strategic configuration of allied interest groups and financial resources. Moral suasion akin to the doctrine of racial justice that drove the civil rights movement of the 1960s no longer works. A medical establishment that has elected not to treat the black health crisis as an emergency, and that has accepted racial health disparities as a fact of life, will not be inclined to remedy this crisis through curricular reforms. It is true that white liberal sentiments recalling the 1960s played an important role in the June 2005 Food and Drug Administration hearing that approved the use of the heart medication BiDil for African American patients only. Certain panelists' testimony made it clear that the approval of this controversial medication was in part an act of reparation and atonement for past medical racism and neglect of the black population. This was, however, a unique situation that allowed white doctors to respond directly, and at no personal or professional cost to themselves, to an urgent appeal from black colleagues. Most importantly, the BiDil decision appeared to be a healing gesture that made its own small contribution toward closing an unhappy chapter in the history of medical race relations. By accepting the recommendation of their black colleagues, the white panelists avoided intramural racial conflict and created an image of racial unanimity among black and white physicians that does not correspond to the realities of interracial medicine in the United States.

These realities include the professional isolation and special stressors with which many black doctors have to cope day in and day out. For most of the twentieth century, and until they were forced to do otherwise, the American Medical Association made a point of telling black physicians that they were marginal men. The tenuous status to which these men had no realistic choice but to adapt forced them to develop the kind of self-possession and self-control the black baseball star Jackie Robinson made famous in the late 1940s. The black medical heroes of the twentieth century have seldom been accorded the credit they deserve for having demonstrated this sort of dedication and fortitude. It is reasonable to assume that the chronic professional insecurity generations of black doctors have endured has made them less inclined to make open demands on behalf of racial education for medical students and doctors. And it is a certainty that many of their white colleagues would regard such a requirement as confrontational and unprofessional conduct. White doctors are not threatened by talk about the medical racism of the past, but they might feel threatened by talk about their own racially motivated behaviors. It is thus hard to imagine that black medical faculty, who live with their own discontents as well as the potential hostility of their white colleagues, are going to campaign for controversial curricular change.

But if black medical faculty do not lead a campaign for effective racial education and "cultural competence" programs in medical schools, who will provide the necessary inspiration and leadership? Even if the small population of black medical students did provide a dynamic vanguard, whom would they lead and how would they persuade white medical students to demand a racial pedagogy that would add to their workloads and challenge their identities as medical humanitarians? We know that today's white medical students, unlike many in this cohort during the 1960s, do not arrive at medical school emotionally burdened (or motivated) by feelings of racial guilt about black suffering. On the contrary, the idea of a "postracial" America has become an emotionally convenient rationale for asserting that racial enlightenment has become irrelevant in today's world. All of these factors suggest that the racial education of American physicians will remain an exceptionally difficult assignment for those who are bold enough to take it on. Perhaps the combination of a wealthy African American philanthropist, an energized Congressional Black Caucus, liberal white allies in the medical establishment, and the reincarnation in medical form of a great African American leader will be able to make black doctors and black interests visible to whites as they never have been before.

Notes

CHAPTER 1

1. See, for example, Ashish K. Jha et al., "Racial Trends in the Use of Major Procedures among the Elderly," *New England Journal of Medicine* 353 (August 18, 2005): 683–691. "More than 600 studies have documented racial and ethnic differences in health care dating back at least to the 1980s. These studies suggested that racial and ethnic differences reflect, in part, underuse by black patients, who fail to receive these procedures when their use is clinically appropriate."

2. H. Jack Geiger, "Race and Health Care," *New England Journal of Medicine* 335 (September 12, 1996): 816.

3. W. Michael Byrd and Linda A. Clayton, *An American Health Dilemma*, vol. II. *Race, Medicine, and Health Care in the United States 1900–2000* (New York and London: Routledge, 2002): 84.

4. Emily Singer, "Beyond Race-Based Medicine," *MIT Technology Review* (January 16, 2009).

5. "Following World War II increasing pressure forced the AMA and its medical establishment to end blatant racial segregation and discrimination. The posture assumed by White organized medicine and its allies was resistance. Other than a few token acknowledgements at its 1950 and 1952 conventions and individual representatives in local and national organizations, the AMA ignored its racial discrimination problem. Taking a cue from national White organized medicine, progress moved at a snail's pace in the desegregation of county and state medical societies, medical specialty organizations, and hospital facilities. Between 1945 and 1965 there was a great deal more racial progress in the areas of nursing and health professions education than in the massive medical practice and services infrastructures themselves... With a background of having barred Blacks throughout most if its 118-year history up to 1965, the AMA 'had its first Black delegate in 1949 and changed its bylaws to ban racial discrimination in 1968', according to Wolinsky." See W. Michael Byrd and Linda A. Clayton, *An American Health Dilemma*, vol. II. *Race, Medicine, and Health Care in the United States 1900–2000* (New York and London: Routledge, 2002): 214, 402.

6. Gunnar Myrdal, *An American Dilemma: The Negro Problem and Modern Democracy*, vol. II [1944] (New Brunswick and London, Transaction Publishers, 1996): 784, 784.

7. Kenneth B. Clark, *Dark Ghetto: Dilemmas of Social Power* (New York and Evanston: Harper Torchbooks, 1965): 75, 76.
8. Maurice Berger, *White Lies: Race and the Myths of Whiteness* (New York: Farrar, Straus & Giroux, 1999): 179.
9. Raj Bhopal, "Racism in Medicine," *BMJ* 322 (June 23, 2001): 1,504.
10. James Baldwin, *Notes of a Native Son* [1955] (Boston: Beacon Press, 1984): 25.
11. James Baldwin, *Notes of a Native Son* [1955] (Boston: Beacon Press, 1984): 41.
12. David Satcher, "Does Race Interfere with the Doctor-Patient Relationship?" *Journal of the American Medical Association* 223 (March 26, 1973): 1,498.
13. David R. Levy, "White Doctors and Black Patients: Influence of Race on the Doctor-Patient Relationship," *Pediatrics* 75 (1985): 639.
14. "Negro Health," *Time* (April 8, 1940).
15. J.W. Jones, "The Frequency of Umbilical Herniae in Negro Infants," *Archives of Pediatrics* 58 (1941): 294.
16. George Devereux, *From Anxiety to Method in the Behavioral Sciences* (The Hague & Paris: Mouton & Co., 1967): 174.
17. "Skin Problems in Blacks Receive Scrutiny," *Journal of the American Medical Association* 242 (December 21, 1979): 2,747–2,748.
18. "U.S. Practices a System of Medicine that Shortchanges Minorities and Women," *Milwaukee Journal Sentinel* (April 16, 2001); "2 Levels of Treatment: Pain Control Lags for Minorities and Women," *Milwaukee Journal Sentinel* (April 23, 2001).
19. Orlando Patterson, "A Job Too Big for One Man" *New York Times* (November 4, 2009).
20. The Journal of the American Medical Association, *A Piece of My Mind: A Collection of Essays*, eds. Bruce B. Dan and Roxanne K. Young (Los Angeles: Feeling Fine Programs, Inc; Toronto Random House of Canada Limited, 1988): 210, 238–239, 100, 100.
21. Paul Austin, *Something for the Pain: Compassion and Burnout in the ER* [2008] (New York: W.W. Norton & Company, 2009): 171, 174, 250–251.
22. John Pekkanen, *M.D.: Doctors Talk About Themselves* (New York: Delacorte Press, 1988): 83, 8, 10.
23. John Pekkanen, *M.D.: Doctors Talk About Themselves* (New York: Delacorte Press, 1988): 222–223.
24. David Leonhardt, "Dr. James Will Make It Better," *New York Times Magazine* (November 8, 2009): 35.
25. David R. Levy, "White Doctors and Black Patients: Influence of Race on the Doctor-Patient Relationship," *Pediatrics* 75 (1985): 640.
26. Sherwin B. Nuland, "Indoctrinology," *The New Republic* (February 19, 2001): 37.
27. Frederic W. Hafferty and Ronald Franks, "The Hidden Curriculum, Ethics Teaching, and the Structure of Medical Education," *Academic Medicine* 69 (November 1994): 868.
28. Paul Austin, *Something for the Pain: Compassion and Burnout in the ER* [2008] (New York: W.W. Norton & Company, 2009): 292, 42, 204.
29. Jane Goldman, "Preventing Malpractice," *Hippocrates* 11 (1997): 27–28, 29–33.
30. David R. Levy, "White Doctors and Black Patients: Influence of Race on the Doctor-Patient Relationship," *Pediatrics* 75 (1985): 642.
31. Brenda L. Beagan, "Teaching Social and Cultural Awareness to Medical Students: "It's All Very Nice to Talk about It In Theory, But Ultimately It Makes No Difference," *Academic Medicine* 78 (June 2003): 605.

32. G. Carlson *et al.*, "Summary of Workshop II: Working Group on Risk Factors," *American Heart Journal* 108 (September 1984): 705.

33. Personal communication on July 29, 2005.

34. Frederic W. Hafferty and Ronald Franks, "The Hidden Curriculum, Ethics Teaching, and the Structure of Medical Education," *Academic Medicine* 69 (November 1994): 869.

35. Douglas S. Massey and Robert J. Sampson, "Introduction: Moynihan Redux: Legacies," in *The Moynihan Report Revisited: Lessons and Reflections after Four Decades, The Annals of The American Academy of Political and Social Science* 621 (January 2009): 17.

36. William Julius Wilson, *More Than Just Race: Being Black and Poor in the Inner City* (New York and London: W.W. Norton & Company, 2009): 16.

37. Reginald L. Peniston, "Further Reflections on a Racial View of Medical Education," *Journal of the National Medical Association* 82 (1990): 325

38. Barry Zuckerman, Deborah A. Frank, and Linda Mayes, "Cocaine-Exposed Infants and Developmental Outcomes," *JAMA* 287 (April 17, 2002): 1991.

39. H. Jack Geiger, "Racial and Ethnic Disparities in Diagnosis and Treatment: A Review of the Evidence and a Consideration of Causes," in *Unequal Treatment: Confronting Racial and Ethnic Disparities in Healthcare* (Washington, DC: The National Academies Press, 2003): 418, 440, 419.

40. Byron M. Roth, *Prescription for Failure: Race Relations in the Age of Social Science* (New Brunswick and London, Transaction Publishers, 1994): 11.

41. See, for example, Sally Satel, *PC, M.D.: How Political Correctness Is Corrupting Medicine* (New York: Basic Books, 2000); "The Indoctrinologists Are Coming," *The Atlantic Monthly* (January 2001): 59–64. For a critical review of *PC, M.D.* by Daniel M. Fox, M.D., see the *New England Journal of Medicine* 344 (February 8, 2001): 462.

42. *Unequal Treatment: Confronting Racial and Ethnic Disparities in Health Care*, Brian D. Smedley, Adrienne Y. Stith, and Alan R. Nelson, eds. (Washington, DC: The National Academies Press, 2003).

43. H. Jack Geiger, "Racial and Ethnic Disparities in Diagnosis and Treatment: A Review of the Evidence and a Consideration of Causes," in *Unequal Treatment: Confronting Racial and Ethnic Disparities in Healthcare* (Washington, DC: The National Academies Press, 2003): 442, 422.

44. Mary-Jo DelVecchio Good et al., "The Culture of Medicine and Racial, Ethnic, and Class Disparities in Healthcare," in *Unequal Treatment: Confronting Racial and Ethnic Disparities in Healthcare* (Washington, DC: The National Academies Press, 2003): 595, 610.

45. Edward M. Hundert, "Characteristics of the Informal Curriculum and Trainees' Ethical Choices," *Academic Medicine* 71 (June 1996): 624.

46. Mary-Jo DelVecchio Good et al., "The Culture of Medicine and Racial, Ethnic, and Class Disparities in Healthcare," in *Unequal Treatment: Confronting Racial and Ethnic Disparities in Healthcare* (Washington, DC: The National Academies Press, 2003): 604.

47. Brenda L. Beagan, "Teaching Social and Cultural Awareness to Medical Students: 'It's All Very Nice to Talk about It in Theory, But Ultimately It Makes No Difference,'" *Academic Medicine* 78 (June 2003): 605–614.

48. Frederic W. Hafferty and Ronald Franks, "The Hidden Curriculum, Ethics Teaching, and the Structure of Medical Education," *Academic Medicine* 69 (November 1994): 865.

49. A curious feature of this and other medical liberal texts is the alternation between soft-pedaling evidence of medical racism and calls for a supposedly unprecedented critical approach to physician behaviors: "When we are

challenged to examine the culture of medicine and of or healthcare institutions, we are also challenged to bring a critical perspective that has largely been ignored by most research to date or that has circumscribed cultural inquiry to the differences between patients and physicians' beliefs." See Mary-Jo DelVecchio Good et al. "The Culture of Medicine and Racial, Ethnic, and Class Disparities in Healthcare," in *Unequal Treatment: Confronting Racial and Ethnic Disparities in Healthcare* (Washington, DC: The National Academies Press, 2003): 620.

50. Alan Nelson, "Unequal Treatment: Confronting Racial and Ethnic Disparities in Health Care," *Journal of the National Medical Association* 94 (August 2002): 667.

51. Sally Satel, "Racist Doctors? Don't Believe the Media Hype," *The Wall Street Journal* (April 4, 2002).

52. W. Michael Byrd and Linda A. Clayton, *An American Health Dilemma*, vol. II. *Race, Medicine, and Health Care in the United States 1900–2000* (New York and London: Routledge, 2002).

53. Jerome Groopman, *How Doctors Think* (Boston and New York: Houghton Mifflin, 2007): 7, 40, 92. Groopman's only (and hypothetical) example of how a white doctor might (not) think about the race factor goes as follows: "When an elderly patient was noncompliant, you generously considered whether this was a sign of early dementia or psychological depression, not a reflection of the severe disadvantages of being a black woman in the rural Mississippi of the 1930s" (92).

CHAPTER 2

1. David Satcher et al., "What If We Were Equal? A Comparison of the Black-White Mortality Gap in 1960 and in 2000," *Health Affairs* 24 (2005): 459.

2. See, for example, Ronald L. Braithwaite and Sandra E. Taylor, eds., *Health Issues in the Black Community* (San Francisco: Jossey-Bass Publishers, 2001): 8–9; Peter T. Kilborn, "Health Gap Grows, With Black Americans Trailing Whites, Studies Say," *New York Times* (January 26, 1998).

3. "A Generation Behind," *Time* (April 7, 1947).

4. Peter T. Kilborn, "Health Gap Grows, with Black Americans Trailing Whites, Studies Say," *New York Times* (January 26, 1998).

5. Daniel S. Greenberg, "Black Health: Grim Statistics," *The Lancet* (March 31, 1990): 780.

6. "The Origins of Racial/Ethnic Disparities," *Health Affairs* 24 (2005): 316.

7. "The National Negro Antituberculosis League," *JAMA* 52 (March 20, 1909): 969–970.

8. Robert A. Hingson, "Comparative Negro and White Mortality during Anesthesia, Obstetrics and Surgery," *Journal of the National Medical Association* 49 (July 1957): 204, 203.

9. John Pekkanen, *M.D.: Doctors Talk about Themselves* (New York: Delacorte Press, 1988): 8.

10. E.C. Ellett, "Diseases of the Ear, Nose, and Throat in the Negro," *JAMA* (December 2, 1899): 1,419–1,420.

11. "Negro Practice," *Journal of the American Medical Association* (May 9, 1908): 1,564.

12. Jarratt P. Robertson and A.B. Lee, "Urology in the Colored Race," *The Urologic and Cutaneous Review* 39 (June 1935): 405.

13. Thomas W. Murrell, "Syphilis and the American Negro," *JAMA* (March 12, 1910): 847.

14. R.A. Vonderlehr et al., "Untreated Syphilis in the Male Negro," *JAMA* 107 (September 12, 1936): 860.
15. S.W. Douglas, "Difficulties and Superstitions Encountered in Practice among the Negroes," *Southern Medical Journal* (October 1926): 736, 737.
16. Charles T. Stone and Frances R. Vanzant, "Heart Disease as Seen in a Southern Clinic," *JAMA* 89 (October 29, 1927): 1,479.
17. James H. Jones, *Bad Blood: The Tuskegee Syphilis Experiment* [1981] (New York: The Free Press, 1993): 43.
18. C.E. Terry, MD, "The Negro: His Relation to Public Health in the South," *American Journal of Public Health* 3 (1913): 304.
19. *Bad Blood*, 22.
20. *Bad Blood*, 59.
21. "Dr. Cartwright on the Caucasians and the Africans," *De Bow's Review* 25 (1858): 49, 47.
22. Robert Wilson, Jr., "Some Medical Aspects of the Negro," *Southern Medical Journal* (January 1, 1915): 3.
23. Frederick L. Hoffman, *Race Traits and Tendencies of the American Negro* (New York: Published for the American Economic Association by the Macmillan Company, 1896): 148.
24. "Some Medical Aspects of the Negro," 4.
25. Charles H. Garvin, "Negro Health," *Opportunity* (November 1924): 341.
26. Franklin O. Nichols, "Social Hygiene in Racial Problems—the Negro," *Journal of Social Hygiene* 18 (1932): 450.
27. Dr. Roscoe C. Brown, "Negro Health IS a Problem," *Opportunity* (June 1941): 164.
28. Paul B. Cornely, "Health Assets and Liabilities of the Negro," *Opportunity* (October–December 1945): 198.
29. Paul B. Cornely, "Segregation and Discrimination in Medical Care in the United States," *American Journal of Public Health* 46 (September 1956): 198–200, 227–228.
30. Quoted in Archie Epps, ed., *Malcolm X: Speeches at Harvard* (New York: Paragon House, 1991): 128. In 1970, 44 percent of black Americans believed that "whites are more apt to catch diseases." See "How It Looks to Blacks," *Time* (April 6, 1970): 65.
31. "Slavery Was 'Great Biological Experiment' Negro MD Claims," *Journal of the American Medical Association* (September 1, 1962).
32. *Journal of the American Medical Association* 196 (June 6, 1966): 9.
33. Paul B. Cornely, "The Health Status of the Negro Today and in the Future," *American Journal of Public Health* 58 (April 1968): 652–653.
34. "You're Black and Sick," *Newsweek* (July 7, 1969): 83.
35. Lawrence Greely Brown, "Experience with Racial Attitudes of the Medical Profession in New Jersey," *JNMA* (January 1963): 66–68.
36. Carter G. Woodson, *The Mis-Education of the Negro* [1933] (Trenton, NJ: Africa World Press, Inc., 1990): 20, 77, 176.
37. "Racially Rationed Medicine," *Time* (April 6, 1970): 91.
38. Sydney Barnwell and Walter F. LaMendola, "A Survey and Analysis of Techniques Used in Attracting the Black Middle-Class Patient," *Journal of the National Medical Association* 77 (1985): 379–384.
39. "Nashville Clinic Offers Case Study of Chronic Gap in Black and White Health," *New York Times* (March 21, 1998).
40. "Filling Special Needs of Minority Patients," *New York Times* (February 14, 1999).
41. John Langston Gwaltney, *Drylongso: A Self-Portrait of Black America* [1980] (New York: Vintage Books, 1981): 241.

42. "How It Looks to Blacks," *Time* (April 6, 1970): 65.
43. "Metabolic Quirk Tied to Blacks' High Diabetes Rate," *Jet* (October 29, 1984): 37.
44. "As Black Men Move into Middle Age, Dangers Rise," *New York Times* (September 23, 2002).
45. Terry L. Mills and Carla D.A. Edwards, "A Critical Review of Research on the Mental Health Status of Older African-Americans," *Aging & Society* 22 (2002): 286.
46. Richard Allen Williams, ed. *Textbook of Black-Related Diseases* (New York: McGraw-Hill Book Company, 1975): 331–332.
47. George S. Schuyler, "Our White Folks," in *Black on White: Black Writers on What It Means to Be White*, ed. David R. Roediger (New York: Schocken Books, 1998): 83, 81.
48. Kenneth B. Clark, *Dark Ghetto: Dilemmas of Social Power* (1965): 6.
49. Ford Fessenden, "A Difference of Life & Death," *Newsday* [Long Island, New York] (November 29, 1998): A5.
50. See Ashish K. Jha et al., "Racial Trends in the Use of Major Procedures among the Elderly," *New England Journal of Medicine* 353 (August 18, 2005): 684, 690.
51. See Rachel L. Johnson et al., "Patient Race/Ethnicity and Quality of Patient-Physician Communication During Medical Visits," *American Journal of Public Health* 94 (December 2004): 2,086–2,087.
52. Thomas Bartlett, "An Ugly Tradition Persists at Southern Fraternity Parties," *Chronicle of Higher Education* (November 30, 2001): A33.
53. Mark B. Wenneker and Arnold M. Epstein, "Racial Inequalities in the Use of Procedures for Patients With Ischemic Heart Disease in Massachusetts," *JAMA* 261 (January 13, 1989): 255.
54. Jeff Whittle et al., "Racial Differences in the Use of Invasive Cardiovascular Procedures in the Department of Veterans Affairs Medical System," *New England Journal of Medicine* 329 (August 26, 1993): 623.
55. H. Jack Geiger, "Race and Health Care—An American Dilemma?" *New England Journal of Medicine* 335 (September 12, 1996).
56. Eric D. Peterson, "Racial Variation in the Use of Coronary-Revascularization Procedures," *New England Journal of Medicine* 336 (February 13, 1997): 484.
57. Saif S. Rathore et al., "Race, Sex, Poverty, and the Medical Treatment of Acute Myocardial Infarction in the Elderly," *Circulation* 102 (August 8, 2000): 647.
58. Viola Vaccarino et al., "Sex and Racial Differences in the Management of Acute Myocardial Infarction, 1994 through 2002," *New England Journal of Medicine* 353 (August 18, 2005): 671–682.
59. Peter B. Bach et al., "Racial Differences in the Treatment of Early-Stage Lung Cancer," *New England Journal of Medicine* 341 (October 14, 1999): 1,198.
60. Christopher S. Lathan, Bridget A. Neville, and Craig C. Earle, "The Effect of Race on Invasive Staging and Surgery in Non-Small-Lung Cancer," *Journal of Clinical Oncology* 24 (January 20, 2006): 413.
61. Ford Fessenden, "A Difference of Life & Death," *Newsday* [Long Island, New York] (November 29, 1998): A4.
62. Marion E. Gornick et al., "Effects of Race and Income on Mortality and Use of Services among Medicare Beneficiaries," *New England Journal of Medicine* 335 (September 12, 1996): 798, 791; Ford Fessenden, "A Difference of Life & Death," *Newsday* [Long Island, New York] (November 29, 1998): A4.
63. Jonathan Skinner et al., "Racial, Ethnic, and Geographic Disparities in Rates of Knee Arthroplasty among Medicare Patients," *New England Journal of Medicine* 349 (October 2, 2003): 1,358.

64. See David S. Strogatz, "Use of Medical Care for Chest Pain: Differences between Blacks and Whites," *American Journal of Public Health* 80 (March 1990): 292.

65. Knox H. Todd, "Ethnicity as a Risk Factor for Inadequate Emergency Department Analgesia," *Journal of the American Medical Association* 269 (March 24/31, 1993): 1,537–1,539.

66. See, for example, David B. Morris, *The Culture of Pain* [1991] (Berkeley: University of California Press, 1993): 54–55.

67. William S. Hunter, "Coronary Occlusion in Negroes," *JAMA* 131 (May 4, 1946): 12.

68. Knox H. Todd, "Ethnicity as a Risk Factor for Inadequate Emergency Department Analgesia," *Journal of the American Medical Association* 269 (March 24/31, 1993): 1,539.

69. Eric D. Peterson, "Racial Variation in the Use of Coronary-Revascularization Procedures," *NEJM* 336 (February 13, 1997): 484.

70. 2005 *National Healthcare Disparities Report* (Rockville, MD: U.S. Department of Health and Human Services, AHRQ Publication No. 06-0017, December 2005): 1, 13.

71. Institute of Medicine. *Unequal Treatment: Confronting Racial and Ethnic Disparities in Health Care* (Washington, DC: National Academies Press, 2002).

72. "Minorities More Likely to Receive Lower-Quality Health Care, Regardless of Income and Insurance Coverage," The National Academies *News* (March 20, 2002).

73. Tom L. Beauchamp and James F. Childress, *Principles of Biomedical Ethics* [Fifth Edition] (New York: Oxford University Press, 2001): 237–239.

74. "U.S. Practices a System of Medicine that Shortchanges Minorities and Women," *Milwaukee Journal Sentinel* (April 16, 2001).

75. M. Gregg Bloche, "Health Care Disparities—Science, Politics, and Race," *New England Journal of Medicine* 350 (April 8, 2004): 1,569.

76. Owen Dyer, "Ethnic Minority Groups Criticize U.S. Report on Healthcare Disparities," *BMJ* 328 (February 7, 2004): 308.

77. M. Gregg Bloche, "Health Care Disparities—Science, Politics, and Race," *New England Journal of Medicine* 350 (April 8, 2004): 1,569.

78. M. Gregg Bloche, "Health Care Disparities—Science, Politics, and Race," *New England Journal of Medicine* 350 (April 8, 2004): 1,568.

79. "Taking Spin Out of Report That Made Bad Into Good," *New York Times* (February 22, 2004).

80. "Taking Spin Out of Report That Made Bad Into Good," *New York Times* (February 22, 2004).

81. Sally Satel, "The Indoctrinologists Are Coming," *The Atlantic Monthly* (January 2001): 59–64. Satel expanded this magazine article into a chapter for her book *PC, M.D.: How Political Correctness Is Corrupting Medicine* (New York: Basic Books, 2000): 155–192. This chapter, like the *Atlantic Monthly* article that announced her book's publication, is lightly researched and unreliable as a basis for thinking about the multiple origins of racial health disparities. Sherwin B. Nuland notes the following in his review of *PC, M.D.*: "Her statistics, and her descriptions of biological differences in disease patterns, read like feeble protests in the face of the experience of anyone who has ever trained in the teaching divisions of a large hospital, by which I mean the great majority of American physicians." See Sherwin B. Nuland, "Indoctrinology," *The New Republic* (February 19, 2001): 34–39. Satel's more recent publication on race and medicine is Jonathan Klick and Sally Satel, The Health Disparities Myth: Diagnosing the

Treatment Gap (Washington, D.C.: The AEI Press, 2006). One reviewer of this pamphlet commented as follows: "What is not clear is why [the authors] feel the need to try to dispel the existence of racism in this country; try to recharacterize the expression of racism in different, more palatable terms; attribute the socioeconomic effects due to racism to other causes; and reframe the discussion in terms of class rather than race." See Barbara Nabrit-Stephens' review in the Journal of the National Medical Association. 99 (July 2007): 852.

82. To watch a socially conscious physician wrestling (I think ineffectually) with these issues, see H. Jack Geiger, "Race and Health Care—An American Dilemma?" *New England Journal of Medicine* 335 (September 12, 1996): 815–816.

83. See Nancy R. Kressin et al., "Racial Differences in Cardiac Catheterization as a Function of Patients' Beliefs," *American Journal of Public Health* 94 (December 2004): 2,096.

84. Richard L. Lichtenstein et al., "Black/White Differences in Attitudes Toward Physician-Assisted Suicide," *Journal of the National Medical Association* 89 (1997): 132.

85. Mark B. Wenneker and Arnold M. Epstein, "Racial Inequalities in the Use of Procedures for Patients with Ischemic Heart Disease in Massachusetts," *JAMA* 261 (January 13, 1989): 257.

86. David Satcher, "Does Race Interfere with the Doctor-Patient Relationship?" *JAMA* 223 (March 26, 1973): 1,498–1,499.

87. John M. Eisenberg, "Sociologic Influences on Decision-Making by Clinicians," *Annals of Internal Medicine* 90 (1979): 957–964.

88. David Levy, "White Doctors and Black Patients: Influence of Race on the Doctor-Patient Relationship," *Pediatrics* 75 (1985): 639–643.

89. John M. Eisenberg, "Sociologic Influences on Decision-Making by Clinicians," *Annals of Internal Medicine* 90 (1979): 957.

90. "Does Race Interfere With the Doctor-Patient Relationship?" *JAMA* 223 (March 26, 1973): 1499.

91. H. Jack Geiger, "Race and Health Care," *New England Journal of Medicine* 335 (September 12, 1996): 816.

92. Talmadge E. King, Jr. and Paul Brunetta, "Racial Disparity in Rates of Surgery for Lung Cancer," *New England Journal of Medicine* 341 (October 14, 1999): 1,231–1,232.

93. "Federal Support Grows for Research on the Role of Race in Public-Health Problems," *Chronicle of Higher Education* (November 24, 2000): A25.

94. Viola Vaccarino et al., "Sex and Racial Differences in the Management of Acute Myocardial Infarction, 1994 through 2002," *New England Journal of Medicine* 353 (August 18, 2005): 680.

95. David Levy, "White Doctors and Black Patients: Influence of Race on the Doctor-Patient Relationship," *Pediatrics* 75 (1985): 640.

96. John Z. Ayanian, "Heart Disease in Black and White," *New England Journal of Medicine* 329 (August 26, 1993): 657.

97. Joseph A. Flaherty and Robert Meagher, "Measuring Racial Bias in Inpatient Treatment," *American Journal of Psychiatry* 137 (1980): 681.

98. Ford Fessenden, "A Difference of Life & Death," *Newsday* [Long Island, New York] (November 29, 1998): A5. The researcher quoted is Michelle van Ryn of the State University of New York at Albany.

99. Jeff Whittle et al., "Racial Differences in the Use of Invasive Cardiovascular Procedures in the Department of Veterans Affairs Medical System," *New England Journal of Medicine* 329 (August 26, 1993): 626.

100. See L. M. Schwartz et al., "Misunderstandings about the Effects of Race and Sex on Physicians' Referrals for Cardiac Catheterization," *New England*

Journal of Medicine 341 (July 22, 1999): 279–283: "Race, Sex, and Physicians' Referrals for Cardiac Catheterization" [letters], New England Journal of Medicine 341 (July 22, 1999): 285–288.

101. Kevin A. Schulman et al., "The Effect of Race and Sex on Physicians' Recommendations for Cardiac Catheterization," New England Journal of Medicine (February 25, 1999): 624–625.

102. Jeffrey N. Katz, "Patient Preferences and Health Disparities," JAMA 286 (September 26, 2001): 1,507.

103. Jonathan Skinner et al., "Racial, Ethnic, and Geographic Disparities in Rates of Knee Arthroplasty among Medicare Patients," New England Journal of Medicine 349 (October 2, 2003): 1,358.

104. Jeffrey N. Katz, "Patient Preferences and Health Disparities," JAMA 286 (September 26, 2001): 1507.

105. John Z. Ayanian et al., "Physicians' Beliefs about Racial Differences in Referral for Renal Transplantation," American Journal of Kidney Disease 43 (February 2004): 350–357.

106. M.L. Margolis et al., "Racial Differences Pertaining to a Belief about Lung Cancer Surgery: Results of a Multi-Center Survey," Annals of Internal Medicine 139 (October 7, 2003): 558–563.

107. Jane V.R. Marsh et al., "Racial Differences in Hormone Replacement Therapy Prescriptions," Obstetrics & Gynecology 93 (1999): 999–1,003.

108. Jeffrey N. Katz, "Patient Preferences and Health Disparities," JAMA 286 (September 26, 2001): 1,507–1,508.

109. Ford Fessenden, "A Difference of Life & Death," Newsday [Long Island, New York] (November 29, 1998): A59.

110. Robert Fresco, "Long, Frustrating Delay for a Kidney," Newsday [Long Island, New York] (December 1, 1998): A44.

111. John Z. Ayanian et al., "The Effect of Patients' Preferences on Racial Differences in Access to Renal Transplantation," New England Journal of Medicine 341 (November 25, 1999): 1,667.

112. M. Gregg Bloche, "Health Care Disparities—Science, Politics, and Race," New England Journal of Medicine 350 (April 8, 2004): 1,568.

113. Michelle D. Holmes, David Hodges, and John Rich, "Racial Inequities in the Use of Procedures for Ischemic Heart Disease" [Letter], JAMA (June 9, 1989): 3,242.

114. Rachel L. Johnson et al., "Patient Race/Ethnicity and Quality of Patient-Physician Communication during Medical Visits," American Journal of Public Health 94 (December 2004): 2,086.

115. The best journalism on the African American health disaster appeared in Newsday (Long Island, New York) in November and December 1998. The first article in this series, titled "The Health Divide," is by Ford Fessenden, "A Difference of Life & Death," Newsday (November 29, 1998).

116. David Levy, "White Doctors and Black Patients: Influence of Race on the Doctor-Patient Relationship," Pediatrics 75 (1985): 642.

117. Dorothy E. Roberts, "Reconstructing the Patient: Starting with Women of Color," in Susan B. Wolf, ed., Feminism & Bioethics (New York: Oxford University Press, 1996): 117–118, 121.

118. Quoted in Roberts, "Reconstructing the Patient: Starting with Women of Color," in Susan B. Wolf, ed., Feminism & Bioethics (New York: Oxford University Press, 1996): 120.

119. Ford Fessenden, "A Difference of Life & Death," Newsday [Long Island, New York] (November 29, 1998): A6, A4.

120. Naaz Coker, ed. Racism in Medicine: An Agenda for Change (London: King's Fund, 2001): 65.

121. See Byron D'Andra Orey, "White Racial Attitudes and Support for the Mississippi State Flag," *American Politics Research* 32 (January 2004): 108.
122. Ken Auletta, *The Underclass* (New York: Random House, 1982): 31.
123. Carl Husemoller Nightingale, *On the Edge: A History of Poor Black Children and Their American Dreams* (New York: Basic Books, 1993): 124.
124. "Ethics Officials to Investigate Drug Experiments on Children," *New York Times* (April 15, 1998).
125. "How Whites Feel about Negroes," *Newsweek* (October 21, 1963): 48.
126. Samuel Cartwright, "Diseases and Peculiarities of the Negro Race," *De Bow's Review* 11 (1851): 68.
127. "Top Health Official Quits Post amid Flak," *Austin American-Statesman* (October 24, 2000).
128. Bob Herbert, "G.O.P. 'Big Tent' Is Shrinking," *New York Times* (May 1, 2000).
129. "Top health official quits post amid flak," *Austin American-Statesman* (October 24, 2000).
130. Susan Richardson, "Racial Reconciliation Requires Practice," *Austin American-Statesman* (July 25, 1988).
131. See, for example, Jacqueline S. Mattis et al., "A Critical Approach to Stress-Related Disorders in African Americans," *Journal of the National Medical Association* 91 (1999): 80–85.
132. "Democrats Attack Radio Host's Remarks on Crime," *New York Times* (September 30, 2005).
133. "Bennett Defends Comment on Blacks, Abortion, Crime," *Austin American-Statesman* (October 1, 2005); Bob Herbert, "Impossible, Ridiculous, Repugnant," *New York Times* (October 5, 2005).
134. Edwin Dorn, "So What Was He Thinking?" *Austin American-Statesman* (October 5, 2005).
135. Quoted in Dan Baum, *Smoke and Mirrors: The War on Drugs and the Politics of Failure* (Boston: Little, Brown, 1996): 268.
136. Jim Sleeper, "The Clash," *The New Republic* (September 19–26, 1994): 51.
137. Linda Chavez, "Coming Soon to a College Near You—Equal Opportunity Enlightenment?" *Jewish World Review* (December 9, 2002), http://www.NewsAnd Opinion.com.
138. "UMass-Rutgers Game Suspended," *The Boston Globe* (February 8, 1995).
139. Personal communication of February 21, 2006.
140. See Delthia Ricks, "Medical Myths," *Newsday* [Long Island, New York] (December 6, 1998): A4, A52–A55.
141. Personal communication of February 28, 2006.
142. Ford Fessenden, "The Health Divide," *Newsday* (November 29, 1998): A55.
143. Personal communication of February 21, 2006.
144. Ritchie Witzig, "The Medicalization of Race: Scientific Legitimization of a Flawed Social Construct," *Annals of Internal Medicine* 125 (October 15, 1996): 677.
145. John Scudder, "Practical Genetic Concepts in Modern Medicine," *Journal of the National Medical Association* (July 1960): 274.
146. "Blood Expert Says Transfusion between Races May Be Perilous," *New York Times* (November 7, 1959).
147. Edward C. Mazique, "The Negro Physician in a Sick Society," *Journal of the National Medical Association* (May 1960): 184. Regarding the laws mentioned in this article, see "Racial Blood Ban Wins," *New York Times* (February 17, 1960).
148. Robert Wilson, Jr., "Some Medical Aspects of the Negro," *Southern Medical Journal* (January 1, 1915): 4.

149. Charles W. Kollock, "Some Interesting Conditions Seen in the Eye of a Negro," *Southern Medical Journal* 10 (1917): 346.
150. Dunbar Roy, "Some Further Observations on Vernal Conjunctivitis in the Negro," *Southern Medical Journal* (October 1, 1915): 897.
151. "Rectal Pathology in the Negro," *JAMA* 84 (January 10, 1925): 97.
152. C. Jeff Miller, "Special Medical Problems of the Colored Woman," *Southern Medical Journal* 25 (1932): 738.
153. "How Whites Feel about Negroes: A Painful American Dilemma," *Newsweek* (October 21, 1963): 55.
154. Lauretta Bender, "Behavior Problems in Negro Children," *Psychiatry* 2 (1939): 214.
155. E.S. Ray and R.C. Cecil, "Infectious Mononucleosis in the Negro," *Southern Medical Journal* 37 (1944): 545.
156. "Anæmia in Africans," *The Lancet* (March 22, 1952): 617.
157. T.C. Redfern, "The Incidence of Exophthalmic Goiter in Negroes," *JAMA* 75 (July 3, 1920): 51.
158. Harry Bakwin, "The Negro Infant," *Human Biology* (1932): 26.
159. Philip F. Williams, "Maternal Care and the Negro," *JAMA* (132 (November 16, 1946): 613.
160. W. Michael Byrd and Linda A. Clayton, *An American Health Dilemma*, vol. II. *Race, Medicine, and Health Care in the United States 1900–2000* (New York and London: Routledge, 2002): 390.
161. George Devereux, *From Anxiety to Method in the Behavioral Sciences* (The Hague & Paris: Mouton & Co., 1967): 173, 174, 174, 175, 175, 175, 174.
162. David Levy, "White Doctors and Black Patients: Influence of Race on the Doctor-Patient Relationship," *Pediatrics* 75 (1985): 642.
163. Wilbur A. Drake, "The Gynecologist: Some of His Problems and His Obligation to the Present and the Future," *Journal of the National Medical Association* (January-March 1920): 18.
164. David Satcher, "Does Race Interfere With the Doctor-Patient Relationship?" *JAMA* 223 (March 26, 1973): 1,499.
165. Charles H. Garvin, "Negro Health," *Opportunity* (November 1924): 342.
166. "Are There Any Blind Babies?" *The Survey* (April 15, 1924): 93.
167. Gunnar Myrdal, *An American Dilemma: The Negro Problem and Modern Democracy* (New York: Harper & Brothers, 1944): 141–142.
168. Frank Dell'Apa, "Medical Screening for Foe Questioned," *Boston Globe* (July 1, 2003).
169. Newton G. Osborne and Marvin D. Feit, "The Use of Race in Medical Research," *JAMA* 267 (January 8, 1992): 278.
170. James Hunt, "On the Negro's Place in Nature," *Memoirs of the Anthropological Society of London* (1863–4): 3.
171. R.W. Alles, "A Comparative Study of the Negro and White Pelvis," *The Journal of the Michigan State Medical Society* 24 (1925): 197.
172. C. Jeff Miller, "A Comparative Study of Certain Gynecologic and Obstetric Conditions as Exhibited in the Colored and White Races," *Transactions of the American Gynecological Society* 53 (1929): 92.
173. Lauretta Bender, "Behavior Problems in Negro Children," *Psychiatry* 2 (1939): 217.
174. Dan Baum, "Jake Leg," *The New Yorker* (September 15, 2003).
175. S.J. Holmes, "The Resistant Ectoderm of the Negro," *American Journal of Physical Anthropology* (1928): 149.
176. Harry Bakwin and Ruth Morris Bakwin, "The Dosage of Ultraviolet Radiation in Infants with Tetany," *JAMA* 95 (August 9, 1930): 399.

177. Milo Hellman, "The Fundamental Pattern of the Human Lower Molar Teeth," *Proceedings of the American Philosophical Society* 67 (1928): 167–169; Julian Herman Lewis, "Diseases of the Eye, Ears, Nose and Throat," in *The Biology of the Negro* (1942): 399.
178. Patrick Buchanan, "Crime and Race," *Conservative Digest* (1989): 37.
179. "Carter's Trip of the Tongue," *Newsweek* 87 (April 19, 1976): 14.
180. Jerome G. Miller, *Search and Destroy: African-American Males in the Criminal Justice System* (Cambridge: Cambridge University Press, 1996): 212–213.
181. "Dispute Threatens U.S. Plan on Violence," *New York Times* (October 23, 1992). For an earlier medical interpretation of the violent black male, see "Role of Brain Disease in Riots and Urban Violence," *JAMA* 202 (September 11, 1967): 895.
182. See, for example, Louis W. Sullivan, "U.S. Violence Studies Are Free of Racial Bias," *New York Times* [letter], October 2, 1992.
183. James Hunt, "On the Negro's Place in Nature," *Memoirs of the Anthropological Society of London* (1863-4): 5, 5, 6, 6, 8–9, 15, 20, 22, 11, 11–12, 18, 19, 19, 23.

CHAPTER 3

1. See Alwyn T. Cohall and Hope E. Bannister, "The Health Status of Children and Adolescents," in *Health Issues in the Black Community*, eds. Ronald L. Braithwaite and Sandra E. Taylor (San Francisco: Jossey-Bass Publishers, 2001): 13–43.
2. L.C. Hayes et al., "The Problem of Prenatal Cocaine Exposure: A Rush to Judgment," *JAMA* 267 (1992): 407.
3. Franz Fanon, *Black Skin, White Masks* (New York: Grove Press, 1967): 167.
4. Frederick L. Hoffman, *Race Traits and Tendencies of the American Negro* (New York: American Economic Association, 1896): 159.
5. Ales Hrdlicka, "Physical Differences between White and Colored Children," *American Anthropologist* 11 (November 1898): 350.
6. Stewart R. Roberts, "Nervous and Mental Influences in Angina Pectoris," *American Heart Journal* 7 (1931–32): 32.
7. Erik H. Erikson, "Ego Development and Historical Change," *Identity and the Life Cycle* (New York: International Universities Press, 1959): 37–38.
8. "Psychology of Africans" [Abstract], *JAMA* 175 (March 18, 1961): 1,018.
9. James Hunt, "On the Negro's Place in Nature," *Memoirs of the Anthropological Society of London* (1863-4): 11.
10. See Stanley M. Garn and Diane C. Clark, "Problems in the Nutritional Assessment of Black Individuals," *American Journal of Public Health* 66 (1976): 264.
11. Janet E. Kilbride et al., "The Comparative Motor Development of Baganda, American White, and American Black Infants," *American Anthropologist* 72 (1970): 1,426.
12. "Smart Pickaninnies," *Time* (April 1, 1940): 56.
13. M.O. Bousfield, "Reaching the Negro Community," *American Journal of Public Health* 24 (1934): 213.
14. "Doctors Pick Prize Pickaninnies at Memphis Tri-State Negro Fair," *Life* 11:19 (November 10, 1941).
15. See http://www3.georgetown.edu/research/nrcbl/hsbioethics/units/cases/unit4_1.html [accessed June 19, 2006].
16. Elazar Barkan, *The Retreat of Scientific Racism: Changing Concepts of Race in Britain and the United States between the World Wars* (New York: Cambridge University Press, 1992): 164.

17. Felice Swados, "Negro Health on the Ante Bellum Plantations," *Bulletin of the History of Medicine* 10 (October 1941): 468.
18. Lee Bivings, "The Negro School Child Compared with the White School Child," *Archives of Pediatrics* 44 (1927): 193.
19. Hildrus A. Poindexter, "Handicaps in the Normal Growth and Development of Rural Negro Children," *AJPH* 28 (1938): 1,048.
20. Hugh Pearson, *Under the Knife: How a Wealthy Negro Surgeon Wielded Power in the Jim Crow South* (New York: The Free Press, 2000): 197.
21. Jeffrey Melnick, *A Right to Sing the Blues: African Americans, Jews, and American Popular Song* (Cambridge, MA: Harvard University Press, 1999): 129.
22. LeRoi Jones, "The Last Days of the American Empire (Including Some Instructions for Black People)," in *Home: Social Essays* (New York: William Morrow & Co., Inc., 1966): 191.
23. Alice Walker, *The Color Purple* [1982] (New York: Pocket Books, 1985): 90.
24. See, for example, Wilma A. Dunaway, "Reproductive Exploitation and Child Mortality," in *The African-American Family in Slavery and Emancipation* (New York: Cambridge University Press, 2003): 113–149.
25. John S. Haller, Jr., "The Negro and the Southern Physician: A Study of Medical and Racial Attitudes 1800–1860," *Medical History* (1972): 240.
26. William F. Brunner, "The Negro Heath Problem in Southern Cities," *American Journal of Public Health* 5 (1915): 185.
27. Marvin L. Graves, "The Negro a Menace to the Health of the White Race," *Southern Medical Journal* 9 (1916): 411.
28. J.H. Mason Knox, "The Health Problem of the Negro Child," *American Journal of Public Health* 16 (1926): 808.
29. J. Ross Snyder, "The Problem of the Negro Child," *Southern Medical Journal* 16 (1923): 9.
30. Mary Robert Baynham and Bertha K. Whipple, "A Nutrition Problem with Special Reference to Negro Children," *The Journal of the Missouri State Medical Association* 22 (1925): 308–309.
31. W.M. Bevis, "Psychological Traits of the Southern Negro with Observations as to Some of His Psychoses," *American Journal of Psychiatry* (1921): 69–78.
32. Ira S. Wile, "The Altered Position of Children as a Factor in Behavior, with Particular Consideration of Negro Children," *Archives of Pediatrics* 49 (1932): 498, 503.
33. L. Bender, "Behavior Problems in Negro Children," *Psychiatry* 2 (1939): 217, 220.
34. H. Reichard Kahle, "Surgical Peculiarities of the Southern Negro," *Tri-State Medical Journal* 13 (1941): 2,683.
35. R.A. Schermerhorn, "Psychiatric Disorders among Negroes: A Sociological Note," *American Journal of Psychiatry* (May 1956): 880.
36. "Negro Schizophrenics Hallucinate More than White Patients," *JAMA* 184 (June 1, 1963): 27.
37. "Sickle-Cell Trait in Africans," *British Medical Journal* (July 5, 1952): 42.
38. Joseph Luder, "Some Pædiatric Problems of Uganda," *British Medical Journal* (November 16, 1957): 1,143.
39. Ira J. Chasnoff et al., "Cocaine Use in Pregnancy," *New England Journal of Medicine* 313 (September 12, 1985): 666–669.
40. Dan Baum, *Smoke and Mirrors: The War on Drugs and the Politics of Failure* (Boston: Little, Brown and Company, 1996): 217.
41. Dan Baum, *Smoke and Mirrors: The War on Drugs and the Politics of Failure* (Boston: Little, Brown and Company, 1996): 268.

42. L.C. Hayes et al., "The Problem of Prenatal Cocaine Exposure: A Rush to Judgment," *JAMA* 267 (1992): 406, 407.

43. Nancy L. Day and Gale A. Richardson, "Cocaine Use and Crack Babies: Science, the Media, and Miscommunication," *Neurotoxicology and Teratology* 15 (1993): 293; quoted in Dorothy Roberts, *Killing the Black Body: Race, Reproduction, and the Meaning of Liberty* (New York: Vintage Books, 1997): 159.

44. Deborah A. Frank et al., "Growth, Development, and Behavior in Early Childhood Following Prenatal Cocaine Exposure," *JAMA* 285 (March 28, 2001): 1,620; Barry Zuckerman, Deborah A. Frank, and Linda Mayes, "Cocaine-Exposed Infants and Developmental Outcomes," *JAMA* 287 (April 17, 2002): 1,990.

45. David C. Lewis, MD, "Stop Perpetuating the 'Crack Baby' Myth," Brown University News Service (March 29, 2004).

46. L.C. Hayes et al., "The Problem of Prenatal Cocaine Exposure: A Rush to Judgment," *JAMA* 267 (1992): 407.

47. Frederick L. Hoffman, *Race Traits and Tendencies of the American Negro* (New York: American Economic Association, 1896): 148.

48. Quoted in John S. Haller, Jr., "The Physician Versus the Negro: Medical and Anthropological Concepts of Race in the Late Nineteenth Century," *Bulletin of the History of Medicine* 44 (March–April 1970): 167.

49. Robert B. Scott, "Sickle-Cell Anemia—High Prevalence and Low Priority," *New England Journal of Medicine* (January 15, 1970): 164.

50. Charles F. Whitten, "Sickle-Cell Programming—An Imperiled Promise," *New England Journal of Medicine* 288 (February 8, 1973): 318–319.

51. Doris Y. Wilkinson, "For Whose Benefit? Politics and Sickle Cell," *The Black Scholar* (May 1974): 30.

52. Dorothy Roberts, *Killing the Black Body: Race, Reproduction, and the Meaning of Liberty* (New York: Vintage Books, 1997): 120.

53. John J. DiIulio, Jr., "My Black Crime Problem, and Ours," *City Journal* 6 (1996).

54. Gideon Koren et al., "Bias against the Null Hypothesis: The Reproductive Hazards of Cocaine," *The Lancet* (December 16, 1989): 1,441.

55. James H. Carter, "Psychosocial Aspects of Aging: The Black Elderly," *JNMA* (1984): 273, 271.

56. Elizabeth D. McKinley et al., "Differences in End-of-Life Decision Making among Black and White Ambulatory Cancer Patients," *Journal of General Internal Medicine* 11 (1996): 651.

57. Rose C. Gibson and James S. Jackson, "The Health, Physical Functioning, and Informal Supports of the Black Elderly," *The Milbank Quarterly* 65 (1987): 444.

58. Marie A. Bernard, "The Health Status of African-American Elderly," *Journal of the National Medical Association* 85 (1993): 524.

59. Rose C. Gibson and James S. Jackson, "The Health, Physical Functioning, and Informal Supports of the Black Elderly," *The Milbank Quarterly* 65 (1987): 444.

60. Robert C. Green et al., "Risk of Dementia among White and African American Relatives of Patients with Alzheimer Disease," *JAMA* 287 (January 16, 2002): 335.

61. Hugh Pearson, *Under the Knife: How a Wealthy Negro Surgeon Wielded Power in the Jim Crow South* (New York: Free Press, 2000): 21.

62. John M. Knox, "Etiological Factors and Premature Aging," *JAMA* (179 (February 24, 1962): 630.

63. Tanya E. Froelich et al., "Dementia and Race: Are There Differences between African Americans and Caucasians?" *Journal of the American Geriatrics Society* 49 (2001): 482.

64. Tanya E. Froelich et al., "Dementia and Race: Are There Differences between African Americans and Caucasians?" *Journal of the American Geriatrics Society* 49 (2001): 477, 478, 482.

65. D.B. Dill, J.W. Wilson, F.G. Hall, and Sid Robinson, "Properties of the Blood of Negroes and Whites in Relation to Climate and Season," *Journal of Biological Chemistry* 136 (October–December 1940): 450–451.

66. D.B. Dill, J.W. Wilson, F.G. Hall, and Sid Robinson, "Properties of the Blood of Negroes and Whites in Relation to Climate and Season," *Journal of Biological Chemistry* 136 (October–December 1940): 457, 459.
Reports of hemoglobin differences between blacks and whites have a long history: "Research on race and anemia (iron status) provides a more current example of the extreme public health implications of assuming that race differences are genetic and pan-racial. For over half a century various investigators have reported differences in mean hemoglobin concentrations between African-Americans and European-Americans (Munday et al. 1938). With the development of national surveys in the U.S., Garn and colleagues in the 1970s were able to present data on the hemoglobin concentration differences between "blacks" and "whites" that purported to support the universality of these differences. . . . This research prompted the recommendation that public health surveillance should work with separate cut-offs for defining anemia in blacks and whites, a suggestion that is still widely supported (Pan and Habicht 1991)." See Alan H. Goodman, "Is Race a Useful Variable in Nutritional Research?" *CommuNicAtor* [American Anthropological Association] 17 (1994): 5.

67. "Remarks by Reagan Doctor on Well-Fed Black Kids Criticized as Insensitive," *Jet* 65 (January 16, 1984): 6.

68. See Jack Olsen, "Pride and Prejudice," *Sports Illustrated* (July 8, 1968): 28–29.

69. "He plays our football and takes our tumbles, but he never damages a cartilage." See W.H. Ogilvie, "Pitfalls of Tropical Surgery," *The Lancet* (November 10, 1945): 586.

70. Personal communication (May 1998).

71. Frank Dell'Apa, "Medical Screening for Foe Questioned," *Boston Globe* (July 1, 2003).

72. See John Hoberman, *Darwin's Athletes: How Sport Has Damaged Black America and Preserved the Myth of Race* (New York: Houghton Mifflin, 1997).

73. See, for example, Helen Elizabeth Sanderson, "Differences in Musical Ability in Children of Different National and Racial Origin," *Journal of Genetic Psychology* XLII (1933): 100–119.

74. Yale S. Nathanson, "The Musical Ability of the Negro," *Annals of the American Academy of Political and Social Science* CXXXX (November 1928): 188, 189.

75. W.E.B. DuBois, ed., *The Health and Physique of the Negro American* [Atlanta University Publications, 1902–1906] (New York: Octagon Books, 1968): 59.

76. James Weldon Johnson, "The Poor White Musician" (1915), in *Black on White: Black Writers on What It Means to Be White*, David R. Roediger, ed. (New York: Schocken Books, 1998): 169.

77. W.M. Bevis, "Psychological Traits of the Southern Negro with Observations as to Some of His Psychoses," *American Journal of Psychiatry* (1921): 71.

78. J.C. Carothers, MB, DPM, "Frontal Lobe Function and the African," *Journal of Mental Science* 97 (1951): 32, 46.

79. Stewart R. Roberts, "Nervous and Mental Influences in Angina Pectoris," *American Heart Journal* 7 (1931–32): 34.
80. "Negro Schizophrenics Hallucinate More Than White Patients," *JAMA* 184 (June 1, 1963): 27.
81. S. Plous and Tyrone Williams, "Racial Stereotypes from the Days of American Slavery: A Continuing Legacy," *Journal of Applied Social Psychology* 25 (1995): 804.
82. Benjamin D. Singer, "Some Implications of Differential Psychiatric Treatment of Negro and White Patients," *Social Science and Medicine* 1 (1967): 81.
83. Thomas Jefferson, "Notes on the State of Virginia, Query XIV: Justice." http://teachingamericanhistory.org/library/index.asp?document=514 (accessed July 7, 2006).
84. Quoted in John S. Haller, Jr., "The Negro and the Southern Physician: A Study of Medical and Racial Attitudes 1800–1860," *Medical History* (1972): 248.
85. Robert Stigler, *Rassenphysiologische Ergebnisse meiner Forschungsreise in Uganda 1911–12* (Vienna: Österreichische Staatsdruckerei, 1952): 25.
86. Quoted in Mia Bay, *The White Image in the Black Mind: African-American Ideas about White People, 1830–1925* (New York and Oxford: Oxford University Press, 2000): 189–190.
87. Langston Hughes, "Slave on the Block" [1934], in *Black on White: Black Writers on What It Means to Be White*, David R. Roediger, ed. (New York: Schocken Books, 1998): 243.
88. George M. Niles, "A Therapeutic Comparison, Medicinal and Otherwise, as between the Caucasian and Afro-American," *Southern Medical Journal* (February 1, 1913): 128, 129.
89. Lauretta Bender, "Behavior Problems in Negro Children," *Psychiatry* 2 (1939): 218.
90. Jeff Miller, "Special Medical Problems of the Colored Woman," *Southern Medical Journal* 25 (1932): 733–739.
91. Julian H. Lewis, "Contribution of an Unknown Negro to Anesthesia," *Journal of the National Medical Association* (January–March 1931): 23.
92. See Robert A. Hingson, "Comparative Negro and White Mortality during Anesthesia, Obstetrics and Surgery," *Journal of the National Medical Association* 49 (July 1957): 203, 208.
93. Stewart R. Roberts, "Nervous and Mental Influences in Angina Pectoris," *American Heart Journal* 7 (1931–32): 31.
94. D. Dowie Dunn, "Medical Practice among Natives," *South African Medical Journal* 13 (1939): 51–53.
95. Chester M. Pierce, "The Ghetto: An Extreme Sleep Environment," *Journal of the National Medical Association* 67 (March 1975): 162–166.
96. Serena Gordon, "Blacks at Raised Risk of Sleep Apnea," MedicineNet.com. http://www.medicinenet.com/script/main/art.asp?articlekey=53540 (2005; accessed July 8, 2006).
97. National Sleep Disorders Research Plan. http://www.nhlbi.nih.gov/health/prof/sleep/res_ plan/section4/section4b.html (accessed July 8, 2006).
98. Terry L. Mills and Carla D.A. Edwards, "A Critical Review of Research on the Mental Health Status of Older African-Americans," *Aging & Society* 22 (2002): 284.
99. "W[ayne] S[tate] U[niversity] School of Medicine to Study Sleep Paralysis, Panic Disorder in African Americans." See http://www.med.wayne.edu/press/2001/press43.htm (accessed July 8, 2006).
100. National Sleep Disorders Research Plan. http://www.nhlbi.nih.gov/health/prof/sleep/res_ plan/section4/section4b.html (accessed July 8, 2006).

101. Serena Gordon, "Blacks at Raised Risk of Sleep Apnea," MedicineNet.com. http://www.medicinenet.com/script/main/art.asp?articlekey=53540 (2005; accessed July 8, 2006).
102. Dr. [Samuel] Cartwright, "Diseases and Peculiarities of the Negro Race," De Bow's Review 11 (1851): 65.
103. James Hunt, "On the Negro's Place in Nature," Memoirs of the Anthropological Society of London 1 (1863–64): 15, 16.
104. Robert J. Terry, "The American Negro," Science 69 (March 29, 1929): 340.
105. Edward H. Schwab and Victor E. Schulze, "Heart Disease in the American Negro of the South," American Heart Journal 7 (1932): 716.
106. I. I. Lemann, "A Study of Disease in the Negro," Southern Medical Journal 27 (1934): 33.
107. L. S. Williams, "Some Aspects of the Native in Disease," South African Medical Journal (March 28, 1936): 214. See also H. L. Heimann, "Disease in Non-European Patients," South African Medical Journal (March 28, 1936): 215–217.
108. Robert C. Moehlig, "The Mesoderm of the Negro," American Journal of Physical Anthropology 22 (1937): 309.
109. "Angina Pectoris in the Negro," JAMA (August 19, 1939). See also Morris M. Weiss, "The Problem of Angina Pectoris in the Negro," American Heart Journal 17 (1939): 711–715.
110. See John Langston Gwaltney, Drylongso: A Self-Portrait of Black America [1980] (New York: Vintage Books, 1981): 268.
111. This is a comment by Dr. W. S. Thayer of Baltimore as quoted in Charles T. Stone and Frances R. Vanzant, "Heart Disease as Seen in a Southern Clinic," JAMA 89 (October 29, 1927): 1,479.
112. William S. Hunter, "Coronary Occlusion in Negroes," JAMA 131 (May 4, 1946): 12.
113. George M. Niles, "A Therapeutic Comparison, Medicinal and Otherwise, as between the Caucasian and Afro-American," Southern Medical Journal (February 1, 1913): 128.
114. W. H. Ogilvie, "Pitfalls of Tropical Surgery," The Lancet (November 10, 1945): 586.
115. James M. Reinhardt, "The Negro: Is He Inferior?" American Journal of Sociology 33 (September 1927): 248–261; R. G. Hoskins, "Hormones and Racial Characteristics," in The Tides of Life: The Endocrine Glands in Bodily Adjustment (New York: W. W. Norton & Company, Inc., 1933): 335–336.
116. Robert C. Moehlig, "The Mesoderm of the Negro," American Journal of Physical Anthropology 22 (1937): 311.
117. Quoted in Robert A. Hingson, "Comparative Negro and White Mortality during Anesthesia, Obstetrics and Surgery," Journal of the National Medical Association 49 (July 1957): 209.
118. Quoted in Robert A. Hingson, "Comparative Negro and White Mortality during Anesthesia, Obstetrics and Surgery," Journal of the National Medical Association 49 (July 1957): 209.
119. H. J. Croot and J. N. P. Davies, "Cancer in Africa" [Letter], The Lancet (January 19, 1952): 158.
120. Robert A. Hingson, "Comparative Negro and White Mortality during Anesthesia, Obstetrics and Surgery," Journal of the National Medical Association 49 (July 1957): 204, 211.
121. On nervous reactivity and hypertension see, for example, N. B. Anderson et al., "Racial Differences in Cardiovascular Reactivity to Mental Arithmetic," International Journal of Psychophysiology 6 (1988): 161–164.
122. M. Packer, "Evolution of the Neurohormonal Hypothesis to Explain the Progression of Chronic Heart Failure," European Heart Journal vol. 16, Issue suppl F, 4.

123. Daniel L. Dries et al., "Racial Differences in the Outcome of Left Ventricular Dysfunction," *NEJM* 340 (February 25, 1999): 616.

124. "Racial Differences in the Outcome of Left Ventricular Dysfunction," *New England Journal of Medicine* 341 (1999): 287–288.

125. David S. Strogatz, "Use of Medical Care for Chest Pain: Differences between Blacks and Whites," *American Journal of Public Health* 80 (March 1990): 290–294.

126. Knox H. Todd et al., "Ethnicity and Analgesic Practice," *Annals of Emergency Medicine* 35 (January 2000): 11–16; "Whites More Often Given Opioid Drugs, Study Finds," *New York Times* (January 8, 2008).

127. M. L. Martin, "Ethnicity and Analgesic Practice: An Editorial," *Annals of Emergency Medicine* 35 (January 2000): 77.

128. R. Sean Morrison et al., "'We Don't Carry That'—Failure of Pharmacies in Predominantly Nonwhite Neighborhoods to Stock Opioid Analgesics," *New England Journal of Medicine* 342 (April 6, 2000): 1,023–1,026.

129. Dr. Gary Dennis of Howard University Hospital, quoted in Nikitta A. Foston, "How to Deal with Chronic Pain," *Ebony* (July 2003): 55.

130. See, for example, Pilar Ossorio and Troy Duster, "Race and Genetics: Controversies in Biomedical, Behavioral, and Forensic Sciences," *American Psychologist* 60 (January 2005): 123.

131. "One Hundred Cases of Heart Disease in the Negro," *JAMA* 65 (December 18, 1915): 2,193.

132. Charles T. Stone and Frances R. Vanzant, "Heart Disease as Seen in a Southern Clinic," *JAMA* 89 (October 29, 1927): 1,474. See also, Edward H. Schwab and Victor E. Schulze, "Heart Disease in the American Negro of the South," *American Heart Journal* 7 (1932): 715.

133. Hal M. Davidson and J. C. Thoroughman, "A Study of Heart Disease in the Negro Race," *Southern Medical Journal* 21 (1928): 467.

134. Eric D. Peterson et al., "Racial Variation in Cardiac Procedure Use and Survival Following Acute Myocardial Infarction in the Department of Veterans Affairs," *JAMA* 271 (April 20, 1994): 1,179.

135. Wallace M. Yater et al., "Coronary Artery Disease in Men Eighteen to Thirty-Nine Years of Age," *American Heart Journal* 36 (1948): 716, 518.

136. Wallace M. Yater et al., "Coronary Artery Disease in Men Eighteen to Thirty-Nine Years of Age," *American Heart Journal* 36 (1948): 517.

137. Richard Allen Williams, "Cardiology," in *Textbook of Black-Related Diseases*, Richard Allen Williams, ed. (New York: McGraw-Hill Book Company, 1975): 332.

138. Richard F. Gillum, "Coronary Heart Disease in Black Populations. I. Mortality and Morbidity," *American Heart Journal* (October 1982): 849.

139. G. Carlson et al., "Summary of Workshop II: Working Group on Risk Factors," *American Heart Journal* 108 (September 1984): 705.

140. "The risk of cardiovascular disease among African Americans is not widely appreciated by many physicians, despite the clearly higher prevalence of essential hypertension," in William W. Dressler, "Health in the African American Community: Accounting for Health Inequalities," *Medical Anthropology Quarterly* 7 (1993): 340.

141. "It is not clear why Negroes, with a higher incidence of hypertension, do not have a correspondingly higher incidence of coronary atherosclerosis, but in fact resist such changes according to the work of Blache and Handler," in John P. Mihaly and Neville C. Whiteman, "Myocardial Infarction in the Negro: Historical Survey as It Relates to Negroes," *American Journal of Cardiology* 2 (October 1958): 468.

142. "The Negro and Heart Disease," *Ebony* 18 (December 1962): 129.
143. Richard F. Gillum, "Coronary heart disease in black populations. I. Mortality and morbidity," *American Heart Journal* (October 1982): 849.
144. Richard F. Gillum and C.T. Grant, "Coronary Heart Disease in Black Populations. II. Risk Factors," *American Heart Journal* 104 (October 1982): 860.
145. Stanislav V. Kasl, "Social and psychologic factors in the etiology of coronary heart disease in black populations: An exploration of research needs," *American Heart Journal* 108 (1984): 661.
146. Charles J. Glueck et al., "High-density lipoprotein cholesterol in blacks and whites: Potential ramifications for coronary heart disease," *American Heart Journal* 108 (1984): 825.
147. See, for example, "Good Cholesterol (HDLs) Provides Human Immunity to Certain Parasites," *Medical News Today* (October 30, 2005) www.medicalnewstoday.com/medicalnews.php?newsid=32807.
148. Personal communication (August 30, 2006).
149. Richard H. Wasserburger, "Observations on the 'Juvenile Pattern' of Adult Negro Males," *American Journal of Medicine* 18 (March 1955): 428.
150. Meyer Friedman and Ray H. Rosenman, "Overt Behavior Pattern in Coronary Disease," *JAMA* 173 (July 23, 1960): 1,320.
151. Robert J. Terry, "The American Negro," *Science* 69 (March 29, 1929): 339.
152. C. Jeff Miller, "A Comparative Study of Certain Gynecologic and Obstetric Conditions as Exhibited in the Colored and White Races," *Transactions of the American Gynecological Society* 53 (1929): 92.
153. Joseph Luder, "Some Pædiatric Problems of Uganda," *British Medical Journal* (November 16, 1957): 1,144.
154. LeRoi Jones, *Blues People* [1968] (New York: Perennial, 2002): 213.
155. James H. Carter, "Frequent Mistakes Made with Black Patients in Psychotherapy," *Journal of the National Medical Association* 71 (1979): 1,008.
156. Stanley Crouch, *The All-American Skin Game, or, The Decoy of Race* [1995] (New York: Vintage Books, 1997): 28.
157. Sherman A. James, "Socioeconomic Influences on Coronary Heart Disease in Black Populations," *American Heart Journal* 108 (1984): 670.
158. Sherman A. James, "Coronary Heart Disease in Black Americans: Suggestions for Research on Psychosocial Factors," *American Heart Journal* 108 (1984): 835.
159. Sherman A. James, "Coronary Heart Disease in Black Americans: Suggestions for Research on Psychosocial Factors," *American Heart Journal* 108 (1984): 836.
160. Sherman A. James, "Socioeconomic Influences on Coronary Heart Disease in Black Populations," *American Heart Journal* 108 (1984): 670–671.
161. "'John Henryism' Key to Understanding Coping, Health Outcomes in African Americans," Duke University Medical Center (March 10, 2006). www.eurekaalert.org/pub_releases/2006-03/dumc-hk031006.php, (accessed September 5, 2006).
162. E.C. Ellett, "Diseases of the Ear, Nose and Throat in the Negro," *JAMA* (December 2, 1899): 1,419–1,420.
163. "Are There Any Blind Babies?" *The Survey* (April 15, 1924): 93.
164. C. Rutherford Morison, "Some Observations on Gynæcology and Obstetrics in Nigeria," *Journal of the Royal Army Medical Corps* 83 (1944): 65.
165. H. Phillip Venable, "Glaucoma in the Negro," *Journal of the National Medical Association* 44 (January 1952): 7, 10–12.
166. "Glaucoma in the Negro," *Journal of the National Medical Association* 44 (May 1952): 196–204.

167. Cited in Charles W. Kollock, "Some Interesting Conditions Seen in the Eye of a Negro," *Southern Medical Journal* 10 (1917): 346.

168. Charles W. Kollock, "Some Interesting Conditions Seen in the Eye of a Negro," *Southern Medical Journal* 10 (1917): 346.

169. Charles W. Kollock, "Some Interesting Conditions Seen in the Eye of a Negro," *Southern Medical Journal* 10 (1917): 347. These two quotations come from two doctors whose statements date from the 1890s and 1917, respectively.

170. Charles W. Kollock, "Some Interesting Conditions Seen in the Eye of a Negro," *Southern Medical Journal* 10 (1917): 346.

171. See M. Roy Wilson, "Glaucoma in Blacks: Where Do We Go From Here?" *JAMA* 261 (January 13, 1989): 281–282; "Blacks, Whites Benefit from Different Surgical Glaucoma Treatments" [NIH News Release] (July 6, 1998); Uday Devgan et al., "Surgical Undertreatment of Glaucoma in Black Beneficiaries of Medicare," *Archives of Ophthalmology* 118 (2000): 253–256.

172. George M. Niles, "A Therapeutic Comparison, Medicinal and Otherwise, as between the Caucasian and Afro-American," *Southern Medical Journal* (February 1, 1913): 128.

173. A. G. Love and C. B. Davenport, "A Comparison of White and Colored Troops in Respect to Incidence of Disease," *Proceedings of the National Academy of Sciences* 5 (1919): 59.

174. Frank R. Freeman, "The Health of the American Slave Examined by Means of Union Army Medical Statistics," *Journal of the National Medical Association* (1985): 50.

175. Thomas B. Hall, "Vegetative Dermatoses in the Negro," *Southern Medical Journal* (1939): 381.

176. "Sweat and Body Odor," *JAMA* (June 1, 1940).

177. Alexander Butchart, *The Anatomy of Power: European Constructions of the African Body* (London and New York: Zed Books, 1998): 56.

178. A. G. Love and C. B. Davenport, "A Comparison of White and Colored Troops in Respect to Incidence of Disease," *Proceedings of the National Academy of Sciences* 5 (1919): 59.

179. C. Leon Wilson, "The Incidence of Syphilis among Pregnant Negro Women," *American Journal of Obstetrics and Gynecology* 18 (1929): 216.

180. J. W. Thompson, "The Clinical Status of a Group of Negro Sharecroppers," *JAMA* 117 (July 5, 1941): 6–8.

181. Frank K. Boland, "Morsus Humanus: Sixty Cases of Human Bites in Negroes," *JAMA* 116 (January 11, 1941): 129.

182. Robert C. Moehlig, "The Mesoderm of the Negro," *American Journal of Physical Anthropology* 22 (1937): 302–303.

183. "Advanced permanent dental eruption in Africans is mainly gene determined . . ." in D. F. Roberts, "Race, Genetics and Growth, "in *Biosocial Aspects of Race* (Oxford and Edinburgh: Blackwell Scientific Publications, 1969) [Journal of Biosocial Science, Supplement No. 1]: 60; "White standards for skeletal maturation and dental development are certainly not appropriate for blacks," in Stanley M. Garn and Diane C. Clark, "Problems in the Nutritional Assessment of Black Individuals," *American Journal of Public Health* 66 (1976): 264.

184. Frantz Fanon, *Black Skin, White Masks* (New York: Grove Press, 1967): 49ftn.

185. Kenneth B. Clark, *Dark Ghetto: Dilemmas of Social Power* (New York: Harper & Row, 1965): 6.

186. Felice Swados, "Negro Health on the Ante Bellum Plantations," *Bulletin of the History of Medicine* 10 (1941): 470.

187. Booker T. Washington, *Up From Slavery* (New York: Penguin Books, 1986): 174–175.

188. M.O. Bousfield, "Reaching the Negro Community," *American Journal of Public Health* 24 (1934): 213.
189. Alice Walker, *The Color Purple* [1982] (New York: Pocket Books, 1985): 155. See also 90, 163.
190. W. Michael Byrd and Linda A. Clayton, *An American Health Dilemma, vol. II. Race, Medicine, and Health Care in the United States 1900–2000* (New York and London: Routledge, 2002): 387.
191. Harrison F. Flippin and O. Norris Smith, "Addison's Disease in the Negro," *American Journal of the Medical Sciences* 192 (1936): 756–757.
192. Charles W. Kollock, "Some Interesting Conditions Seen in the Eye of a Negro," *Southern Medical Journal* 10 (1917): 347.
193. Dr. [Samuel] Cartwright, "The Diseases of Negroes—Pulmonary Congestions, Pneumonia, etc." *De Bow's Review* 11 (1851): 209–213.
194. George M. Niles, "A Therapeutic Comparison, Medicinal and Otherwise, as between the Caucasian and Afro-American," *Southern Medical Journal* (February 1, 1913): 129.
195. "Peptic Ulcer in Africans," *British Medical Journal* (February 13, 1960): 506.
196. Charles H. Garvin, "Negro Health," *Opportunity* (November 1924): 342.
197. I.I. Lemann, "Diabetes Mellitus in the Negro Race," *Southern Medical Journal* (July 1921): 523.
198. Curtis Rosser, "Rectal Pathology in the Negro," *Journal of the American Medical Association* (January 10, 1925): 94.
199. "Disease, Race, and Civilization," *British Medical Journal* (June 13, 1953): 1,320.
200. Howard J. Osofsky, MD, "The Walls Are Within: An Exploration of Barriers between Middle-Class Physicians and Poor Patients," in *Among the People: Encounters with the Poor*, Irwin Deutscher and Elizabeth J. Thompson, eds. (New York: Basic Books, 1968): 239.
201. Stewart R. Roberts, "Nervous and Mental Influences in Angina Pectoris," *American Heart Journal* 7 (1931–32): 34.
202. Laura Briggs, "The Race of Hysteria: 'Overcivilization' and the 'Savage' Woman in Late Nineteenth-Century Obstetrics and Gynecology," *American Quarterly* 52 (June 2000): 260, 258.
203. C. Jeff Miller, "A Comparative Study of Certain Gynecologic and Obstetric Conditions as Exhibited in the Colored and White Races," *Transactions of the American Gynecological Society* 53 (1929): 94.
204. Judith B. Kaplan and Trude Bennett, "Use of Race and Ethnicity in Biomedical Publication," *JAMA* 289 (May 28, 2003): 2,712.
205. William F. Mengert, "Racial Contrasts in Obstetrics and Gynecology," *Journal of the National Medical Association* 58 (November 1966): 414.
206. Crystal Hlaing, "Race and Obstetrics and Gynecology" (University of Texas, 2005).
207. Lyle J. Breitkopf, MD, and Marion Gordon Bakoulis, *Coping with Endometriosis* (New York: Prentice Hall Press, 1988): xxiv.
208. E. Ann Kaplan, "Resisting Pathologies of Age and Race: Menopause and Cosmetic Surgery in Films by Rainer and Tom," in Paul Komesaroff, Philipa Rothfield, and Jeanne Daly, eds., *Reinterpreting Menopause: Cultural and Philosophical Issues* (New York & London: Routledge, 1997): 116–117.
209. Tracee Cornforth, "Menopause Worse for African American Women," About .com-Women's Health (accessed August 3, 2008). This report refers to a study published in the January/February 2001 issue of *Menopause, the Journal of the North American Menopause Society;* "Menopause and Midlife: Health Risks: Black Women's Views," Yale University School of Nursing (2004), accessed August 3, 2008.

210. Hilde Bruch, "Anorexia Nervosa and its Differential Diagnosis," *The Journal of Nervous and Mental Disease* 141 (1966): 556, 563.
211. Tomas J. Silber, "Anorexia in Black Adolescents," *Journal of the National Medical Association* 76 (1984): 29.
212. Denise Brodey, "Blacks Join the Eating-Disorder Mainstream," *New York Times* (September 20, 2005).
213. "Lyrica Lightens Up, DTCwise," Pharma Marketing Blog (July 24, 2008), accessed on August 6, 2008, at http://pharmamkting.blogspot.com/2008/07/lyrica-lightens-up-dtcwise.html.
214. "Fibromyalgia/Lyrica Commercial #3," Bee's Eclectic Life (July 21, 2008), accessed on August 6, 2008, at http://eclecticwoman.wordpress.com/2008/07/21/fibromyalgialyrica-commercial-3/.
215. Raymond Prince, "The 'Brain Fag' Syndrome in Nigerian Students," *The Journal of Mental Science (The British Journal of Psychiatry)* 106 (January 1960): 566.
216. See http://www.thefreedictionary.com/yuppie+flu. See also David Tuller, "Chronic Fatigue No Longer Seen as 'Yuppie Flu'," *New York Times* (July 17, 2007).
217. Tracy Hampton, "Researchers Find Genetic Clues to Chronic Fatigue Syndrome," *Journal of the American Medical Association* 295 (June 7, 2006): 2,467.
218. Jerome Groopman, "Hurting All Over," *The New Yorker* (November 13, 2000).
219. "No More 'Yuppie Flu'," ImmuneSupport.com. Accessed on August 8, 2008 at http://www.immunesupport.com/library/showarticle.cfm/ID/1205/t/CFIDS_FM.
220. Leonard A. Jason et al., "A Community-Based Study of Chronic Fatigue Syndrome," *Annals of Internal Medicine* 159 (October 11, 1999): 2,136.
221. "Chronic Fatigue Syndrome," Intelihealth.com. Accessed on August 8, 2008 at http://www.intelihealth.com/IH/ihtIH/WSIHW000/9339/9715.html.
222. Dag Album and Steinar Westin, "Do Diseases Have a Prestige Hierarchy? A Survey among Physicians and Medical Students," *Social Science & Medicine* 66 (January 2008).
223. Lee Rainwater, "The Lower Class: Health, Illness, and Medical Institutions," in *Among the People: Encounters with the Poor*, Irwin Deutscher and Elizabeth J. Thompson, eds. (New York: Basic Books, 1968): 263, 270.
224. Lee Rainwater, "The Lower Class: Health, Illness, and Medical Institutions," in *Among the People: Encounters with the Poor*, Irwin Deutscher and Elizabeth J. Thompson, eds. (New York: Basic Books, 1968): 261, 262, 265, 270.
225. A.G. Love and C.B. Davenport, "A Comparison of White and Colored Troops in Respect to Incidence of Disease," *Proceedings of the National Academy of Sciences* 5 (1919): 60.
226. S.W. Douglas, "Difficulties and Superstitions Encountered in Practice among the Negroes," *Southern Medical Journal* (1926): 737.
227. S.J. Holmes, "The Resistant Ectoderm of the Negro," *American Journal of Physical Anthropology* (1928): 150.
228. C. Jeff Miller, "A Comparative Study of Certain Gynecologic and Obstetric Conditions as Exhibited in the Colored and White Races," *Transactions of the American Gynecological Society* 53 (1929): 102.
229. S.W. Douglas, "Difficulties and Superstitions Encountered in Practice among the Negroes," *Southern Medical Journal* (1926): 736.
230. W. Winwood Reade, *Savage Africa* (London: Smith, Elder, and Co., 1864): 528; "The Nutrition of the African Native," *The Lancet* (July 25, 1936) 235.
231. Frederick L. Hoffman, *Race Traits and Tendencies of the American Negro* (New York: American Economic Association, 1896): 164.

232. Charles H. Garvin, "Negro Health," *Opportunity* (November 1924): 341.
233. W. Montague Cobb, "An Anatomist's View of Human Relations," *Journal of the National Medical Association* (May 1975): 192.
234. "Slavery Was 'Great Biological Experiment' Negro MD Claims," *Journal of the American Medical Association* (September 1, 1962): 58, 59.
235. Chester M. Pierce, MD, "Is Bigotry the Basis of the Medical Problems of the Ghetto?" in John C. Norman, ed., *Medicine in the Ghetto* (New York: Appleton-Century-Crofts, 1969): 301.
236. Mia Bay, *The White Image in the Black Mind: African-American Ideas about White People, 1830–1925* (New York and Oxford: Oxford University Press, 2000): 60.
237. George S. Schuyler, "Our White Folks," in *Black on White: Black Writers on What It Means to Be White*, ed. David R. Roediger, (New York: Schocken Books, 1998): 78, 83.
238. John Langston Gwaltney, *Drylongso: A Self-Portrait of Black America* [1980] (New York: Vintage Books, 1981): 241.
239. Hugh Pearson, *The Shadow of the Panther: Huey Newton and the Price of Black Power in America* (New York: Addison-Wesley Publishing Company, 1994): 285.
240. Louis I. Dublin, "The Problem of Negro Health as Revealed by Vital Statistics," *Journal of Negro Education* 6 (1937): 275.
241. Linda Villarosa, "THE RACIAL DIVIDE; As Black Men Move Into Middle Age, Dangers Rise," *New York Times* (September 23, 2002).
242. Floyd P. Allen, "Physical Impairment among One Thousand Negro Workers," *American Journal of Public Health* 22 (June 1932): 586.
243. Alyce C. Gullattee, "The Negro Psyche: Fact, Fiction and Fantasy," *Journal of the National Medical Association* 61 (1969): 124.
244. Carl C. Bell and Harshad Mehta, "The Misdiagnosis of Black Patients with Manic Depressive Illness," *Journal of the National Medical Association* 72 (1980): 145.
245. James H. Carter, "Recognizing Psychiatric Symptoms in Black Americans," *Geriatrics* (November 1974): 96.
246. Jacobo E. Mintzer and Carol A. Macera, "Prevalence of Depressive Symptoms among White and African-American Caregivers of Demented Patients," *American Journal of Psychiatry* 149 (April 1992): 576.
247. Terry L. Mills and Carla D.A. Edwards, "A Critical Review of Research on the Mental Health Status of Older African-Americans," *Aging & Society* 22 (2002): 291.
248. See, for example, Trudier Harris, "This Disease Called Strength: Some Observations on the Compensating Construction of Black Female Character," *Literature and Medicine* (Spring 1995): 109–126.
249. K. Danielle Edwards, "Polarized: Bi-Polar Disorder and the Ghosts That Haunt." The Black Commentator, accessed at http://www.blackcommentator.com/221/221_polarized_edwards_guest.html on August 17, 2008.
250. Arthur J. Prange, Jr. and M.M. Vitols, "Cultural Aspects of the Relatively Low Incidence of Depression in Southern Negroes," *International Journal of Social Psychiatry* 8 (Spring 1962): 108.
251. Carl C. Bell and Harshad Mehta, "The Misdiagnosis of Black Patients with Manic Depressive Illness," *Journal of the National Medical Association* 72 (1980): 141.
252. Arthur J. Prange, Jr. and M.M. Vitols, "Cultural Aspects of the Relatively Low Incidence of Depression in Southern Negroes," *International Journal of Social Psychiatry* 8 (Spring 1962): 108. This article can be read as a systematic presentation of the sources of emotional hardiness in the southern black person.

253. See, for example, Douglas Staley and R. Roxburgh Wand, "Obsessive-Compulsive Disorder: A Review of the Cross-Cultural Epidemiological Literature," *Transcultural Psychiatry* 32 (1995): 103–136; Marjorie L. Hatch et al., "Behavioral Treatment of Obsessive-Compulsive Disorder in African Americans," *Cognitive and Behavioral Practice* 3 (Winter 1996): 303–315.

254. Raymond Prince, "The 'Brain Fag' Syndrome in Nigerian Students," *The Journal of Mental Science* (*The British Journal of Psychiatry*) 106 (January 1960): 568.

255. "Black Hang-Ups," *Time* 95 (April 6, 1970): 64.

256. Meyer Friedman and Ray H. Rosenman, "Overt Behavior Pattern in Coronary Disease," *JAMA* 173 (July 23, 1960): 1,320.

257. Sherman A. James, "Socioeconomic Influences on Coronary Heart Disease in Black Populations," *American Heart Journal* 108 (1984): 670.

258. Louis A. Lurie, "The Endocrine Factor in Homosexuality: Report of Treatment of 4 Cases with Androgen Hormone," *American Journal of Medical Sciences* (1944): 176.

259. A.T. Childers, "Some Notes on Sex Mores among Negro Children," *The American Journal of Orthopsychiatry* 6 (1936): 444–445.

260. Lauretta Bender, "Behavior Problems in Negro Children," *Psychiatry* 2 (1939): 224.

261. Chandak Sengoopta, *The Most Secret Quintessence of Life: Sex, Glands, and Hormones, 1850–1950* (Chicago and London: The University of Chicago Press, 2006): 318.

262. Cathy J. Cohen, *The Boundaries of Blackness: AIDS and the Breakdown of Black Politics* (Chicago and London: The University of Chicago Press, 1999): 328.

263. "Sex Experts and Medical Scientists Join Forces against a Common Foe: AIDS," *JAMA* 259 (February 5, 1988): 641–642.

264. Benoit Denizet-Lewis, "Double Lives on the Down Low," *The New York Times Magazine* (August 3, 2003): 30.

265. L.M. Lothstein and Howard Roback, "Black Female Transsexuals and Schizophrenia: A Serendipitous Finding," *Archives of Sexual Behavior* 13 (1984): 383–384.

266. Robert E. House, "The Use of Scopolamine in Criminology," *The American Journal of Police Science* (1931): 329, 332.

267. See M.M. Vitols, H.G. Waters, and M.H. Keeler, "Hallucinations and Delusions in White and Negro Schizophrenics," *American Journal of Psychiatry* 120 (1963): 472–476; "Negro Schizophrenics Hallucinate More Than White Patients," *JAMA* 184 (June 1, 1963): 27; Victor R. Adebimpe et al., "Hallucinations and Delusions in Black Psychiatric Patients," *Journal of the National Medical Association* 73 (1981): 517–520; Carl C. Bell et al., "Prevalence of Isolated Sleep Paralysis in Black Subjects," *Journal of the National Medical Association* 76 (1984): 507.

268. William B. Lawson, "The Art and Science of the Psychopharmacology of African Americans," *The Mount Sinai Journal of Medicine* 63 (October/November 1996): 302.

269. Judy C. Davison, "Perceptions of Attention Deficit Hyperactivity Disorder in One African American Community," *Journal of Negro Education* (Fall 2001): 264–274.

270. Julie B. Mallinger, "Racial Disparities in the Use of Second-Generation Antipsychotics for the Treatment of Schizophrenia," *Psychiatric Services* 57 (January 2006): 133–136.

271. Julie Magno Zito et al., "Racial Disparity in Psychotropic Medications Prescribed for Youth with Medicaid Insurance in Maryland," *Journal of the American Academy of Child and Adolescent Psychiatry* 37 (1998): 180.

272. See *Unequal Treatment: Confronting Racial and Ethnic Disparities in Health Care*, Brian D. Smedley, Adrienne Y. Stith, and Alan R. Nelson, eds. (Washington, DC: The National Academies Press, 2003).

273. Julie Magno Zito et al., "Racial Disparity in Psychotropic Medications Prescribed for Youth with Medicaid Insurance in Maryland," *Journal of the American Academy of Child and Adolescent Psychiatry* 37 (1998): 180, 181.

274. Amy M. Kilbourne and Harold Alan Pincus, "Patterns of Psychotropic Medication Use by Race among Veterans with Bipolar Disorder," *Psychiatric Services* 57 (January 2006): 123–126.

275. See, for example, Knox H. Todd, "Ethnicity as a Risk Factor for Inadequate Emergency Department Analgesia," *JAMA* 269 (March 24/31, 1993): 1,537–1,539; B. Ng et al., "Ethnic Differences in Analgesic Consumption for Postoperative Pain," *Psychosomatic Medicine* 58 (1996): 125–129.

276. David A. Sclar et al., "Antidepressant Prescribing Patterns: A Comparison of Blacks and Whites in a Medicaid Population," *Clinical Drug Investigation* 16 (1998): 135–140.

277. Julie Magno Zito et al., "Racial Disparity in Psychotropic Medications Prescribed for Youth with Medicaid Insurance in Maryland," *Journal of the American Academy of Child and Adolescent Psychiatry* 37 (1998): 183.

278. David A. Sclar et al., "Antidepressant Prescribing Patterns: A Comparison of Blacks and Whites in a Medicaid Population," *Clinical Drug Investigation* 16 (1998): 135–140.

279. "ACE Inhibitors Prevent Diabetes in African Americans with Hypertensive Kidney Disease," *Heartwire* (April 13, 2006). *Archives of Internal Medicine* (April 10, 2006).

280. See, for example, Derek V. Exner et al., "Lesser Response to Angiotensin-Converting-Enzyme Inhibitor Therapy in Black as Compared with White Patients with Left Ventricular Dysfunction," *New England Journal of Medicine* 344 (May 3, 2001): 1,351–1,357.

281. See, for example, Clyde W. Yancy et al., "Race and the Response to Adrenergic Blockade with Carvedilol in Patients with Chronic Heart Failure," *New England Journal of Medicine* 344 (May 3, 2001): 1,358.

282. James S. Kalus and Jean M. Nappi, "Role of Race in the Pharmacotherapy of Heart Failure," *The Annals of Pharmacotherapy* 36 (March 2002): 474, 475.

283. Stephen B. Liggett et al., "A GRK5 Polymorphism that Inhibits B-Adrenergic Receptor Signaling Is Protective in Heart Failure," *Nature Medicine* (April 20, 2008): 1–8.

284. Pascal Bovet and Fred Paccaud, "Race and Responsiveness to Drugs for Heart Failure" [Letter], *New England Journal of Medicine* 345 (September 6, 2001): 766.

285. "Black Patients Not Uniquely Unresponsive to ACE Inhibitor Monotherapy," *Medscape Cardiology* 8 (2004).

286. "Beta-Blocker Shown to Be Ineffective in Patients with Advanced Heart Failure," *Science Blog* (University of Texas Southwestern Medical Center, May 2001).

287. "Beta Blocker Controls High Blood Pressure in Blacks," healthSCOUT.com (July 16, 2005).

288. Alastair J.J. Wood, "Racial Difference in the Response to Drugs—Pointers to Genetic Differences," *New England Journal of Medicine* 344 (May 3, 2001): 1,394.

289. Frederick A. Masoudi and Edward P. Havranek, "Race and Responsiveness to Drugs for Heart Failure" [Letter], *New England Journal of Medicine* 345 (September 6, 2001): 766.

290. Marion M. Torchia, "Tuberculosis among American Negroes: Medical Research on a Racial Disease, 1830–1950," *Journal of the History of Medicine and Allied Sciences* 32 (July 1977): 269.

291. "Use of Antibiotics in Different Races," *JAMA* (January 29, 1955): 486.

292. Robert C. Moehlig, "The Mesoderm of the Negro," *American Journal of Physical Anthropology* 22 (1937): 309.

293. A.Q. Adigun et al., "Chronotropic Dose Response of Atropine in Nigerians with Congestive Heart Failure: Assessment of Ethnic Variation and Reversibility of Parasympathetic Dysfunction," *Ethnicity & Disease* 10 (June 2000): 203–207.

294. Louis Lasagna et al., "Drug-Induced Changes in Man. 1. Observations on Healthy Subjects, Chronically Ill Patients, and 'Postaddicts,'" *Journal of the American Medical Association* 157 (March 19, 1955): 1,019.

295. Allen Raskin and Thomas H. Crook, "Antidepressants in Black and White Inpatients," *Archives of General Psychiatry* 32 (May 1975): 643.

296. "There is no ready explanation for the poor response to chlorpromazine in the black men. However, a lead that might be pursued stems from a report by DiMascio that individuals whose personalities were organized about the use of physical activity and self-assertiveness experienced the drug-induced sedation and psychomotor retarding properties of chlorpromazine as more disruptive and uncomfortable than individuals whose personality structures were organized around intellectual activities and introspective concerns. Most of the black men in the study were in their 20s and 30s when interest in physical activities is still strong and they were drawn primarily from the lower social class where there is presumably a low level of interest in intellectual pursuits; and they also rated themselves higher than either the black women or the white men and women on the outspokenness . . . and assault . . . factors of the Hostility-Guilt Inventory." See Allen Raskin and Thomas H. Crook, "Antidepressants in Black and White Inpatients," *Archives of General Psychiatry* 32 (May 1975): 647–648.

297. Laurence O. Watkins, "Epidemiology of coronary heart disease in black populations: Methodologic proposals," *American Heart Journal* 108 (September 1984): 638.

298. David Satcher, "Does Race Interfere with the Doctor-Patient Relationship?" *Journal of the American Medical Association* [henceforth *JAMA*] 223 (March 26, 1973): 1,499.

299. "Rarity of Pelvic Endometriosis in Negro Women," *JAMA* 147 (September 22, 1951): 343.

300. C. Jeff Miller, "A Comparative Study of Certain Gynecologic and Obstetric Conditions as Exhibited in the Colored and White Races," *Transactions of the American Gynecological Society* 53 (1929): 91–106.

301. Carl Henry Davis, "Obstetrics and Gynecology in General Practice," *JAMA* 93 (September 28, 1929): 961–963.

302. "Relief of Pain in Midwifery," *British Medical Journal* (February 14, 1948): 318.

303. "U.S. Senate Committee on Education and Labor," *JAMA* 120 (November 21, 1942): 944.

304. C. Jeff Miller, "Special Medical Problems of the Colored Woman," *Southern Medical Journal* 25 (1931): 738, 739.

305. "South African Negro or Bantu as a Parturient," *JAMA* 133 (April 5, 1947): 1,037.

306. C. Rutherford Morison, "Some Observations on Gynæcology and Obstetrics in Nigeria," *Journal of the Royal Army Medical Corps* 83 (1944): 60–65.

307. "Rectal Pathology in the Negro," *JAMA* 84 (January 10, 1925): 94.
308. Harry Bakwin, "The Negro Infant," *Human Biology* (1932): 26.
309. "Pelvic Measurements of Western Women," *British Medical Journal* (April 13, 1946): 595.
310. William F. Mengert, "Racial Contrasts in Obstetrics and Gynecology," *Journal of the National Medical Association* 58 (November 1966): 413.
311. W.Z. Bradford and Wallace B. Bradford, "A Comparative Study of Pregnancy in the White and Colored Races," *American Journal of Obstetrics and Gynecology* 42 (1941): 886.
312. J.R. McCord, "The Results Obtained in a Conservative Teaching Clinic among 2500 Negro Patients," *American Journal of Obstetrics and Gynecology* 8 (1924): 726.
313. C.H. Peckham, "The Influence of Age and Race on the Duration of Labor," *American Journal of Obstetrics and Gynecology* 24 (1932): 745–746, 750.
314. C. Rutherford Morison, "Some Observations on Gynæcology and Obstetrics in Nigeria," *Journal of the Royal Army Medical Corps* 83 (1944): 64.
315. Duncan E. Reid and Mandel E. Cohen, "Evaluation of Present Day Trends in Obstetrics," *JAMA* 142 (March 4, 1950): 622.
316. See Dorothy Roberts, *Killing the Black Body: Race, Reproduction, and the Meaning of Liberty* (New York: Vintage Books, 1999).
317. George A. Williams, "Elliott Therapy of Pelvic Inflammations in the Negress," *Southern Medical Journal* 31 (1938): 1,171. "Pelvic inflammatory disease is rampant in the colored and is much more frequent and severe than in the white," in "A Comparative Obstetrical and Gynecological Study of the White and Colored Races," 419.
318. Thomas H. Green, Jr., "Symposium on Endometriosis," *Clinical Obstetrics and Gynecology* 9 (1966): 269; quoted in Richard Allen Williams, ed., *Textbook of Black-Related Diseases* (New York: McGraw-Hill Book Company, 1975): 120.
319. Richard Allen Williams, ed. *Textbook of Black-Related Diseases* (New York: McGraw-Hill Book Company, 1975): 120–121.
320. William F. Mengert, "Racial Contrasts in Obstetrics and Gynecology," *Journal of the National Medical Association* 58 (November 1966): 414.
321. Lyle J. Breitkopf, MD, and Marion Gordon Bakoulis, *Coping with Endometriosis* (New York: Prentice Hall Press, 1988): xxiv.
322. Dorothy Roberts, *Killing the Black Body: Race, Reproduction, and the Meaning of Liberty* (New York: Vintage Books, 1997): 255.
323. See Dorothy Roberts, Killing the Black Body: Race, Reproduction, and the Meaning of Liberty (New York: Vintage Books, 1999).
324. See, for example, Knox H. Todd et al., "Ethnicity and Analgesic Practice," *Annals of Emergency Medicine* 35 (January 2000): 11–16; M.L. Martin, "Ethnicity and Analgesic Practice: An Editorial," *Annals of Emergency Medicine* 35 (January 2000): 77–79; L.R. Goldfrank and R.K. Knopp, "Racially and Ethnically Selective Oligoanesthesia: Is This Racism?" *Annals of Emergency Medicine* 35 (January 2000): 79–82.
325. Deborah A. Frank et al., "Growth, Development, and Behavior in Early Childhood Following Prenatal Cocaine Exposure," *JAMA* 285 (March 28, 2001): 1,613–1,614.
326. "Anesthesia Measure Passes," *New York Times* (September 21, 1998).
327. Kimberly D. Gregory et al., "Variation in Vaginal Breech Delivery Rates by Hospital Type," *Obstetrics and Gynecology* 97 (March 2001): 385–390.
328. "Age of Loss of Potency—Menopause," *JAMA* 107 (December 26, 1936): 2,153.

CHAPTER 4

1. Andrew Hacker, *Two Nations: Black and White, Separate, Hostile, Unequal* (New York: Ballantine Books, 1992): 3, 4.
2. Dorothy E. Roberts, "The Social and Moral Coast of Mass Incarceration in African American Communities," *Stanford Law Review* 56 (2003–2004): 1273, 1279, 1287.
3. Orlando Patterson, "A Job Too Big for One Man," *New York Times* (November 4, 2009).
4. "The Pediatrician and the Public," *Pediatrics* 3 (June 1949): 857.
5. Durado D. Brooks et al., "Medical Apartheid: An American Perspective," *JAMA* 266 (November 20, 1991): 2,747.
6. W. Michael Byrd and Linda A. Clayton, *An American Health Dilemma*, vol. II. *Race, Medicine, and Health Care in the United States 1900–2000* (New York and London: Routledge, 2002): 409.
7. Franz Fanon, "Medicine and Colonialism," in *A Dying Colonialism* (New York: Grove Press, 1959): 130.
8. Carter G. Woodson, *The Mis-Education of the Negro* [1933] (Trenton, NJ: Africa World Press, Inc., 1990): 193.
9. E. Franklin Frazier, *Black Bourgeoisie: The Rise of a New Middle Class in the United States* [1957] (New York: Collier Books, 1962): 86.
10. Alex Hrdlicka, "The Full-Blood American Negro," *American Journal of Physical Anthropology* 12 (1928): 15.
11. P.W. Laidler, "The Relationship of the Native to South Africa's Health," *South African Medical Journal* 6 (1932): 617.
12. Thomas F. Pettigrew, *A Profile of the Negro American* (Princeton: D. van Nostrand Company, Inc., 1964): 10.
13. Franz Fanon, "Medicine and Colonialism," in *A Dying Colonialism* [1959] (New York: Grove Press, 1967): 121–145.
14. Charles E. Silberman, *Crisis in Black and White* (New York: Random House, 1964): 314.
15. Charles E. Silberman, *Crisis in Black and White* (New York: Random House, 1964): 317.
16. Harlan L. Dalton, "AIDS in Blackface," *Daedalus* 118 (Summer 1989): 209–210.
17. *The Negro Family: A Case for National Action* (Washington, DC: Office of Policy Planning and Research, United States Department of Labor, 1965).
18. Ralph Ellison, "Introduction," *Shadow and Act* (New York: Vintage Books, 1972): xvii, xx.
19. Albert Murray, *The Omni-Americans: Black Experience & American Culture* (New York: Da Capo Press, 1970): 37, 69, 82.
20. Kenneth B. Clark, *Dark Ghetto: Dilemmas of Social Power* [1965] (New York and Evanston: Harper Torchbooks, 1967): 11.
21. Harold Cruse, *The Crisis of the Negro Intellectual* [1967] (New York: Quill, 1984): 334, 433.
22. Stokely Carmichael and Charles V. Hamilton, *Black Power: The Politics of Liberation in America* (New York: Random House, 1967): 31.
23. Quoted in Stokely Carmichael and Charles V. Hamilton, *Black Power: The Politics of Liberation in America* (New York: Random House, 1967): 2–3.
24. William Ryan, "Savage Discovery: The Moynihan Report" [*The Nation*, November 22, 1965], in Lee Rainwater and William L. Yancey, *The Moynihan Report and the Politics of Controversy* (Cambridge, MA and London: The MIT Press, 1967): 225.

25. Robin D.G. Kelley, *Yo Mama's Dysfunktional: Fighting the Culture Wars in Urban America* (Boston: Beacon Press, 1997): 19–20.

26. Quoted in Lee Rainwater and William L. Yancey, *The Moynihan Report and the Politics of Controversy* (Cambridge, MA and London: The MIT Press, 1967): 409, 418.

27. C. Eric Lincoln, "Mood Ebony: The Acceptance of Being Black," in *Children and Poverty: Some Sociological and Psychological Perspectives*, ed. Nona Y. Glazer and Carol F. Creedon (Chicago: Rand McNally & Company, 1968): 51.

28. Richard Majors and Janet Mancini Billson, *Cool Pose: The Dilemmas of Black Manhood in America* (New York: Touchstone Books, 1993): 3.

29. Quoted in Charles E. Silberman, *Crisis in Black and White* (New York: Random House, 1964): 321.

30. Theodore H. White, *The Making of the President, 1960* (New York: Atheneum Publishers, 1965): 225, 227, 229, 230.

31. Charles F. Whitten, "Sickle-Cell Programming—an Imperiled Promise," *New England Journal of Medicine* 288 (February 8, 1973): 318–319.

32. M. Tapper, "Sickling and the Paradoxes of African American Citizenship," in *In the Blood: Sickle Cell Anemia and the Politics of Race* (Philadelphia: University of Pennsylvania Press, 1999): 112.

33. Howard Markel, "Appendix 6. Scientific Advances and Social Risks: Historical Perspectives of Genetic Screening Programs for Sickle Cell Disease, Tay-Sachs Disease, Neural Tube Defects and Down Syndrome, 1970–1977." Accessed June 26, 2007 from LSU Law Center's Medical and Public Health Law Site, http://biotech.law.lsu.edu/research/fed/tfgt/appendix6.htm.

34. M. Tapper, "Sickling and the Paradoxes of African American Citizenship," in *In the Blood: Sickle Cell Anemia and the Politics of Race* (Philadelphia: University of Pennsylvania Press, 1999): 116.

35. R.W. Alles, "A Comparative Study of the Negro and the White Pelvis," *Journal of the Michigan State Medical Society* 24 (1925): 197.

36. Curtice Rosser, "Rectal Pathology in the Negro," *JAMA* 84 (January 10, 1925): 96.

37. S.J. Holmes, "The Resistant Ectoderm of the Negro," *American Journal of Physical Anthropology* (1928): 149; Milo Hellman, "The Fundamental Pattern of the Human Lower Molar Teeth," *Proceedings of the American Philosophical Society* 67 (1928): 158–174.

38. C. Jeff Miller, "A Comparative Study of Certain Gynecologic and Obstetric Conditions as Exhibited in the Colored and White Races," *Transactions of the American Gynecological Society* 53 (1929): 92.

39. See, for example, Knox H. Todd et al., "Ethnicity and Analgesic Practice," *Annals of Emergency Medicine* 35 (January 2000): 11–16; L.R. Goldfrank and R.K. Knopp, "Racially and Ethnically Selective Oligoanesthesia: Is This Racism?" *Annals of Emergency Medicine* 35 (January 2000): 79–82; Nikitta A. Foston, "How to Deal with Chronic Pain," *Ebony* (July 2003): 52–59.

40. Franz Fanon, *Black Skin, White Masks* [1952] (New York: Grove Press, 1967): 165.

41. P.W. Laidler, "The Relationship of the Native to South Africa's Health," *South African Medical Journal* 6 (1932): 618.

42. Paul Gilroy, *There Ain't No Black in the Union Jack* [1987] (Chicago: The University of Chicago Press, 1991): 226.

43. See John Hoberman, *Darwin's Athletes: How Sport Has Damaged Black America and Preserved the Myth of Race* (New York: Houghton Mifflin, 1997).

44. See John Hoberman, "Race and Athletics in the 21st Century," in *Physical Culture, Power, and the Body*, Jennifer Hargreaves and Patricia Vertinsky, eds. (London and New York: Routledge, 2007): 208–231.

45. Jane P. Sheldon, Toby Epstein Jayaratne, and Elizabeth M. Petty, "White Americans' Genetic Explanations for a Perceived Race Difference in Athleticism," *Athletic Insight* (in press).

46. E.M. Green, "Psychoses among Negroes—a Comparative Study," *Journal of Nervous and Mental Disease* 41 (1914): 708.

47. W.G. Smillie and D.L. Augustine, "Vital Capacity of Negro Race," *JAMA* 87 (December 18, 1926): 2,087.

48. C. Jeff Miller, "A Comparative Study of Certain Gynecologic and Obstetric Conditions as Exhibited in the Colored and White Races," *Transactions of the American Gynecological Society* 53 (1929): 103.

49. Laurence O. Watkins, "Epidemiology of Coronary Heart Disease in Black Populations: Methodologic Proposals," *American Heart Journal* 108 (1984): 638.

50. Alfred Maund, "New Day Dawning: The Negro and Medicine," *The Nation* (May 9, 1953): 396.

51. John E. Lind, "The Dream as a Simple Wish-Fulfillment in the Negro," *The Psychoanalytic Review* 1 (1913–14): 295, 300.

52. E.M. Green, "Psychoses among Negroes—a Comparative Study," *Journal of Nervous and Mental Disease* 41 (1914): 703, 706, 708.

53. W.M. Bevis, "Psychological Traits of the Southern Negro With Observations as to Some of His Psychoses," *American Journal of Psychiatry* (1921): 69.

54. W.M. Bevis, "Psychological Traits of the Southern Negro with Observations as to Some of His Psychoses," *American Journal of Psychiatry* (1921): 69, 70, 71, 72.

55. Harvey C. Lehman and Paul A. Witty, "Some Compensatory Mechanisms of the Negro," *Journal of Abnormal and Social Psychology* 23 (1928–29): 29.

56. James A. Brussel, "Father Divine: Holy Precipitator of Psychoses," *American Journal of Psychiatry* (1935): 219.

57. Erwin Wexberg, "The Comparative Racial Incidence (White and Negro) of Neuropsychiatric Conditions in a General Hospital," *Tri-State Medical Journal* 13 (1941): 2,696.

58. Richard L. Jenkins, *Breaking Patterns of Defeat: The Effective Readjustment of the Sick Personality* (Philadelphia: J.B. Lippincott Company, 1954): 216.

59. Rutherford B. Stevens, "Racial Aspects of Emotional Problems of Negro Soldiers," *American Journal of Psychiatry* 103 (1947): 497.

60. "The Negro—A Venereal Disease Problem," *Southern Medical Journal* 12 (1919): 109.

61. Herbert S. Ripley and Stewart Wold, "Mental Illness among Negro Troops Overseas," *American Journal of Psychiatry* 103 (January 1947): 507.

62. Rutherford B. Stevens, "Racial Aspects of Emotional Problems of Negro Soldiers," *American Journal of Psychiatry* 103 (1947): 497.

63. On the American psychiatric profession and African American soldiers during the Second World War, see Ellen Dwyer, "Psychiatry and Race during World War II," *Journal of the History of Medicine and Allied Sciences* 61 (2006): 117–143.

64. Rutherford B. Stevens, "Racial Aspects of Emotional Problems of Negro Soldiers," *American Journal of Psychiatry* 103 (1947): 493, 497.

65. Lieutenant Colonel Herbert S. Ripley and Major Stewart Wolf, "Mental Illness among Negro Troops Overseas," *American Journal of Psychiatry* (January 1947): 509, 510, 511.

66. For a more enlightened account of these relationships by a white psychiatrist, see Major Jerome D. Frank, "Adjustment Problems of Selected Negro Soldiers," *The Journal of Nervous and Mental Disease* 105 (June 1947): 647–660.

67. John E. Lind, "The Dream as a Simple Wish-Fulfillment in the Negro," *The Psychoanalytic Review* 1 (1913–14): 295–300.
68. Lieutenant Colonel Herbert S. Ripley and Major Stewart Wolf, "Mental Illness among Negro Troops Overseas," *American Journal of Psychiatry* (January 1947): 507, 508, 509.
69. Rutherford B. Stevens, "Racial Aspects of Emotional Problems of Negro Soldiers," *American Journal of Psychiatry* 103 (1947): 493, 496, 497.
70. Jerome D. Frank, "Adjustment Problems of Selected Negro Soldiers," *Journal of Nervous and Mental Disease* 105 (1947): 654.
71. Ralph G. Martin, "A Doctor's Dream in Harlem," *The New Republic* (June 3, 1940): 798–799; "Psychiatry in Harlem," Time (December 1, 1947).
72. Harvey R. St. Clair, "Psychiatric Interview Experiences with Negroes," *American Journal of Psychiatry* (1951): 116.
73. Walter A. Adams, "The Negro Patient in Psychiatric Treatment," *American Journal of Orthopsychiatry* 20 (1950): 305.
74. Morton Shane, "Some Subcultural Considerations in the Psychotherapy of a Negro Patient," *Psychiatric Quarterly* (1960): 9.
75. Ralph Mason Dreger and Kent S. Miller, "Comparative Psychological Studies of Negroes and Whites in the United States," *Psychological Bulletin* 70 (September 1968): 39.
76. Brian L. Weiss and David J. Kupfer, "The Black Patient and Research in a Community Mental Health Center: Where Have All the Subjects Gone?" *American Journal of Psychiatry* 131 (1974): 417.
77. Leonard J. Duhl, "The Psychiatrist's Role in Dealing with Social Turmoil," *American Journal of Psychiatry* 127 (1970): 225–226.
78. "The Psychiatrist, the APA, and Social Issues: A Symposium," *American Journal of Psychiatry* 128 (1971): 677, 678, 679, 687.
79. H. Warner Johnson and John Snibbe, "The Selection of a Psychiatric Curriculum for Medical Students: Results of a Survey," *American Journal of Psychiatry* 132 (1975): 513–516.
80. Edward F. Foulks, "The Concept of Culture in Psychiatric Residency Education," *American Journal of Psychiatry* 137 (1980): 812.
81. James H. Carter, "Applause for the End of a 'Drought'" [Letter], *American Journal of Psychiatry* 136 (1979): 734.
82. See Melvin Sabshin et al., "Dimensions of Institutional Racism in Psychiatry," *American Journal of Psychiatry* 127 (December 1970): 787–793; Wendell R. Lipscomb, "Drug Use in a Black Ghetto," *American Journal of Psychiatry* 127 (1971): 1,166–1,169; Jonathan F. Borus et al., "Racial Perceptions in the Army: An Approach," *American Journal of Psychiatry* 128 (1972): 1,369–1,374; Jeanne E. Fish and Charlotte J. Larr, "A Decade of Change in Drawings by Black Children," *American Journal of Psychiatry* 129 (1972): 421–426; Brian L. Weiss and David J. Kupfer, "The Black Patient and Research in a Community Mental Health Center: Where Have All the Subjects Gone?" *American Journal of Psychiatry* 131 (1974): 415–418; Alfred M. Bloch, "Combat Neurosis in Inner-City Schools," *American Journal of Psychiatry* 135 (1978): 1,189–1,192; Jesse O. Cavenar and Jean G. Spaulding, "When the Psychotherapist Is Black," *American Journal of Psychiatry* 135 (1978): 1,084–1,087; Walter H. Bradshaw, Jr., "Training Psychiatrists for Working with Blacks in Basic Residency Programs," *American Journal of Psychiatry* 135 (1978): 1,520–1,524; Victor B. Adebimpe et al., "MMPI Diagnosis of Black Psychiatric Patients," *American Journal of Psychiatry* 136 (1979): 85–87; Judith Godwin Babkin, "Ethnic Density and Psychiatric Hospitalization: Hazards of Minority Status," *American Journal of Psychiatry*

136 (1979): 1,562–1,566; Eric Lager and Israel Zwerling, "Time Orientation and Psychotherapy in the Ghetto," *American Journal of Psychiatry* 137 (1980): 1,279; Carl C. Bell, "Time Orientation and Ghetto Patients" [Letter], *American Journal of Psychiatry* 137 (1980): 1,279.

83. Melvin Sabshin et al., "Dimensions of Institutional Racism in Psychiatry," *American Journal of Psychiatry* 127 (December 1970): 787, 788, 790.

84. Daniel Patrick Moynihan, *The Negro Family: The Case for National Action* (Washington, DC: Office of Policy Planning and Research, United States Department of Labor, 1965): 29, 47.

85. Daryl Michael Scott, *Contempt and Pity: Social Policy and the Imager of the Damaged Black Psyche 1880–1996* (Chapel Hill and London: University of North Carolina Press, 1997): 157, 245.

86. Lee Rainwater and William L. Yancey, *The Moynihan Report and the Politics of Controversy* (Cambridge, MA and London: The MIT Press, 1967): 201, 263.

87. Melvin Sabshin et al., "Dimensions of Institutional Racism in Psychiatry," *American Journal of Psychiatry* 127 (December 1970): 789, 790.

88. "The delusion of the 'white liberal,'" Kenneth Clark wrote, is the "fantasy of purity" that succeeds his "fantasy of *tolerance*," in Kenneth B. Clark, *Dark Ghetto: Dilemmas of Social Power* (New York and Evanston: Harper & Row, Publishers, 1965): 228.

89. Lee Rainwater and William L. Yancey, *The Moynihan Report and the Politics of Controversy* (Cambridge, MA and London: The MIT Press, 1967): 411.

90. Daniel Patrick Moynihan, *The Negro Family: The Case for National Action* (Washington, DC: Office of Policy Planning and Research, United States Department of Labor, 1965): 5, 6, 29, 30.

91. Melvin Sabshin et al., "Dimensions of Institutional Racism in Psychiatry," *American Journal of Psychiatry* 127 (December 1970): 787, 788, 790, 791.

92. Kenneth B. Clark, *Dark Ghetto: Dilemmas of Social Power* (New York and Evanston: Harper & Row, Publishers, 1965): 81, 82.

93. Daniel Patrick Moynihan, *The Negro Family: The Case for National Action* (Washington, DC: Office of Policy Planning and Research, United States Department of Labor, 1965): 47.

94. William H. Grier and Price M. Cobbs, *Black Rage* (New York: Basic Books, 1968): 24, 26, 83–84.

95. Alvin F. Poussaint, "The Negro American: His Self-Image and Integration," *Journal of the National Medical Association* 58 (1966): 419.

96. Charles A. Pinderhughes, "Pathogenic Social Structure: A Prime Target for Preventive Psychiatric Intervention," *Journal of the National Medical Association* 58 (1966): 427.

97. James H. Carter, "Recognizing Psychiatric Symptoms in Black Americans," *Geriatrics* (November 1974): 98.

98. Alvin F. Poussaint, "The Negro American: His Self-Image and Integration," *Journal of the National Medical Association* 58 (1966): 421; Sidney B. Jenkins, "The Impact of the Black Identity Crisis on Community Psychiatry," *Journal of the National Medical Association* 61 (1969): 425.

99. William H. Grier and Price M. Cobbs, *Black Rage* (New York: Basic Books, 1968): 4.

100. Lee Rainwater and William L. Yancey, *The Moynihan Report and the Politics of Controversy* (Cambridge, MA and London: The MIT Press, 1967): 407.

101. Alvin F. Poussaint, "The Negro American: His Self-Image and Integration," *Journal of the National Medical Association* 58 (1966): 420.

102. William H. Grier, "Some Special Effects of Negroeness on the Oedipal Conflict," *Journal of the National Medical Association* 58 (1966): 418.

103. Paul B. Cornely, "The Health Status of the Negro Today and in the Future," *American Journal of Public Health* 58 (1968): 647.

104. James H. Carter, "Recognizing Psychiatric Symptoms in Black Americans," *Geriatrics* (November 1974): 95.

105. Abram Kardiner and Lionel Ovesey, *The Mark of Oppression: Explorations in the Personality of the American Negro* [1951] (Cleveland and New York: Meridian Books, 1962): ix, xviii.

106. Alyce C. Gullattee, "The Negro Psyche: Fact, Fiction and Fantasy," *Journal of the National Medical Association* 61 (1969): 120.

107. Frantz Fanon, *Black Skin, White Masks* (New York: Grove Press, 1967): 30, 50.

108. Frantz Fanon, "Medicine and Colonialism," in *A Dying Colonialism* (New York: Grove Press, 1967): 130.

109. Joseph H. Douglass, "Racial Integration in the Psychiatric Field," *Journal of the National Medical Association* 57 (1965): 2. According to this author, there were "approximately 250 Negro psychiatrists in the United States in 1965."

110. Carl C. Bell, "Review of *Black Psychiatrists and American Psychiatry*," *Journal of the American Medical Association* 282 (September 8, 1999): 993.

111. George M. Niles, "A Therapeutic Comparison, Medicinal and Otherwise, as between the Caucasian and Afro-American," *Southern Medical Journal* (February 1, 1913): 127–129.

112. D.H. Sandell, "Some Surgical Aspects of the African Soldier," *Journal of the Royal Army Medical Corps* (1945): 14.

113. George S. Schuyler, "Our White Folks" [1927], in *Black on White: Black Writers on What It Means to Be White*, ed. David R. Roediger, (New York: Schocken Books, 1998): 81.

114. John E. Lind, "The Dream as a Simple Wish-Fulfillment in the Negro," *The Psychoanalytic Review* 1 (1913–14): 295.

115. E.M. Green, "Psychoses among Negroes—A Comparative Study," *Journal of Nervous and Mental Disease* 41 (1914): 706.

116. Raymond Prince, "The 'Brain Fag' Syndrome in Nigerian Students," *The Journal of Mental Science (The British Journal of Psychiatry)* 106 (January 1960): 566.

117. See John Langston Gwaltney, *Drylongso: A Self-Portrait of Black America* [1980] (New York: Vintage Books, 1981): 5, 7, 59, 67, 166.

118. John Langston Gwaltney, *Drylongso: A Self-Portrait of Black America* [1980] (New York: Vintage Books, 1981): xxii, 15, 28, 66, 242.

119. John Langston Gwaltney, *Drylongso: A Self-Portrait of Black America* [1980] (New York: Vintage Books, 1981): 45, 53, 67, 102, 127, 220.

120. Harvey R. St. Clair, "Psychiatric Interview Experiences with Negroes," *American Journal of Psychiatry* (August 1951): 113.

121. John Langston Gwaltney, *Drylongso: A Self-Portrait of Black America* [1980] (New York: Vintage Books, 1981): 46.

122. William H. Grier, "Some Special Effects of Negroness on the Oedipal Conflict," *Journal of the National Medical Association* 58 (1966): 418.

123. Chester M. Pierce, MD, "Is Bigotry the Basis of the Medical Problems of the Ghetto?" in John C. Norman, ed., *Medicine in the Ghetto* (New York: Appleton-Century-Crofts, 1969): 308.

124. Joel Fischer, "Negroes and Whites and Rates of Mental Illness: Reconsideration of a Myth," *Psychiatry* 32 (1969):

125. James H. Carter, "Psychiatry's Insensitivity to Racism and Aging," *Psychiatric Opinion* 10 (December 1973): 21.

126. Eva Rose-Towns, "The Underprivileged Adolescent in an Underprivileged Community," *Journal of the National Medical Association* 57 (1965): 147.

127. William H. Grier, "Some Special Effects of Negroeness on the Oedipal Conflict," *Journal of the National Medical Association* 58 (1966): 418.
128. Benjamin D. Singer, "Some Implications of Differential Psychiatric Treatment of Negro and White Patients," *Social Science &d Medicine* 1 (1967): 80.
129. Walter H. Bradshaw, Jr., "Training Psychiatrists for Working with Blacks in Basic Residency Programs," *American Journal of Psychiatry* 135 (1978): 1,522.
130. Gerald Gregory Jackson, "Is Behavior Therapy A Threat to Black Clients?" *Journal of the National Medical Association* 68 (1976): 365.
131. Guy B. Johnson, "The Stereotype of the American Negro," in Otto Klineberg, ed., *Characteristics of the American Negro* (New York: Harper & Brothers Publishers, 1944): 3.
132. LeRoi Jones, *Blues People* [1968] (New York: Perennial, 2002): 213.
133. Stanley Crouch, *The All-American Skin Game, or, The Decoy of Race* [1995] (New York: Vintage Books, 1997): 28.
134. Eric Lager and Israel Zwerling, "Time Orientation and Psychotherapy in the Ghetto," *American Journal of Psychiatry* 137 (1980): 306, 307.
135. James H. Carter, "Frequent Mistakes Made with Black Patients in Psychotherapy," *Journal of the National Medical Association* 71 (1979): 1,009.
136. Carl C. Bell, "Time Orientation and Ghetto Patients" [Letter], *American Journal of Psychiatry* 137 (1980): 1,279.
137. Carl C. Bell, "Time Orientation and Ghetto Patients" [Letter], *American Journal of Psychiatry* 137 (1980): 1,279.
138. "Physicians treating Negro and white schizophrenic patients in the state hospital system of North Carolina were of the impression that the incidence of hallucinations was considerably higher in the Negro than in the white group," in M.M. Vitols, H.G. Waters, and M.H. Keeler, "Hallucinations and Delusions in White and Negro Schizophrenics," *American Journal of Psychiatry* 120 (1963): 472.
139. M.M. Vitols, H.G. Waters, and M.H. Keeler, "Hallucinations and Delusions in White and Negro Schizophrenics," *American Journal of Psychiatry* 120 (1963): 474.
140. Arrah B. Evarts, "The Ontogenetic against the Phylogenetic Elements in the Psychoses of the Colored Race," *Psychoanalytic Review* 3 (1916): 286, 287.
141. Herbert S. Ripley and Stewart Wold, "Mental Illness among Negro Troops Overseas," *American Journal of Psychiatry* 103 (January 1947): 507.
142. Herbert S. Ripley and Stewart Wold, "Mental Illness among Negro Troops Overseas," *American Journal of Psychiatry* 103 (January 1947): 509.
143. Victor R. Adebimpe et al., "Hallucinations and Delusions in Black Psychiatric Patients," *Journal of the National Medical Association* 73 (1981): 519.
144. Benjamin D. Singer, "Some Implications of Differential Psychiatric Treatment of Negro and White Patients," *Social Science and Medicine* 1 (1967): 81.
145. M.M. Vitols, H.G. Waters, and M.H. Keeler, "Hallucinations and Delusions in White and Negro Schizophrenics," *American Journal of Psychiatry* 120 (1963): 473.
146. Kenneth B. Clark, *Dark Ghetto: Dilemmas of Social Power* (New York: Harper Torchbooks, 1965): 83.
147. Ralph Mason Dreger and Kent S. Miller, "Comparative Psychological Studies of Negroes and Whites in the United States," *Psychological Bulletin* 70 (September 1968): 41.
148. Linda K. Susman et al., "Treatment-Seeking for Depression by Black and White Americans," *Social Science and Medicine* 24 (1987): 195.
149. "Black Hang-Ups," *Time* 95 (April 6, 1970): 64.

150. Harvey R. St. Clair, "Psychiatric Interview Experiences with Negroes," *American Journal of Psychiatry* (1951): 113–114.
151. James H. Carter, "Recognizing Psychiatric Symptoms in Black Americans," *Geriatrics* (November 1974): 95–96.
152. On the history of ideas about the disorderly black male, see John Hoberman, "Athleticizing the Black Criminal," in *Darwin's Athletes: How Sport Has Damaged Black America and Preserved the Myth of Race* (New York: Houghton Mifflin, 1997): 208–220.
153. Ronald L. Braithwaite, "The Health Status of Black Men," in *Health Issues in the Black Community*, Ronald L. Braithwaite and Sandra E. Taylor, eds. (San Francisco: Jossey-Bass Publishers, 2001): 62.
154. Jerome G. Miller, *Search and Destroy: African-American Males in the Criminal Justice System* (Cambridge and New York: Cambridge University Press, 1996): 90–91.
155. V.H. Mark et al., "Role of Brain Disease in Riots and Urban Violence," *JAMA* 202 (September 11, 1967): 895. On Mark's psychosurgeries, see "Neurosurgeon Cites Work with Epileptic Patients," *Journal of the American Medical Association* 225 (August 20, 1973): 917.
156. Seymour L. Pollack, "Role of Brain Disease in Riots and Urban Violence," *JAMA* 202 (November 13, 1967): 211.
157. Mitchell Cohen, "Beware the Violence Initiative Project," *Z Magazine* (April 2000): 36.
158. Melvin Sabshin et al., "Dimensions of Institutional Racism in Psychiatry," *American Journal of Psychiatry* 127 (December 1970): 790.
159. See "Ethics Officials to Investigate Drug Experiments on Children," *New York Times* (April 15, 1998); "U.S. Criticizes Mount Sinai and CUNY over Psychiatric Experiments," *New York Times* (June 12, 1999).
160. "Dispute Threatens U.S. Plan on Violence," *New York Times* (October 23, 1992).
161. Benjamin D. Singer, "Some Implications of Differential Psychiatric Treatment of Negro and White Patients," *Social Science and Medicine* 1 (1967): 78; John M. Eisenberg, "Sociologic Influences on Decision-Making by Clinicians," *Annals of Internal Medicine* 90 (1979): 958.
162. James H. Carter, "Psychosocial Aspects of Aging: The Black Elderly," *Journal of the National Medical Association* (1984): 274.
163. John Dunn and Thomas A. Fahy, "Police Admissions to a Psychiatric Hospital: Demographic and Clinical Differences between Ethnic Groups," *British Journal of Psychiatry* 156 (1990): 377; Glyn Lewis et al., "Are British Psychiatrists Racist?" *British Journal of Psychiatry* 157 (1990): 410.
164. Aneez Esmail, "The Prejudices of Good People," *British Medical Journal* 328 (June 19, 2004): 1,449.
165. Rahn K. Bailey and Dion L. Owens, "Overcoming Challenges in the Diagnosis and Treatment of Attention-Deficit/Hyperactivity Disorder in African Americans," *Journal of the National Medical Association* [Supplement to October 2005, Volume 97, No. 10]: 8S.
166. Benjamin D. Singer, "Some Implications of Differential Psychiatric Treatment of Negro and White Patients," *Social Science and Medicine* 1 (1967): 78; John M. Eisenberg, "Sociologic Influences on Decision-Making by Clinicians," *Annals of Internal Medicine* 90 (1979): 958.
167. Rahn K. Bailey and Dion L. Owens, "Overcoming Challenges in the Diagnosis and Treatment of Attention-Deficit/Hyperactivity Disorder in African Americans," *Journal of the National Medical Association* [Supplement to October 2005, Volume 97, No. 10]: 8S; Julie Magno Zito et al., "Racial Disparity in Psychotropic Medications Prescribed for Youth with Medicaid Insurance in

Maryland," *Journal of the American Academy of Child and Adolescent Psychiatry* 37 (1998): 182.

168. John Langston Gwaltney, *Drylongso: A Self-Portrait of Black America* [1980] (New York: Vintage Books, 1981): 127.

169. "Colonial Medical Service," *British Medical Journal* (August 7, 1948): 314.

170. Sheryl Thorburn Bird and Laura M. Bogart, "Birth Control Conspiracy Beliefs, Perceived Discrimination, and Contraception among African Americans: An Exploratory Study," *Journal of Health Psychology* 8 (2003): 263–276; Laura M. Bogart and Sheryl Thorburn Bird, "Exploring the Relationship of Conspiracy Beliefs About HIV/AIDS to Sexual Behaviors and Attitudes Among African-American Adults," *Journal of the National Medical Association* 95 (November 2003): 1057–1065.

171. Tamar Jacoby, *Someone Else's House: America's Unfinished Struggle for Integration* (New York: Basic Books, 1998): 374–375.

172. Jonathan Brent, "Political Perversity in Chicago," *The New Republic* (August 8 and 15, 1988): 17.

173. Jeffrey Goldberg, "I'm Going to Kill You, Cracker, and Other Greetings of the Day," *Forward* (September 11, 1998).

174. Sheryl Thorburn Bird and Laura M. Bogart, "Birth Control Conspiracy Beliefs, Perceived Discrimination, and Contraception among African Americans: An Exploratory Study," *Journal of Health Psychology* 8 (2003): 263–276.

175. Laura M. Bogart and Sheryl Thorburn Bird, "Exploring the Relationship of Conspiracy Beliefs about HIV/AIDS to Sexual Behaviors and Attitudes among African-American Adults," *Journal of the National Medical Association* 95 (November 2003): 1058.

176. Benoit Denizet-Lewis, "Double Lives on the Down Low," *The New York Times Magazine* (August 3, 2003): 52.

177. "South Africa in a Furor over Advice about AIDS," *New York Times* (March 19, 2001); "A President Misapprehends a Killer," *New York Times* (May 14, 2000); "Merging the First and Third Worlds," *The Economist* (May 2, 1998); "Mbeki's Visit to U.S. Puts AIDS Activists in a Quandary," *New York Times* (May 21, 2000).

178. Kenneth B. Clark, "Candor about Negro-Jewish Relations," *Commentary* (1946): 9.

179. Abram Kardiner and Lionel Ovesey, *The Mark of Oppression: Explorations in the Personality of the American Negro* [1951] (New York: Meridian Books, 1962): xviii.

180. Quoted in Lee Rainwater and William L. Yancey, *The Moynihan Report and the Politics of Controversy* (Cambridge, MA and London: The MIT Press, 1967): 410.

181. Chester M. Pierce, "Possible Social Science Contributions to the Clarification of the Negro Self-Image," *Journal of the National Medical Association* 60 (1968): 100.

182. Alyce C. Gullattee, "The Negro Psyche: Fact, Fiction and Fantasy," *Journal of the National Medical Association* 61 (1969): 120.

183. Wendell R. Lipscomb, "Drug Use in a Black Ghetto," *American Journal of Psychiatry* 127 (1971): 1,166.

184. Alexander Thomas and Samuel Sillen, "The Mark of Oppression," in *Racism and Psychiatry* (New York: BRUNNER/MAZEL, Publishers, 1972): 46.

185. Irving Howe, "Why Should Negroes Be above Criticism?" *Saturday Evening Post* 241 (December 14, 1968): 14.

186. See, for example, Daryl Michael Scott, *Contempt and Pity: Social Policy and the Image of the Damaged Black Psyche, 1880–1996* (Chapel Hill and London: The University of North Carolina Press, 1997).
187. William Julius Wilson, "The Truly Disadvantaged Revisited: A Response to Hochschild and Boxill," *Ethics* 101 (April 1991): 598.

CHAPTER 5

1. Jean M. Goodwin et al., "Psychiatric Symptoms in Disliked Medical Patients," *JAMA* 241 (March 16, 1979): 1,117.
2. Ronald M. Davis, "Achieving Racial Harmony for the Benefit of Patients and Communities," *JAMA* 300 (July 16, 2008): 323.
3. Ford Fessenden, "Blacks Passed By," *Newsday* (November 29, 1998): A55.
4. "Nashville Clinic Offers Case Study of Chronic Gap in Black and White Health," *New York Times* (March 21, 1998).
5. Ronald M. Davis, "Achieving Racial Harmony for the Benefit of Patients and Communities," *JAMA* 300 (July 16, 2008): 324.
6. Molly Cooke et al., "American Medical Education 100 Years after the Flexner Report," *New England Journal of Medicine* 355 (September 28, 2006): 1,341, 1,342. On the "hidden curriculum," see *inter alia* Frederic W. Hafferty and Ronald Franks, "The Hidden Curriculum, Ethics Teaching, and the Structure of Medical Education," *Academic Medicine* 69 (November 1994): 861–871.
7. Peter B. Bach et al., "Racial Differences in the Treatment of Early-Stage Lung Cancer," *NEJM* 341 (October 14, 1999): 1,198–1,205. "Both unadjusted and adjusted analyses showed that black patients who underwent surgical resection had a five-year survival rate similar to that of white patients who underwent resection, and we estimated that of the 77 more deaths per 1,000 black patients, the majority (44) could be attributed to the lack of surgical treatment" (1,202).
8. "New for Aspiring Doctors, the People Skills Test," *New York Times* (July 10, 2011).
9. L.J. Henderson, "Physician and Patient as a Social System," *New England Journal of Medicine* 212 (May 2, 1935): 821, 822, 823.
10. Rael D. Strous et al., "The Hateful Patient Revisited: Relevance for 21st Century Medicine," *European Journal of Internal Medicine* 17 (2006): 388.
11. Barbara Gerbert, "Perceived Likeability and Competence of Simulated Patients: Influence on Physicians' Management Plans," *Social Science and Medicine* 18 (1984): 1,053.
12. Elizabeth H.B. Lin et al., "Frustrating Patients: Physician and Patient Perspectives among Distressed High Users of Medical Services," *Journal of General Internal Medicine* 6 (1991): 241.
13. James E. Groves, "Taking Care of the Hateful Patient," *New England Journal of Medicine* 298 (April 20, 1978): 883.
14. Douglas A. Drossman, "The Problem Patient: Evaluation and Care of Medical Patients with Psychosocial Disturbances," *Annals of Internal Medicine* 88 (1978): 368.
15. Richard Gorlin and Howard D. Zucker, "Physicians' Reactions to Patients: A Key to Teaching Humanistic Medicine," *New England Journal of Medicine* 308 (May 5, 1983): 1,059.
16. Sam Smith, "Dealing with the Difficult Patient," *Postgraduate Medical Journal* 71 (1995) 653.

17. Steven R. Hahn et al., "The Difficult Patient: Prevalence, Psychopathology, and Functional Impairment," *Journal of General Internal Medicine* 11 (1996): 7.
18. Richard Gorlin and Howard D. Zucker, "Physicians' Reactions to Patients: A Key to Teaching Humanistic Medicine," *New England Journal of Medicine* 308 (May 5, 1983): 1,059.
19. Solomon Papper, "The Undesirable Patient," in *Dominant Issues in Medical Sociology*, Howard D. Schwartz, ed. (New York: Random House, 1987): 260.
20. William M. Zinn, "Doctors Have Feelings Too," *JAMA* 259 (June 10, 1988): 3,296.
21. Dennis H. Novack et al., "Calibrating the Physician: Personal Awareness and Effective Patient Care," *JAMA* 278 (August 13, 1997): 502.
22. Dennis H. Novack et al., "Calibrating the Physician: Personal Awareness and Effective Patient Care," *JAMA* 278 (August 13, 1997): 502.
23. David R. Levy, "White Doctors and Black Patients: Influence of Race on the Doctor-Patient Relationship," *Pediatrics* 75 (1985): 642.
24. See James E. Groves, "Taking Care of the Hateful Patient," *New England Journal of Medicine* 298 (April 20, 1978): 883; Frederic W. Hafferty and Ronald Franks, "The Hidden Curriculum, Ethics Teaching, and the Structure of Medical Education," *Academic Medicine* 69 (November 1994): 865.
25. James E. Groves, "Taking Care of the Hateful Patient," *New England Journal of Medicine* 298 (April 20, 1978): 884, 885, 886.
26. Jean M. Goodwin et al., "Psychiatric Symptoms in Disliked Medical Patients," *JAMA* 241 (March 16, 1979): 1,118.
27. William M. Zinn, "Doctors Have Feelings Too," *JAMA* 259 (June 10, 1988): 3,297, 3,298.
28. Dennis H. Novack et al., "Calibrating the Physician: Personal Awareness and Effective Patient Care," *JAMA* 278 (August 13, 1997): 502, 503, 504.
29. Sandra Turbes et al., "The Hidden Curriculum in Multicultural Medical Education: The Role of Case Examples," *Academic Medicine* 77 (March 2002): 214.
30. Mary-Jo DelVecchio Good, Cara James, Byron J. Good, Anne E. Becker, "The Culture of Medicine and Racial, Ethnic, and Class Disparities in Healthcare," in *Unequal Treatment: Confronting Racial and Ethnic Disparities in Healthcare* (Washington, DC: The National Academies Press, 2003): 620.
31. Nancy R. Kressin et al., "Racial Differences in Cardiac Catheterization as a Function of Patients' Beliefs," *American Journal of Public Health* 94 (December 2004): 2,091.
32. Frederic W. Hafferty and Ronald Franks, "The Hidden Curriculum, Ethics Teaching, and the Structure of Medical Education," *Academic Medicine* 69 (November 1994): 867.
33. Lisa Soleymani Lehmann et al., "A Survey of Medical Ethics Education at U.S. and Canadian Medical Schools," *Academic Medicine* 79 (July 2004): 682, 688.
34. Nisha Dogra and Niranjan Karnik, "First-Year Medical Students' Attitudes toward Diversity and its Teaching: An Investigation at One U.S. Medical School," *Academic Medicine* 78 (November 2003): 1,191–1,192.
35. Frederic W. Hafferty and Ronald Franks, "The Hidden Curriculum, Ethics Teaching, and the Structure of Medical Education," *Academic Medicine* 69 (November 1994): 868.
36. Samuel L. Bloom, "Structure and Ideology in Medical Education: An Analysis of Resistance to Change," *Journal of Health and Social Behavior* 29 (December 1988): 297, 298, 301.

37. Billy E. Jones et al., "Problems of Black Psychiatric Residents in White Training Institutes," *American Journal of Psychiatry* 127 (December 1970): 799.

38. Mary-Jo DelVecchio Good, Cara James, Byron J. Good, Anne E. Becker, "The Culture of Medicine and Racial, Ethnic, and Class Disparities in Healthcare," in *Unequal Treatment: Confronting Racial and Ethnic Disparities in Healthcare* (Washington, DC: The National Academies Press, 2003): 604.

39. H. Jack Geiger, "Racial and Ethnic Disparities in Diagnosis and Treatment: A Review of the Evidence and a Consideration of Causes," in *Unequal Treatment: Confronting Racial and Ethnic Disparities in Healthcare* (Washington, DC: The National Academies Press, 2003): 443.

40. Mary Anne C. Johnston, "A Model Program to Address Insensitive Behaviors toward Medical Students," *Academic Medicine* 67: 4 (April 1992): 236.

41. K. Harnett Sheehan et al., "A Pilot Study of Medical Student 'Abuse': Student Perceptions of Mistreatment and Misconduct in Medical School," *JAMA* 263 (January 26, 1990): 535.

42. Brenda L. Beagan, "Teaching Social and Cultural Awareness to Medical Students: "It's All Very Nice to Talk about It In Theory, But Ultimately It Makes No Difference," *Academic Medicine* 78 (June 2003): 611.

43. See, for example, Henry K. Silver, "Medical Students and Medical School," *JAMA* 247 (1982): 309–310; D.A. Rosenberg and Henry K. Silver, "Medical Student Abuse: An Unnecessary and Preventable Cause of Stress," *JAMA* 251 (1984): 739–742; Val I. Robichaux, "Medical Student Abuse," *JAMA* 252 (1984): 2,958; J. Paul Carlson, "Medical Student Abuse," *JAMA* 252 (1984): 2,959; Henry K. Silver and Anita Duhl Glicken, "Medical Student Abuse: Incidence, Severity, and Significance," *JAMA* 263 (January 26, 1990): 527–532. K. Harnett Sheehan et al., "A Pilot Study of Medical Student 'Abuse': Student Perceptions of Mistreatment and Misconduct in Medical School," *JAMA* 263 (January 26, 1990): 533–537; De Witt C. Baldwin et al., "Student Perceptions of Mistreatment and Harassment during Medical School: A Survey of Ten United States Schools," *Western Journal of Medicine* 155 (August 1991): 140–145; Mary Anne C. Johnston, "A Model Program to Address Insensitive Behaviors toward Medical Students," *Academic Medicine* 67: 4 (April 1992): 236–237; R. S. Mangus et al., "Prevalence of Harassment and Discrimination among 1996 Medical School Graduates: A Survey of Eight U.S. Schools," *JAMA* 280 (September 2, 1998): 851–853; D. Kassebaum and E. Cutler, "On the Culture of Student Abuse in Medical School," *Academic Medicine* 73 (November 1988): 1,149–1,158; Paul E. Ogden et al., "Do Attending Physicians, Nurses, Residents, and Medical Students Agree on What Constitutes Medical Student Abuse?" *Academic Medicine* 80 (October 2005 Supplement): S80–S83; David Michael Elnicki et al., "Medical Student Abuse from Multiple Perspectives," *The Clinical Teacher* 4 (published online August 17, 2007): 153–158 (accessed April 11, 2010).

44. Martin Luther King, Jr., "The Role of the Behavioral Scientist in the Civil Rights Movement," *American Psychologist* 23 (March 1968): 180.

45. "How Whites Feel about Negroes: A Painful American Dilemma," *Newsweek* (October 21, 1963): 50.

46. Victor R. Adebimpe et al., "Symptomatology of Depression in Black and White Patients," *Journal of the National Medical Association* 74 (1982): 185.

47. See, for example, Maria Krysan, "Privacy and the Expression of White Racial Attitudes," *Public Opinion Quarterly* 62 (1998): 506–544.

48. Victoria J. Balenger et al., "Racial Attitudes among Incoming White Students: A Study of 10-Year Trends," *Journal of College Student Development* 33 (May 1992): 251.

49. Mary C. Howell, "What Medical Schools Teach about Women," *New England Journal of Medicine* 291 (August 8, 1974): 304, 306. See also Mary C. Howell, "The New Feminism and the Medical School Milieu," *Annals of the New York Academy of Sciences* (1979): 210–214.

50. "Women have long been excluded from the population considered at high risk for cardiovascular disease," in Theresa A. Beery, "Gender Bias and Diagnosis and Treatment of Coronary Artery Disease," *Heart & Lung* 24 (1995): 427.

51. "In the late 1960s, medical schools across the United States began recognizing the effects of racism and how racism might lead to cultural insensitivity in medicine. Since then, how to teach medical students to understand and contend with race and culture has been a critical focus for medical education reform," in Nisha Dogra and Niranjan Karnik, "First-Year Medical Students' Attitudes toward Diversity and its Teaching: An Investigation at One U.S. Medical School," *Academic Medicine* 78 (November 2003): 1,191. The claim here that teaching medical students about race and culture "has been a critical focus for medical education reform" ever since strikes me as an exaggeration of the effort that has been invested in this aspect of medical education.

52. Billy E. Jones et al., "Problems of Black Psychiatric Residents in White Training Institutes," *American Journal of Psychiatry* 127 (December 1970): 799–800, 802, 803.

53. Richard Gorlin and Howard D. Zucker, "Physicians' Reactions to Patients: A Key to Teaching Humanistic Medicine," *New England Journal of Medicine* 308 (May 5, 1983): 1,061.

54. Barbara Gerbert, "Perceived Likeability and Competence of Simulated Patients: Influence on Physicians' Management Plans," *Social Science and Medicine* 18 (1984): 1,054.

55. William M. Zinn, "Doctors Have Feelings Too," *JAMA* 259 (June 10, 1988): 3,298.

56. Frederic W. Hafferty and Ronald Franks, "The Hidden Curriculum, Ethics Teaching, and the Structure of Medical Education," *Academic Medicine* 69 (November 1994): 861.

57. H. Jack Geiger, "Race and Health Care," *NEJM* 335 (September 12, 1996): 815–816.

58. "Teaching and Learning of Cultural Competence in Medical School," Contemporary Issues in Medical Education [One-page bulletin published by the AAMC] (1998): 1(5). Cited in Sandra Turbes et al., "The Hidden Curriculum in Multicultural Medical Education: The Role of Case Examples," *Academic Medicine* 77 (March 2002): 209.

59. Lisa Soleymani Lehmann et al., "A Survey of Medical Ethics Education at U.S. and Canadian Medical Schools," *Academic Medicine* 79 (July 2004): 687.

60. Sunil Kripalani et al., "A Prescription for Cultural Competence in Medical Education," *Journal of General Internal Medicine* 21 (October 2006): 1,118.

61. "A survey of GLB physicians found that 88% had heard medical colleagues disparage GLB patients, and 57% had observed colleagues provide diminished care or deny care to patients because of sexual orientation," in Sandra Turbes et al., "The Hidden Curriculum in Multicultural Medical Education: The Role of Case Examples," *Academic Medicine* 77 (March 2002): 213.

62. "Cultural Competence Education" (Association of American Medical Colleges, Washington, D.C., 2005): 1–18.

63. "Furthermore, although the majority of deans agreed that being a physician was not sufficient background to be an effective teacher of ethics, many deans also reported a lack of funding for ethics teaching at their institutions,"

from Lisa Soleymani Lehmann et al., "A Survey of Medical Ethics Education at U.S. and Canadian Medical Schools," *Academic Medicine* 79 (July 2004): 687.

64. "Cultural Competence Education" (American Association of Medical Colleges, 2005): 5.

65. Cindy Brach and Irene Fraserirector, "Can Cultural Competency Reduce Racial and Ethnic Health Disparities? A Review and Conceptual Model," *Medical Care Research and Review* 57 (November 2000): 184.

66. Jack Coulehan and Peter C. Williams, "Vanquishing Virtue: The Impact of Medical Education," *Academic Medicine* 76 (June 2001): 598–605.

67. Sunil Kripalani et al., "A Prescription for Cultural Competence in Medical Education," *Journal of General Internal Medicine* 21 (October 2006): 1,116–1,120.

68. Jonathan M. Metzl, *The Protest Psychosis: How Schizophrenia Became a Black Disease* (Boston: Beacon Press, 2009): xviii.

69. John Z. Ayanian et al., "Physicians' Beliefs about Racial Differences in Referral for Renal Transplantation," *American Journal of Kidney Diseases* 43 (February 2004): 350–357.

70. Diana J. Burgess et al., "Why Do Providers Contribute to Disparities and What Can Be Done about It?," *Journal of Health Care for the Poor and Underserved* 21 (2004): 1,156.

71. Nicole Lurie et al., "Racial and Ethnic Disparities in Care: The Perspectives of Cardiologists," *Circulation* 111 (2005): 1265, 1266.

72. Stephanie L. Taylor et al., "Racial and Ethnic Disparities in Care: The Perspectives of Cardiovascular Surgeons," *Annals of Thoracic Surgery* 81 (2006): 535.

73. Rose Clark-Hitt et al., "Doctors' and Nurses' Explanations for Racial Disparities in Medical Treatment," *Journal of Health Care for the Poor and Underserved* 21 (2010): 387, 390.

74. Jennifer Malat et al., "White Doctors and Nurses on Racial Inequality in Health Care in the USA: Whiteness and Colour-Blind Racial Ideology," *Ethnic and Racial Studies* (2010): 13, 16; Rose Clark-Hitt et al., "Doctors' and Nurses' Explanations for Racial Disparities in Medical Treatment," *Journal of Health Care for the Poor and Underserved* 21 (2010): 392, 396–397.

75. Arthur Schatzkin and John Yergan, "The Case for Minority Admissions," *New England Journal of Medicine* 297 (September 8, 1977): 556.

76. Nicole Lurie et al., "Racial and Ethnic Disparities in Care: The Perspectives of Cardiologists," *Circulation* 111 (2005): 1,267.

77. Elisabeth Wilson et al., "Medical Student, Physician, and Public Perceptions of Health Care Disparities," *Medical Student Education* 36 (November–December 2004): 715, 718.

78. For example, "fewer than 20% of cardiovascular surgeons felt that increasing provider awareness about racial/ethnic disparities or improving the cultural competence of either the provider or the institution would be likely to be useful in addressing disparities," from Stephanie L. Taylor et al., "Racial and Ethnic Disparities in Care: The Perspectives of Cardiovascular Surgeons," *Annals of Thoracic Surgery* 81 (2006): 534.

79. Elisabeth Wilson et al., "Medical Student, Physician, and Public Perceptions of Health Care Disparities," *Medical Student Education* 36 (November–December 2004): 718.

80. John Z. Ayanian et al., "Physicians' Beliefs about Racial Differences in Referral for Renal Transplantation," *American Journal of Kidney Diseases* 43 (February 2004): 350–356.

81. David R. Levy, "White Doctors and Black Patients: Influence of Race on the Doctor-Patient Relationship," *Pediatrics* 75 (1985): 640.
82. Nicholas D. Kristof, "Two Men and Two Paths," *New York Times* (June 13, 2012).
83. Vonnie C. McLoyd, "The Impact of Economic Hardship on Black Families and Children: Psychological Distress, Parenting, and Socioemotional Development," *Child Development* 61 (1990): 326.
84. Allen Raskin and Thomas H. Crook, "Antidepressants in Black and White Inpatients," *Archives of General Psychiatry* 32 (May 1975): 647–648.
85. Dr. John Maupin, quoted in "Nashville Clinic Offers Case Study of Chronic Gap in Black and White Health," *New York Times* (March 21, 1998).
86. David R. Levy, "White Doctors and Black Patients: Influence of Race on the Doctor-Patient Relationship," *Pediatrics* 75 (1985): 641.
87. David R. Levy, "White Doctors and Black Patients: Influence of Race on the Doctor-Patient Relationship," *Pediatrics* 75 (1985): 641.
88. Loudell F. Snow, "Folk Medical Beliefs and Their Implications for Care of Patients," *Annals of Internal Medicine* 81 (1974): 82.
89. S. Underwood, "Cancer Risk Reduction and Early Detection Behaviors among Black Men: Focus on Learned Helplessness," *Journal of Community Health and Nursing* 9 (1992): 21–31, cited in Barbara D. Powe, "Cancer Fatalism among African-Americans: A Review of the Literature," *Nursing Outlook* 44 (1996): 19.
90. Barbara D. Powe, "Cancer Fatalism among African-Americans: A Review of the Literature," *Nursing Outlook* 44 (1996): 20.
91. B. Lee Green et al., "Powerlessness, Destiny, and Control: The Influence on Health Behaviors of African Americans," *Journal of Community Health* 29 (February 2004): 15–27. The quotation is from the Abstract on p. 15.
92. "Multiple Stigmas Keep Blacks Away from MH System," *Psychiatric News* (October 19, 2001).
93. Arthur Kleinman and Peter Benson, "Anthropology in the Clinic: The Problem of Cultural Competency and How to Fix It," *PLoS Medicine* 3 (October 2006): 1,673, 1,674.
94. Francis W. Peabody, "The Care of the Patient," *JAMA* 88 (March 19, 1927).
95. I. C. McManus, "Humanity and the Medical Humanities," *Lancet* 346 (1995): 1,143.
96. "The use of humanities and arts in medical education has also grown in the last 40 years, to the extent that over half to three-quarters of all U.S. and Canadian medical schools (depending on one's definition) have some sort of curricular offering in the medical humanities," from Johanna Shapiro, "A Sampling of the Medical Humanities," *Journal for Learning through the Arts* 2 (2006): 1.
97. Alan Petersen et al., "The Medical Humanities Today: Humane Health Care or Tool of Governance?" *Journal of the Medical Humanities* 29 (2008): 1.
98. Trudier Harris, "This Disease Called Strength: Some Observations on the Compensating Construction of Black Female Character," *Literature and Medicine* 14 (1995): 109–126.
99. Robert Haas, "Might Zora Neale Hurston's Janie Woods Be Dying of Rabies? Considerations from Historical Medicine," *Literature and Medicine* 19 (2000): 205–228.
100. Jennifer Yee, "Malaria and the Femme Fatale: Sex and Death in French Colonial Africa," *Literature and Medicine* 21 (2002): 201–215; Jessica Howell, "'Self Rather Seedy': Climate and Colonial Pathography in Conrad's African Fiction," *Literature and Medicine* 27 (Fall 2008): 223–247.

101. This list does not include the following book review: "Review of J. Elizabeth Clark, *Bodies in a Broken World: Women Novelists of Color and the Politics of Medicine*," *Literature and Medicine* 24 (2005): 142–45.
102. Cynthia Ryan, "'Am I Not a Woman?' The Rhetoric of Breast Cancer Stories in African American Women's Popular Periodicals," *Journal of the Medical Humanities* 25 (2004): 129–150; Naa Oyo A. Kwate, "The Heresy of African-Centered Psychology," *Journal of the Medical Humanities* 26 (2005): 215–235.
103. Lawrence Hammar, "The Dark Side to Donovanosis: Color, Climate, Race and Racism in American South Venereology," *Journal of Medical Humanities* 18 (1997): 29–57; Britt Rusert, "'A Study in Nature': The Tuskegee Experiments and the New South Plantation," *Journal of the Medical Humanities* 30 (2009): 155–171.
104. Lawrence Hammar, "The Dark Side to Donovanosis: Color, Climate, Race and Racism in American South Venereology," *Journal of Medical Humanities* 18 (1997): 29–57; Britt Rusert, "'A Study in Nature': The Tuskegee Experiments and the New South Plantation," *Journal of the Medical Humanities* 30 (2009): 155–171.
105. Sheryl Nestel, "(Ad)Ministering Angels: Colonial Nursing and the Extension of Empire in Africa," *Journal of Medical Humanities* 19 (1998): 257–277.
106. Olivia McNeely Pass, "Toni Morrison's *Beloved*: A Journey through the Pain of Grief," *Journal of Medical Humanities* 27 (2006): 117–124.
107. Delese Wear and Julie M. Aultman, "The Limits of Narrative: Medical Student Resistance to Confronting Inequality and Oppression in Literature and Beyond," *Medical Education* 39 (2005): 1,057, 1,058.
108. Proposals for social activism in medicine seldom appear in the medical humanities literature. "The putative existence of an obligation for social and political activism constitutes one of the most interesting, yet poorly developed themes in medical ethics. Perhaps this subject strays too far from the doctor-patient relationship that constitutes the focus of most ethical discussions," from T. Forcht Dagi, "Physicians and Obligatory Social Activism," *The Journal of Medical Humanities and Bioethics* 9 (Spring/Summer 1988): 51. The behavioral scientist Delese Wear may be the only medical humanist who has directly challenged physicians to think seriously about changing the status quo they have established and continue to dominate. As she declared in 1992: "... if the language seems excessive or even hostile to my medical colleagues, I apologize again, but stand by its use because of its confrontive and startling metaphors that may move us to look at our thinking and practice problematically." See Delese Wear, "The Colonization of the Medical Humanities: A Confessional Critique," *The Journal of Medical Humanities* 13 (1992): 200. See also: Delese Wear and Julie M. Aultman, "The Limits of Narrative: Medical Student Resistance to Confronting Inequality and Oppression in Literature and Beyond," *Medical Education* 39 (2005): 1,056–1,065.
109. Robert A. Hahn and Arthur Kleinman, "Biomedical Practice and Anthropological Theory: Frameworks and Directions," *Annual Review of Anthropology* 12 (1983): 306.
110. Susan E. Cayleff, "Teaching Women's History in a Medical School: Challenges and Possibilities," *Women's Studies Quarterly* (1988): 99
111. Delese Wear, "The Colonization of the Medical Humanities: A Confessional Critique," *The Journal of Medical Humanities* 13 (1992): 202.
112. Quoted in John Langone, *Harvard Med: The Story Behind America's Premier Medical School and the Making of American Doctors* (Holbrook, MA: Adams Media Corporation, 1995): 67. "But for all the comforting commentary on

the humanities—and all the dire warnings from educators about medical students in peril of becoming slaves to rampant technology—science is still necessarily king, and don't believe anybody who tells you otherwise" (67).

113. Emily Bazelon, "The New Abortion Providers," *New York Times Magazine* (July 18, 2010): 32.

114. Emily Bazelon, "The New Abortion Providers," *New York Times Magazine* (July 18, 2010): 33.

115. See Susan Hunt, "The Flexner Report and Black Academic Medicine: An Assignment of Place," *Journal of the National Medical Association* 85 (1993): 152, 154.

116. W. Michael Byrd and Linda A Clayton, *An American Health Dilemma: Race, Medicine, and Healthcare in the United States, 1900–2000* (New York & London: Routledge, 2002).

117. Samuel C. Bullock and Earline Houston, "Perceptions of Racism by Black Medical Students Attending White Medical Schools," *Journal of the National Medical Association* 79 (1987): 604, 606. See also Henry T. Frierson, "Black Medical Students' Perceptions of the Academic Environment and of Faculty and Peer Interactions," *Journal of the National Medical Association* 79 (1987): 737–743.

Index

abortion training, curriculum changes in, 229–33

Academic Medicine, 11, 15, 209, 212, 216

Accreditation Council for Graduate Medical Education, 230, 232

ACE inhibitors, racial pharmacology in use of, 135–39

African American population: colonialism and medical status of, 193–97; conspiracy theories concerning medicine in, 194–97; cultural competence of white physicians concerning, development of, 212–16; disparities in health care for, 4–7; emotional hardiness myth in, 125–30; "internal colonialism" for, 148–54; medical humanities omission of, 227; medical vulnerability of, 24–32; military service in Second World War by, 162–65; myths and conspiracy theories about medicine in, 49–52; perceptions of racial pharmacology in, 133–39; physical hardiness myth among, 121–25; racial disparities in management of, 33–37; silence concerning health crisis in, 18–24; skin color variations in, stereotypes concerning, 55–66; therapeutic fatalism and misdiagnoses of, 222–24

Africanization of African Americans: black image and, 154–58; "internal colonialism" and, 150–54; medical humanities curriculum discussion of, 227–29

Agency for Healthcare Research and Quality (AHRQ), 37–41

aging, racial interpretations of elderly black patients and, 81–83

AIDS epidemic: in African American population, 18–19, 129–30; conspiracy theories concerning, 194–97; "internal colonialism" and, 151–54; psychiatric assessments of African Americans and, 162; racial interpretations of black infants and children and, 77–81; therapeutic fatalism and misdiagnoses and, 224

"AIDS in Blackface," 162

American Association of Physical Anthropology, 195

American Dilemma, An (Myrdal), 4–7, 65

American Heart Journal: heart disease in black patients discussed in, 100–101; loss of consciousness in African Americans discussed in, 89, 92; racial pharmacology in, 139; racism in, 3, 12

American Journal of Orthopsychiatry, 128–29

American Journal of Physical Anthropology, 67, 93–94, 121, 150

American Journal of Psychiatry: black infants and children discussed in, 74, 77; black psychiatry and, 187–88, 211–12; medical racism in, 196; racial primitive discussed in, 160, 162–68; stereotypes of black musical aptitude in, 86–87

American Journal of Public Health, 76, 125

American Journal of Sociology, 94

American Medical Association (AMA): apology to African Americans by, 198; collaboration with NMA, 199–200; medical racism research by, 37–41; racist exclusionary policies of, 3–7, 27, 232–33, 235n.5

American Nervousness, 114

American Psychiatric Association, Task Force on Cultural and Ethnic Issues in Psychiatry, 168

American Public Health Association, 23–24

American Social Hygiene Association, 26

Andy, Orlando J., 191

anesthesia: loss of consciousness and, racial stereotypes concerning, 89–92; nervous system in black patients, racial interpretations of, 93–97

"Angina Pectoris in the Negro," 93

Annals of Internal Medicine, 42, 59–60

anthropological research: black dental health and disease in, racial interpretations of, 111–12; *Drylongso* testimonies and, 179–80; loss of consciousness, racial stereotypes concerning, 88–92; medical racism and, 66–70; nervous system in black patients, racial interpretations of, 92–97; organ systems and disorders, racialized interpretations based on, 106–30; racial stereotypes and fantasies and, 55–66

antipsychotic drugs, racial pharmacology and, 133–39, 192–93

Archer, William (Reyn) III, 55–56, 58

Archives of Pediatrics, 75–77

Association of American Medical Colleges, 212, 214

athletics. *See* black athletes

attention deficit/hyperactivity disorder (ADHD), racial pharmacology and, 133, 192

Austin, Paul, 7

avoidance of racism, 3–7

Baldwin, James, 5, 151

Baldwin, Kenneth, 39

Beard, George, 114

behavioral control, racial pharmacology and, 132–39

behavior patterns in physicians: aversion to race issues and, 204–7; evidence of medical racism in, 32–37; "halo effect" and, 8–11; judgments about, 7–8; medical literature on, 41–52; privacy issues and, 8–11, 52–55; problem patients and, 202–4; racialized differences in, 62–66; racial obstetrics and gynecology and, 139–40; resistance to charges of racism in, 47–52

"Behavior Problems in Negro Children," 88

Bell, Carl C., 125, 185–87, 224

Bell Curve, The, 58

Bennett, William J., 57, 68

Berger, Maurice, 4–5

beta-blockers, racial pharmacology in use of, 135–39

Better Babies Contests, 74

BiDil medication, FDA approval of, for African American patients, 136–39, 232

Biology of the Negro, The (Lewis), 89

biomedical ethics: cultural competence and, 208–9, 212–16; resistance to medical racism critiques and, 38–41

bio-underclass concept, racial interpretations of black infants and children and, 81

bipolar disorder: emotional hardiness myth and, 127–30; racial stereotypes concerning, 93–97 birth control: conspiracy theories concerning, 194–97; racialized stereotypes concerning black sexuality and fertility and, 144–45

"Birth of a Nation" (film), 179

black athletes: racial interpretations concerning, 83–85; racial pharmacology and, 138–39

blackface, African American racial defamation and, 33–37

black "hardiness." *See* medical "hardiness" doctrine

black image, Africanization of, 154–58

black intellectualism, 153–54, 173–76

Black Panther Party, 124

black physicians: history of education and training of, 230–33; invisibility in medical literature of, 199–200; marginalization of, 28–32, 232–33; medical education curriculum and involvement of, 217–21

Black Power movement, 153, 176

Black Power: The Politics of Liberation in America (Carmichael), 153

black psychiatry: colonialism and, 194–97; evolution of, 176–93; race syllabus and influence of, 210–12

Black Rage (Grier and Cobbs), 173–74

Black Scholar, The, 80–81

Black Skin, White Masks (Fanon), 72–73, 111, 146

black women: anthropological stereotypes concerning, 55–57; dental health and disease in, racial interpretations of, 110–11; emotional hardiness myth and, 129–30; racial interpretations of disease in, 114–20; racial obstetrics and gynecology medicine and, 139–45; therapeutic fatalism and misdiagnoses of, 222–24; white physicians' attitudes concerning, 64

Bloche, M. Gregg, 39–41, 50

blood composition, racial differences in, 249n.66

"Blood Expert Says Transfusion Between Races May Be Perilous," 60

Bloom, Samuel L., 208

Blues People (Jones), 184

body odor, racial interpretations concerning, 110

Bonhomme, Jean, 124–25

Briggs, Laura, 114

British Journal of Psychiatry, 179, 191

British Medical Journal, 77, 112–13, 140–41, 191

Brown, Roscoe C., 26

Buchanan, Patrick, 68

Buffett, Warren, 230

Bunche, Ralph, 4

Bush, George W., 55

Byrd, W. Michael, 231

Calloway, N. O., 123

cancer: racial disparities in treatment of, 35–37; racial stereotypes concerning, 61–62, 113–20; therapeutic fatalism and misdiagnoses of African Americans and, 223–24

cardiology: heart disease in black patients, racial interpretations of, 97–106; history of medical racism in, 218–21; loss of consciousness and, racial stereotypes concerning, 89–92; racial bias in practice of, 12, 23–24, 47–48, 65–66

Carmichael, Stokely, 153

Carothers, J. C., 86–87

Carter, James H.: on black elderly patients, 82; on black hardiness stereotype, 126; on black psychiatry, 182, 184, 190–92; on oppression, 175; on pathological ideology, 168; on racial steretypes about time, 104

Carter, Jimmy, 68

Cartwright, Samuel, 88, 92, 112, 131

CBS Evening News, 78–79

Characteristics of the American Negro (Klineberg), 184

Chase, Carolyn, 180

Chasnoff, Ira J., 78–79

childbirth. *See* obstetrics and gynecology

cholesterol levels in black patients, racial interpretations of heart disease and, 101–6

chronic fatigue syndrome (CFS), racial interpretations of, 117–19
Chronicle of Higher Education, 44
civil rights movement: black physicians' participation in, 28–32; influence on psychiatry of, 167; medical racism and, 196–97
Clark, Kenneth B.: on African American health care disparities, 4, 111; as black intellectual, 173–75; on black psychiatry, 188–89; on conspiracy theories of African Americans, 195; on "internal colonialism" of African Americans, 153, 169–70
class status: black psychiatry and role of, 181–93; "internal colonialism" and, 148–54; misdiagnoses and therapeutic fatalism and, 222–24; racial interpretations of disease and, 112–20
Clayton, Linda A., 231
Cobb, W. Montague, 122
Cobbs, Price M., 153–54, 169–76
"Cocaine Use in Pregnancy," 78–79
cognitive function, loss of consciousness, racial stereotypes concerning, 87–92
colonialism: African American medical status and, 193–97; Africanization of the black image and, 154–58; black psychiatry and, 177–93; heart disease in black patients, racial interpretations based on, 104–6; "internal colonialism" and medical apartheid, 148–54; medical humanities curriculum discussion of, 227; medical science and, 69–70; nervous system in black patients, racial interpretations of, 94–97; racial obstetrics and gynecology and, 142–45; racial primitive in psychiatry and, 160–76
"Colored People's Time." *See* time, racial stereotypes concerning perceptions of
Color Purple, The (Walker), 76, 112
"Committee on the Negro," 195

Committee on Understanding and Eliminating Racial and Ethnic Disparities in Health Care, 16
Committee on Urban Conditions among Negroes, 64
complexity principle, racialization of medicine and, 224–25
consciousness, loss of: racial interpretations of, 87–92; racial pharmacology and, 131–39
conservatism: colonial medicine and, 196–97; denial of medical racism and, 14–16, 39–41
conspiracy theories: medical colonialism and, 193–97; therapeutic fatalism and misdiagnoses and, 224
Cornely, Paul B., 26–28
"crack babies," stereotypes and fantasies concerning, 57, 78–81
crime: incarceration of African Americans and, 147–54, 190–91; stereotypes of African Americans and, 55–57, 68, 81
Crisis in Black and White (Silberman), 151, 176
Crisis of the Negro Intellectual, The (Cruse), 153
crossover effect, in black elderly patients, 82–83
Crouch, Stanley, 184
Cruse, Harold, 153
cultural competence: black physicians' involvement in, 233; curriculum development for, 218–21; history of racism as part of, 230–33; knowledge of stereotypes and, 224–26; race syllabus in medical education and development of, 207–12; racially different versions of, 212–16
"Cultural Competence Education," 214–16
cultural relativism, black psychiatry and, 185–93
Cunningham, Velma, 180

Dalton, Harlon, 162
Dark Ghetto (Clark), 4, 173, 188–89

Darwinian fitness, racial interpretations of black infants and children and, 74–81
Davenport, Charles B., 74, 109–10, 121
Davis, Ronald M., 198–200
De Kruif, Paul, 141
Delany, Martin, 123
dentistry: racial folklore in, 67–68; racial interpretations of human teeth and, 110–12
depression. *See also* psychiatry and psychology: African American stoic approach to, 30–32; emotional hardiness myth and, 125–30; loss of consciousness and, racial stereotypes concerning, 89–92; racial pharmacology in treatment of, 134–39
Devereux, George, 6, 63
diabetes mellitus, racial interpretations of disease and, 113–20
diagnostic habits: misdiagnoses and therapeutic fatalism and, 222–24; racial stereotypes and, 59–66
DiIulio, John J., 81
"Dimensions of Institutional Racism in Psychiatry" (Sabshin), 168–70, 173–74
diseases and disorders. *See also* specific diseases and disorders: black "hardiness" concept and, 120–21; racialized identification of human types and traits and, 71, 106–30; racial stereotypes concerning incidence and prevalence of, 61–63; "white" *vs.* "black" disorders, racial interpretations of, 112–20
doctor-patient relationship: cultural competence and, 208–10; development of cultural competence and, 207–12; medical racism and, 198–200; problem patient and, 202–4; race syllabus in medical education for, 200–202; racism's impact on, 5–6, 51–52
"Doctors Have Feelings Too" (Zinn), 203, 206
Doctors Talk About Themselves, 7

dream analysis, racialized interpretations in, 163
Drossman, Douglas A., 202–4
drug effects: loss of consciousness and, racial stereotypes concerning, 88–92; neurohormonal antagonists, impact on black patients of, 96–97; pain sensitivity in black patients, racial interpretations of, 97–98; racial folklore and genetics in pharmacology and, 130–39; racial stereotypes concerning, 55–57, 65–66, 260n.296; therapeutic fatalism, misdiagnoses and race and, 222–24
Drylongso: A Self-Portrait of Black America, 30, 123–24, 179–80
DuBois, W. E. B., 86–87, 88
dyspepsia, racial interpretations of, 112

eating disorders, racial interpretations of, 115–16
Ebony magazine, 101
economic status: black psychiatry and role of, 181–82; racial interpretations of disease and, 112–20
Edwards, Christopher L., 106
"Effect of Race and Sex on Physicians' Recommendations for Cardiac Catheterization, The," 47–48
Eisenberg, John, 42–43
elderly black patients, racial interpretations of, 81–83
Elkins, Stanley, 73
Ellison, Ralph, 153
emergency room analgesia, racial disparities in management of, 35–37, 65–66
emotional excitability: nervous system in black patients, racial interpretations of, 94–97; racialized psychiatric assessment and, 165–66
emotional hardiness, racial stereotype of, 125–30
endometriosis: racial interpretations of, 114–15; racial obstetrics and gynecology and treatment of, 140–45

Epstein, Arnold, 198–99
Erikson, Erik H., 73
ethics. *See* biomedical ethics
eugenics: African American medical
vulnerability and, 30–32; black skin
health and disease, racial interpretations based on, 109–10; racial
interpretations of black infants and
children and, 74–81
evasion concerning racism, 3–7
evolutionary theory: Africanization
of the black image and, 157–58;
medical racism and, 66–70; racial
interpretations of black infants and
children and, 75–81
examination procedures, racialized
behavior concerning, 62–63
extinction theory: African American
medical vulnerability and predictions of, 25–32; "crack" baby crisis
and, 79–81
eyes and vision disorders, racial
interpretations of, 107–9

families of African Americans: black
psychiatry and, 183–93; "internal
colonialism" and pathologization
of, 153–54, 169–76; stereotypes
concerning, 78–81
Fanon, Frantz, 72–73, 75, 111, 146,
158, 176–77, 193
Farmer, James, 171, 196
fenfluramine experiments, 191–92;
on relatives of juvenile delinquents,
54–55
fibromyalgia (FMS), racial
interpretations of, 117–19
*Flexner Report on Medical Education
in the United States and Canada,
The*, 230–31
Foe, Marc-Vivien, 85
folkloric beliefs, racial interpretations based on: about black athletes,
83–85; about black elderly patients,
82–83; black infants and children
and, 71–81; black psychiatry and,
183–93; emotional hardiness myth
and, 125–30; generation of racial

stereotypes from, 57–66; heart
disease in black patients, 97–106;
human organs and disorders and,
106–30; knowledge of, cultural
competence and, 224–26; loss of
consciousness in black patients,
stereotypes concerning, 85–92; in
medical specialties, 130–45; obstetrics and gynecology and, 139–45;
physical hardiness myth and,
121–25; psychiatry and, 165–76;
racialized medicine and, 66–70,
224–25; therapeutic fatalism and
misdiagnoses and, 223–24
Frank, Jerome D., 164–65
Franks, Ronald, 207–8
Frazier, E. Franklin, 150
Freud, Sigmund, 182
"Full-Blood American Negro, The"
(Hrdlicka), 150

Gaffney, Kathleen, 53
Garvin, Charles H., 113, 122
Gaston, Robert (Dr.), 49–50
Geiger, H. Jack, 1, 13, 17, 34, 44, 209
general population, racial beliefs in,
12–14
genetic hypothesis: racial interpretations of heart disease and, 101–6;
racial pharmacology and, 130–39
"Genetics and 'Race' in *The Merchant
of Venice*", 227
George, Theodore R., 108
Gerbert, Barbara, 201–2
ghetto environment: black psychiatry
and, 185–93; "internal colonialism"
and medical apartheid and, 148–54;
medical practice in, 7; psychiatric
analysis of, 168–76; riots of 1960s
and, 191; sleep patterns and, racial
stereotypes concerning, 90–92
Gillum, Richard F., 101
Gilroy, Paul, 158
"gland theory," nervous system in
black patients, racial interpretations
of, 94–97
glaucoma in black patients, racial
interpretation of, 107–9

"Glaucoma in the Negro," 107–8
Goodwin, Frederick K., 68
Gorlin, Richard, 202–4
Graham, George E., 84
Gregory, Dick, 194
Grier, William H., 153–54, 169–76, 181
Groopman, Jerome, 7, 16–17, 118, 229
Groves, James E., 202–5
Gullattee, Alyce, C., 125, 176, 196
Gwaltmey, Judith, 59
Gwaltney, John Langston, 30, 180, 193–94

Hacker, Andrew, 147
Hafferty, Frederic W., 207–8
hallucinations: black psychiatry and role of, 187–93; racial pharmacology and, 131–39; racial stereotypes concerning, 87–92
"halo effect," medical racism and, 8–11, 14
Hannan, Ed, 49–50
hard labor: black skin health and disease and, racial interpretations concerning, 110; disease and disorders, racial interpretations of, 112–20; heart disease in black patients, racial interpretations of, 99–106; medical racism concerning, 159–60
Havranek, Edward, 102–3
Hawthorne, Nathaniel, 228
Health Affairs journal, 19
Health and Human Services, Department of, 68; medical racism research by, 37–41
Health and Physique of the Negro American (Du Bois), 86–87
health care disparities of African Americans, 4–7, 24–32
heart disease in black patients: in black athletes, stereotypes concerning, 85; in black infants and children, 73; nervous system and pain awareness, racial stereotypes concerning, 93–97; racial disparities in treatment of, 12, 23–24, 34–37, 47–48, 65–66, 97–106; racial interpretations of, 113–20; racial pharmacology in

management of, 136–39; stereotypes of black musical aptitude and, 86–87
Henderson, L. J., 200
Hingson, Robert A., 20, 95, 97
Hispanic patients: pain sensitivity and, racial interpretations of, 98; racial disparities in management of, 35–37
history of medical racism, 16–17; absence in medical literature of, 42–52; in medical education curriculum, 217–21, 230–33
Hoffman, Frederick L., 25, 73, 80, 121–22
homosexuality among African Americans, emotional hardiness myth and, 128–30
hormone replacement therapy, racial interpretations in use of, 115
House, Robert E., 131–32
How Doctors Think (Groopman), 7, 16–17, 229
Howe, Irving, 197
Howell, Mary C., 210
"How Much Can We Boost I.Q. and Scholastic Achievement?", 74
Hrdlicka, Alex, 73, 150
Hughes, Langston, 88
human types and traits, racial interpretations of, 71–106
Hunt, James, 66–69, 74, 92
hyperfertility, racial stereotypes concerning, 144–45
hypertension: incidence in black patients of, 95–97, 113–20; racial disparities in treatment of, 65–66; racial pharmacology in management of, 135–39
hypnosis, loss of consciousness and, racial stereotypes concerning, 90–92
hypochondria, racial interpretations of, 119–20

incarceration of African Americans: black psychiatry and, 190–91; "internal colonialism" and medical apartheid and, 147–54
infants and children, racial interpretations of, 71–81

insomnia, incidence in African
Americans of, 90–92
Institute of Medicine, 214–16
intelligence: loss of consciousness,
racial stereotypes concerning,
87–92; nervous system in black
patients, racial interpretations of,
92–97; psychiatry as medical racism and, 159–60; racial stereotypes
concerning, 57–59, 73–74
"internal colonialism": African
American health crisis and, 146–54;
Africanization of the black image
and, 154–58; black psychiatry and,
176–93; racialized physicality of
African Americans and, 158–60; racial
primitive in psychiatry and, 160–76
isolated sleep paralysis, incidence in
African Americans of, 90–92

James, Sherman A., 105
Jefferson, Thomas, 88
Jenkins, Sidney B., 175
Jensen, Arthur C., 74
"John Henryism" coping style, 105–6
Johnson, James Weldon, 86–87
Johnson, Lyndon, 169
Jones, LeRoi, 76, 184
Journal of Biological Chemistry, 83–84
*Journal of the American Medical
Association* (JAMA): on African
American health crisis, 19–21;
African American homosexuality
discussed in, 129; aversion to race
issues in articles of, 206–7; on black
dental health and disease, 110–11;
black elderly patients in, 83; black
infants and children, racial interpretations of, 73–74, 77; black skin health
and disease, racial interpretations of,
110; "crack" baby coverage in, 79–80;
heart disease in black patients, racial
interpretations of, 99; "internal colonialism" and medical apartheid discussed in, 148–49; nervous system in
black patients, racial interpretations
of, 93; psychiatry as medical racism
in, 159–60; racial folklore in, 67;

racial obstetrics and gynecology
discussed in, 139–40; racial pharmacology discussed in, 137–39; on racial
stereotyping of patients, 61; racism in
articles in, 3, 6–7, 42, 50–51; stereotypes of black musical aptitude in, 87;
urban violence discussed in, 191
Journal of the Medical Humanities,
227–28
*Journal of the Michigan State Medical
Society,* 67
*Journal of the National Medical
Association:* African American vision
disorders discussed in, 108–9; black
psychiatry discussed in, 190; medical
racism discussed in, 42–43, 199–200;
racial interpretation of disease
discussed in, 114–15; stereotypes and
misdiagnoses discussed in, 60

Kardiner, Abram, 175–76
Katz, Jeffrey N., 49–50
Kelley, Robin D. G., 154
King, Martin Luther Jr., 27, 55,
154, 175, 209
Kleinman, Arthur, 228–29
Klineberg, Otto, 184
Krauthammer, Charles, 57

Lancet, The, 81, 84–85, 95, 121
Lawrence, Francis, 57–58, 68
Lee, Spike, 182
Levy, David: doctors' recognition of
their negative racial attitudes,
51–52; on medical racism, 5–6,
42–43, 45–46; on misdiagnoses
and therapeutic fatalism, 222–23;
on problem patients, 204; on racial
folkloric beliefs, 63
Lewis, Julian H., 89
liberalism: in American psychiatry,
165–76; aversion to race issues
in medical literature and, 204–7;
medical literature and, 41–52,
237n.49; in medical profession,
14–17; medical racism research
and, 38–41; race syllabus in medical
education and role of, 230–23

Lincoln, C. Eric, 155
Lincoln, Mabel, 180
Literature and Medicine journal, 227
longevity: African American disparities in, 19; of black elderly patients, 82–83; physical hardiness myth and, 123–25
Losing Ground (Murray), 196
lung cancer, racial disparities in treatment of, 35–37
Lurie, Louis, 128

Making of the President, 1960, The (White), 155–56
Malcolm X, 27
Mark, Vernon, 191
Mark of Oppression, The (Kardiner and Ovesey), 175–76, 195–96
Maugham, Somerset, 226
Mbeki, Thabo, 195
media coverage of African American health issues: Africanization of black image and, 155–58; black psychiatry and, 179; "crack" baby story and, 78–80; racial health disparities coverage, 49–52
medical apartheid: black psychiatry and, 182–93; "internal colonialism" and, 147–54
medical education: beliefs about racial differences in curriculum for, 216–17; curriculum development on race in, 217–21, 229–33; denigration of black medical students in, 230–33; development of cultural competence in, 207–12; hidden curriculum, 16–17; marginalization of black physicians in, 28–32; raceless humanism in, 226–29; race syllabus for, 198–233; racial folkloric beliefs and, 59; racial integration of, 230–31; racially different versions of cultural competence and, 212–16; racism in, 12, 15
medical "hardiness" doctrine: black athletes' pain and injury and, 84–85; black "hardiness" concept and, 120–21, 224–25; emergency room analgesia management and, 35–37, 65–66; emotional hardiness

stereotype and, 125–30; heart disease in black patients, racial interpretations of, 99–106; nervous system in black patients, racial interpretations of, 93–97; obstetrics and gynecology medicine and, 139–45; physical hardiness myths and, 121–25
medical humanities curriculum, evasion of difference and, 226–29
medical literature: absence of black physicians in, 199; absence of social activism in, 277n.108; aversion to race issues in, 199, 204–7; doctor-patient relationship discussed in, 200–201; heart disease in black patients, differing racial interpretations of, 100–106; liberalism and, 41–52; problem patient discussed in, 202–4
medical racism: avoidance and evasion concerning, 3–7; evidence of, 32–37; folkloric beliefs and, 58–66; liberals and, 14–17; medical humanities curriculum discussion of, 227–29; medical liberals, 14–17; oral tradition in medical training and, 11–12; origins and consequences, 1–3; pervasiveness of, 12–14; physician behavior and, 7–8; practical advice concerning, 221–22; privacy issues and, 52–55; in psychiatry, 158–60; racial folklore and, 66–70; resistance to critiques of, 37–41; silence surrounding, 18–24, 198–99
medical research, absence of critique of medical racism in, 42–52
medical specialties. See also specific specialties: racial folklore in, 130–45
medical students: abortion training for, 229–33; behavior toward African American patients of, 62–63; development of cultural competence and, 207–12; discrimination against black medical students, 230–33; evidence of medical racism in, 33–37; history of medical racism for, 218–21; medical students, abuse of, 273n.43; medical students, female, exclusion of, 210; race syllabus for, 198–233; racism among, 12, 15

Medical Students for Choice, 229–33
Meharry Medical College, 29, 199, 222
Mengert, William F., 60, 114, 143
menopause, racial interpretations
of, 115
mental illness. See psychiatry and
psychology
"Mental Illness among Negro Troops
Overseas," 162–63
Metzl, Jonathan M., 216
micro-aggressions: African American
experience of, 56; black psychiatry
and role of, 181–82
Miller, Jerome G., 191
Millington, Porter, 180
Million Man March, 18
misdiagnoses, race and class and,
222–24
Mis-Education of the Negro, The
(Woodson), 149–50
misogyny, in medical practice, 210–12
Mississippi Medical Monthly, 22
Morrison, Toni, 227
Moynihan, Daniel Patrick, 57, 81,
153–54, 169–74
Moynihan Report. See Negro Family:
A Case for National Action, The
(Moynihan Report)
Murray, Albert, 153
Murray, Charles, 196
musical aptitude, racial interpretations
of, 85–87
myopia in black patients, racial
interpretations of, 108–9, 112
Myrdal, Gunnar, 4, 65, 161

narrative medicine, in medical
education, 228
National Abortion Federation, 230
National Academies' Institute of
Medicine, 37–41
National Association for the Advance-
ment of Colored People (NAACP),
169–70
National Black Men's Health
Network, 124
National Health Disparities Report
(NHDR), 37–41

National Medical Association, 27,
199–200
National Negro Health Week, 74,
112, 122
National Research Council, 195
Negro Family: A Case for National
Action, The (Moynihan Report),
153–54, 169–74, 185–86, 197
"Negro Patient in Psychiatric
Treatment, The," 166
Nelson, Alan (Dr.), 15–16
"Nervous and Mental Influences in
Angina Pectoris," 86–87
nervous system in black patients,
racial interpretations of, 92–97
neurohormonal antagonists, impact on
black patients of, 96–97, 135–39
neurohormonal doctrine, nervous
system in black patients, racial
interpretation of, 94–97
neurology, nervous system in black
patients, racial interpretations of,
92–97
New England Journal of Medicine, 34,
47–48, 79; doctor-patient relationship
discussed in, 200–201; mandatory
testing for sickle cell disease in,
156–57; racial pharmacology
discussed in, 96–97, 136–37
New Negro movement, 178
New Republic, The, 165
Newsday, 49–50
Newsweek magazine, 27, 55, 61, 209
Newton, Huey P., 124
New Yorker magazine, 182
New York Times, 55–57, 60
Notes on the State of Virginia
(Jefferson), 88
Novack, Dennis H., 203–4
Nuland, Sherwin, 9, 241n. 81

Obama, Barack, 155
obesity, racial interpretations of, 116–20
obsessive-compulsive personality
disorder (OCPD), racial interpretations of, 127–30
obstetrics and gynecology: black
infants and children, racial

interpretations of health of, 72–81; physical hardiness myth and, 121–25; racial folklore in, 139–45; racial stereotypes in practice of, 60, 67–70, 114–20

obstructive sleep apnea (OSA), incidence in African Americans of, 90–92

Oedipus complex, African American view of, 181

Of Human Bondage (Maugham), 226

Oldham, John, 192

Oliver, John, 180

"On the Negro's Place in Nature" (Hunt), 66–67, 92

opinion surveys, medical racism research and, 53–55

oral tradition, racial beliefs and, 11–12

organ systems, racial interpretations of, 106–30

out-of-wedlock births, racial stereotypes concerning, 57

overmedication, racial pharmacology and, 133–39, 192–93

Ovesey, Lionel, 175–76

Owens, Jesse, 83–84

Oxford Handbook of Bioethics, The, 39

pain sensitivity in black patients: in black athletes, racial interpretations of, 84–85; emergency room analgesia management and, 35–37, 65–66; glaucoma surgery and, 107; nervous system in black patients, racial interpretations of, 93–97; racial interpretations of, 97–98

Papper, Solomon, 203

paternalism, racial interpretations of black infants and children and, 74–81

pathological ideology, medical racism and use of, 168–76

"patient preferences" paradigm, medical racism and, 50–52

patient's racial identification, clinical practice and assumptions linked to, 59–60

patients rights, black psychiatry and, 184–93

Patterson, Orlando, 6–7, 147

Pauling, Linus, 157

Peabody, Francis W., 226

pediatric medicine: racial interpretations of black infants and children and, 71–81

Pediatrics journal, 42–43, 63, 148

pelvic inflammatory disease (PID), racial interpretations of, 115, 143

pelvic measurements, racial obstetrics and gynecology and, 141–45

"Personal Awareness and Effective Patient Care," 206–7

personality traits: cultural competence and knowledge of stereotypes concerning, 224–26; emotional hardiness myth and, 127–30; heart disease in black patients, racial interpretations based on, 103–6; racial interpretations of, 73

Pettigrew, Thomas F., 151

pharmacology, racial folklore and genetics in, 130–39

Phillips, U. B., 74

physical hardiness myth, medical "hardiness" doctrine and, 121–25

"Physician and Patient as a Social System" (Henderson), 200

"Physicians' Beliefs about Racial Differences in Referral for Renal Transplantation," 217

physiology: of black athletes, stereotypes concerning, 83–85; of elderly black patients, 81–83; heart disease in black patients, racial interpretations of, 99–106; nervous system in black patients, racial interpretations of, 92–97; organ systems and disorders, racial interpretations of, 106–30; physical hardiness myth and, 121–25; psychiatry as medical racism and, 158–60; racial interpretations of black infants and children and, 72–81; racial pharmacology and, 137–39; racial stereotypes concerning, 55–57, 65–66, 69–70

Pierce, Chester M., 90–92, 123, 181–83, 196

290 / Index

Pinderhughes, Charles A., 174–75
Pollack, Seymour L., 191
"Poor White Musician, The"
    (Johnson), 86–87
Potts, James L., 199
Poussaint, Alvin, 128, 174–75
poverty: African American vulner-
    ability and, 20–21, 29–32; disease
    and disorders, racial interpretations
    of, 112–20; racial interpretations
    of black infants and children and,
    74–81; therapeutic fatalism, misdi-
    agnoses and race and, 222–24
precocity: racial interpretations of
    black musical aptitude and, 85–87;
    racial stereotypes concerning
    intelligence and, 74
pregnancy and delivery. See obstetrics
    and gynecology
prenatal development, racial interpre-
    tations of black infants and children
    and, 72–81
primitivism: "internal colonialism,"
    152; racial primitive in psychiatry
    and, 160–76
Principles of Biomedical Ethics
    (Beauchamp and Childress), 38–39
privacy issues: "halo effect" in, 8–11;
    mandatory sickle cell anemia testing
    and, 156–57; medical racism and,
    52–55
problem patient: race syllabus
    concerning, 202–4; racial
    interpretations of, 204–7
Proctor, Malcolm, 108
professional conduct: judgment
    concerning, 7–8; privacy and
    "halo effect" and, 8–11
"protective factors" hypothesis, racial
    interpretations of heart disease and,
    99–106
"Psychiatrist's Role in Dealing with
    Social Turmoil," 167
psychiatry and psychology: African
    American military service in Second
    World War and, 162-165; African
    American patients and, 31–32,
    61–62, 67–70; in black elderly

patients, 83; black psychiatry and,
    176–93; emotional hardiness myth
    and, 125–30; "internal colonialism"
    and, 146–54; loss of consciousness,
    racial stereotypes concerning, 87–92;
    medical humanities curriculum and,
    227–28; nervous system in black
    patients, racial interpretations of,
    92–97; physical hardiness myth and,
    123–25; problem patient and role
    of, 203–4; racial interpretations of
    disease and, 113–20; racialized inter-
    pretations of black children and, 73,
    77; as racial medicine, 158–60; racial
    pharmacology and, 131–39; racial
    primitive in, 160–76; stereotypes of
    black musical aptitude and, 86–87
Psychiatry journal, 67
Psychoanalytic Review, The, 160, 179
public health statistics: on African
    American health crisis, 19–20;
    "internal colonialism" and medi-
    cal apartheid and, 148–54; racial
    interpretations of black infants and
    children and, 72–81

"Race and Health Care—An American
    Dilemma?" (Geiger), 44
"Race and Sport in African-American
    Life," 84–85
raceless humanism, in race syllabus,
    226–29
race syllabus for medical education,
    198–233; aversion to race issues in
    medical literature and, 204–7; beliefs
    about racial differences in, 216–17;
    curriculum changes and, 229–33;
    development of cultural competence
    and, 207–12; doctor-patient relation-
    ship in, 200–202; ethics education in,
    208–9; history of medical racism in,
    217–21; knowledge of stereotypes
    and, 224–26; problem patient in,
    202–4; raceless humanism in,
    226–29; two different official ver-
    sions of cultural competence and,
    212–16; therapeutic fatalism, misdi-
    agnoses and social class in, 222–24

Race Traits and Tendencies of the American Negro (Hoffman), 25, 73
"Racial Aspects of Emotional Problems of Negro Soldiers" (Stevens), 162
"Racial Contrasts in Obstetrics and Gynecology" (Mengert), 60
racial defamation, African American medical vulnerability and, 24–32
"Racial Disparity in Rates of Surgery for Lung Cancer," 44
racialization. *See also* stereotypes: Africanization of black images and, 156–58; in psychiatry, 168–76; "white" vs. "black" disease and, 66–70, 112–20, 224–25
Racism and Psychiatry (Thomas and Sillen), 196–97
"Racist Doctors? Don't Believe the Media Hype," 16
Rainwater, Lee, 119–20
"Rectal Pathology in the Negro," 61
renal disease, racial disparities in treatment of, 48–52, 217
Report of the Secretary's Task Force on Black and Minority Health (HHS), 37–41
reproductive disorders, racial interpretations of, 114–20
Richardson, Susan, 56
Ripley, Herbert S., 162
Ritalin, racial pharmacology and administration of, 133, 137
Roberts, Dorothy, 52, 79, 147
Robinson, Jackie, 233
"Role of Brain Disease in Riots and Urban Violence" (Mark), 191
Roth, Byron M., 14
Rustin, Bayard, 154
Ryan, William, 154

Sabshin, Melvin, 168–70, 174, 191
Sandell, D. H., 178
Satcher, David, 5–6, 42–43, 64, 139–40
Satel, Sally, 14, 16, 40–41, 242n.81
SAT scores, racial stereotypes concerning, 57
Saunders, Elijah, 136

Schuyler, George, 31–32, 123, 178–79, 181
Schweitzer, Albert, 77, 165
Science magazine, 92
scopolamine trial, racial pharmacology and history of, 131–32
Second World War, African American military service in, 162–76
segregation, impact on American medicine of, 6–7
self-analysis: aversion to race issues and, 206–7; doctor-patient relationship, 201–2
sensuality and sexuality: emotional hardiness myth and, 128–30; racialized stereotypes concerning, 55–57, 64, 73, 144–45; syphilis-related blindness, racial stereotypes concerning, 108–9
Sharpton, Al, 32
Shays, Ruth, 179–80
sickle-cell anemia: mandatory testing for, 80–81, 156–57; patient's racial identification and, 59–60
Sickle Cell Anemia Control Act, 80–81
Silberman, Charles, 151, 176
Sillen, Samuel, 196
skin and skin disorders, racial interpretations of, 109–10
"Slave on the Block" (Hughes), 88
slavery: African American medical vulnerability and, 25–32; nervous system in black patients linked to, 95–96; physical hardiness myth and, 121–25; psychological impact of, 73; racial obstetrics and gynecology and, 142–45
sleep disordered breathing (SDB), incidence in African Americans of, 90–92
sleep patterns in black patients: racial pharmacology and, 131–39; racial stereotypes concerning, 88–92
Smith, Grant, 180
social activism, absence in medical literature of, 277n.108

social Darwinism, African American medical vulnerability and, 25–32

social history, absence of critique of medical racism in, 44–52

social science research: lack of interest in medical racism and, 54–55; racial attitudes of citizens and, 12–14; racialization of psychiatry and, 169–76

"Sociologic Influences on Decision-Making by Clinicians" (Eisenberg), 42–43

Something for the Pain (Austin), 7

South Africa, conspiracy theories concerning AIDS in, 194–97

South African Medical Journal, 92–93, 99

Southern Medical Journal, 25, 76, 88, 92, 110, 112, 161, 178

Steggerda, Morris, 74

Steinauer, Jody, 229–33

stereotypes: of African American patients, 22–24; amateur anthropology and perpetuation of, 55–66; of black infants and children, 71–81; black psychiatry and, 178–93; of black teeth, 110–12; cultural competence and knowledge of, 224–26; racialization of American psychiatry and, 168–76; racial pharmacology and, 138–39; racism in medicine based on, 5–7; in whites' perceptions of African Americans, 53–55

Stevens, Rutherford B., 161–64, 187

stoicism of African American patients, 31–32. See also medical "hardiness" doctrine; emotional hardiness myth and, 126–30; nervous system in black patients, racial interpretations of, 93–97; pain sensitivity and, racial interpretations of, 97–98; physical hardiness myth and, 121–25; racial obstetrics and gynecology and, 141–45

Stone, I. F., 153–54

superlongevity phenomenon, in black elderly patients, 82–83

surgery, African American patients' fears of, 47–48

Surry, Ellen Turner, 124, 180

"survival of the fittest" ideology: physical hardiness myth and, 123–25; racial interpretations of black infants and children and, 74–81

syphilis: Africanization of the black image and racialization of, 156–58; blindness from, racial interpretations of, 107–9; medical humanities curriculum, 228; racial stereotypes about African American patients and, 25–32, 61, 64–65

"Taking Care of the Hateful Patient" (Groves), 202–4

Tarzan of the Apes, 151

"Teaching Cultural Competence in Health Care: A Review of Current Concepts, Policies and Practices," 212–16

teeth and dental disorders: folkloric stereotypes concerning, 67–68; racial interpretations of, 110–12

Textbook of Black-Related Diseases, 143

therapeutic fatalism, misdiagnoses and, 222–24

Thomas, Alexander, 196

Thompson, Tommy, 39–41

time, racial stereotypes concerning perceptions of: black psychiatry and, 184–93; heart disease in black patients linked to, 104–6

Time magazine, 6, 28, 74, 128, 165, 189–90

Tool for Assessing Cultural Competence Training, 214–16

Transactions of the American Gynecological Society, 67, 159

transfusion procedures, racial stereotypes concerning, 60

transplant technology, African American fear of, 49–50

traumatized black children, racialized images of, 74–76

tricyclic antidepressants, racial pharmacology in use of, 134–39
tuberculosis: racial defamation of African American patie[n]... 25–32; racial pharmacol[ogy] treatment of, 137–39
Tuskegee Syphilis Experi[ment], 43–44, 228
Two Nations: Black and ... *rate, Hostile, Unequal* (Ha... type A/type B personality dich..., emotional hardiness myth and, 128–30; heart disease in black patients, racial interpretations based on, 103–6

UCLA Law Review, 157
undermedication, racial pharmacology and, 133–39
Unequal Treatment: Confronting Racial and Ethnic Disparities in Health Care, 14–15, 214–16
UNESCO Statement on Race, 138
Urban League: African American medical vulnerability and, 26; on stereotypes about syphilis in African Americans, 64–65
urban poverty, African American health crisis and, 20–21, 29–32

Venable, H. Phillip, 107
violence: black psychiatry and, 191–93; racial interpretations of eye injuries and stereotypes concerning, 108–9; racial pharmacology and, 132–39; white stereotypes of African Americans and, 54–55, 68–69
Violence and the Brain (Mark), 191
Violence Initiative, 68–69
vision. *See* eyes and vision disorders
Vonderlehr, R. A., 22–23

Walker, Alice, 76, 112
Wall Street Journal, The, 16
Walters, Ronald, 69, 192
Ward, Benjamin, 152

Washington, Book... –12
Wear, Delese, 27...
Wertham, Fr[edric]...
...56
...ck Patients"
...
...[ph]ys[ici]ans: African American ...[t]rust of, 180–93; awareness of ...[m]edical racism among, 7–8, 32–37; [b]lack psychiatry and role of, 181–93; conspiracy theories concerning, 194–97; development of cultural competence in, 207–12; "internal colonialism" and, 147–54; lack of cultural competence among, 209–10; physical hardiness myth and, 121–25; practical advice for, 221–22; psychiatry as medical racism and, 158–60, 162–76; racial attitudes of, 200, 204–7, 216–17; racial obstetrics and gynecology and, 139–40; racial stereotypes and fantasies of, 55–66; racism in medical literature and, 51–52, 204–7; therapeutic fatalism and misdiagnoses by, 222–24
white women: racial interpretations of disease in, 114–20; racial obstetrics and gynecology and, 140–45
Whitten, Charles F., 80–81, 156–57
Williams, Reginald, 152
Williams, Richard Allen, 31–32, 100
Wilson, William Julius, 12–14
Wolf, Stewart, 162
women patients. *See* black women; white women
Woodson, Carter G., 28, 149–50

Yancy, Clyde, 3
Yo Mama's Dysfunktional: Fighting the Culture Wars in Urban America (Kelley), 154

Zinn, William M., 203, 206, 211
Zucker, Howard D., 202–4

Text: 10/13 Aldus
Display: Aldus
Compositor: MPS Limited, a Macmillan Company
Indexer: Diana Witt
Printer and Binder: Maple-Vail Book Manufacturing Group